Teaching Health Humanities

Teaching Health Humanities

Edited by
Olivia Banner
Nathan Carlin
and
Thomas R. Cole

OXFORD
UNIVERSITY PRESS

OXFORD
UNIVERSITY PRESS

Oxford University Press is a department of the University of Oxford. It furthers the University's objective of excellence in research, scholarship, and education by publishing worldwide. Oxford is a registered trade mark of Oxford University Press in the UK and certain other countries.

Published in the United States of America by Oxford University Press
198 Madison Avenue, New York, NY 10016, United States of America.

Library of Congress Cataloging- in- Publication Data
Names: Banner, Olivia, Carlin, Nathan, Cole, Thomas R. editor.
Title: Teaching health humanities / [edited by] Olivia Banner,
Nathan Carlin, and Thomas R. Cole
Description: New York, NY : Oxford University Press, 2019. | Includes
bibliographical references.
Identifiers: LCCN 2018018336| ISBN 9780190636890 (cloth : alk. paper) |
ISBN 9780190636906 (updf) | ISBN 9780190636913 (epub) |
ISBN 9780190636920 (online content)
Subjects: | MESH: Humanities—education | Education, Medical | Teaching |
Cultural Competency
Classification: LCC R834 | NLM W 18 | DDC 610.71/1—dc23
LC record available at https://lccn.loc.gov/2018018336

9 8 7 6 5 4 3 2 1

Printed by Sheridan Books, Inc., United States of America

CONTENTS

CONTRIBUTORS

Olivia Banner is an assistant professor of critical media studies at the University of Texas Dallas. Her book, *Communicative Biocapitalism: The Voice of the Patient in Digital Health and the Health Humanities*, was published in 2017 by University of Michigan Press, and she is working on a second book, *Screening "Madness," 1949–2020*. Her articles have appeared in *Literature and Medicine, Signs, Discourse*, and the collections *Identity Technologies, Endemic: Essays in Contagion Theory,* and *Interdisciplinary Approaches to Disability Studies*. She teaches courses on humanities and health and critical disability media studies.

Michael Blackie is associate professor of health humanities in the Department of Medical Education in the College of Medicine at the University of Illinois, Chicago. He has published widely in health humanities pedagogy and medical education. He is associate editor of the *Journal of Medical Humanities,* book review editor for *Literature and Medicine*, and editor of the Literature and Medicine book series published by Kent State University Press. He is a recipient of a Mapping the Landscape Gold Foundation grant and is the co-editor of *From Reading to Healing: Teaching Medical Professionalism Through Literature*.

Marcia Brennan is the Carolyn and Fred McManis Professor of Humanities at Rice University and artist in residence in the Department of Palliative Care and Rehabilitation Medicine at the University of Texas M. D. Anderson Cancer Center. Her research areas include modernist aesthetics and curatorial studies and clinical aesthetics within the medical humanities. Her art historical books include *Curating Consciousness: Mysticism and the Modern Museum; Modernism's Masculine Subjects: Matisse, The New York School, and Post-Painterly Abstraction*; and *Painting Gender, Constructing Theory: The Alfred Stieglitz Circle and American Formalist Aesthetics*. Her medical humanities monographs include *Life at the End of Life: Finding Words Beyond Words* and *A Rose from Two Gardens: Saint Thérèse of Lisieux and Images of the End of Life*.

Nathan Carlin holds the Samuel Karff Chair and is Associate Professor in the McGovern Center for Humanities and Ethics at The University of Texas Health Science Center at Houston (UTHealth). Dr. Carlin has published over 100 chapters, articles, book reviews, and commentaries. He also is the author or co-author of five previous books. These include: *Living in Limbo: Life in* *the Midst of Uncertainty; 100 Years of Happiness: Insights and Findings from the Experts; Religious Mourning: Reversals and Restorations in Psychological Portraits of Religious Leaders; Medical Humanities: An Introduction*; and *The Gift of Sublimation: A Psychoanalytic Study of Multiple Masculinities*.

Andrea Charise is an assistant professor in the Department of English and the Interdisciplinary Centre for Health & Society at the University of Toronto Scarborough. She is the recipient of the John Charles Polanyi Prize for Literature and brings fifteen years of experience as a medical researcher (primarily in geriatrics) to her teaching and scholarship in literary studies. Her award-winning research is published in venues including *Journal of the American Geriatrics Society, Academic Medicine, Journal of Medical Humanities, Modern Drama*, and *English Literary History*. She is the principal investigator of SCOPE: The Health Humanities Learning Lab and the founder of Canada's first undergraduate program in health humanities.

Thomas R. Cole is the McGovern Chair in Medical Humanities and Director of the McGovern Center for Humanities and Ethics at The University of Texas Health Science Center at Houston (UTHealth). Dr. Cole has published many articles and books on the history of aging and humanistic gerontology. His book *The Journey of Life: A Cultural History of Aging in America* was nominated for a Pulitzer Prize. His most recent book is *A Country for Old Men: My Search Among the Elders*.

Sayantani DasGupta, originally trained in pediatrics and public health, teaches at the Master's Program in Narrative Medicine, the Institute for Comparative Literature and Society, and the Center for the Study and Ethnicity, all at Columbia University. She is the author, co-author, or co-editor of several academic books, including *Stories of Illness and Healing: Women Write Their Bodies; Globalization and Transnational Surrogacy in India: Outsourcing Life*; and *Principles and Practices of Narrative Medicine*. DasGupta is also a children's book author, and her Bengali folktale-inspired series from Scholastic, Kiranmala and the Kingdom Beyond, includes *The Serpent's Secret* (2018) *Game of Stars* (2019), and *The Chaos Curse* (2020).

Maria de Bruyn, a medical anthropologist, works on patient choice in medical care and sexual and reproductive health and rights in developing countries. She has done consultancies for national and international non-governmental organizations and multilateral agencies such as the World Health Organization, UNAIDS, the United Nations Trust Fund on Violence against Women, the United Nations Population Fund, and the European Union. Her publications include *Young Lives at Risk: Adolescents and Sexual Health; HIV, Sexual and Reproductive Health: Understanding and Claiming Rights*; and *Women, Gender and HIV/AIDS: Where Are We Now & Where Are We Going?*

Lisa Diedrich is professor of women's, gender, and sexuality studies at Stony Brook University. Her research and teaching interests include critical medical studies, disability studies, feminist science studies, and interdisciplinary feminist and queer theories and methodologies. She is the author of *Indirect Action: Schizophrenia, Epilepsy, AIDS, and the Course of Health Activism* and *Treatments: Language, Politics, and the Culture of Illness*.

Rebecca Garden is associate professor of bioethics and humanities at SUNY Upstate Medical University in Syracuse, New York. She has published widely in journals such as *New Literary History, Disability Studies Quarterly*, the *Journal of General Internal Medicine*, and the *Journal of Clinical Ethics*, as well as in the *Journal of Medical Humanities* and *Literature and Medicine*. She teaches medical students and residents, directs the healthcare ethics and humanities course for nursing and health professions students at SUNY Upstate, and is executive director of the Consortium for Culture and Medicine, an interinstitutional collaboration in Syracuse.

Amy M. Haddad is professor and the Dr. C. C. and Mabel L. Criss Endowed Chair in the Health Sciences at Creighton University. She is also the former director for the Center for Health Policy & Ethics at Creighton University (1995–2016), where she also served as program director for a fully online graduate program in healthcare ethics. Her publications include *Health Professional and Patient Interaction* with Drs. Ruth Purtilo and Regina Doherty, *Case Studies in Pharmacy Ethics* with Drs. Robert Veatch and E. J. Last, and *Case Studies in Biomedical Ethics—Decision-Making, Principles, and Cases* with Drs. Robert Veatch and Dan English. Her poetry and short stories have appeared in the *American Journal of Nursing, Fetishes: Literary Journal of Colorado Health Sciences Center, Janus Head, Journal of Medical Humanities, Touch*, and the *Bellevue Literary Review*.

John Hoberman is a medical historian who works in two primary areas: the history of male hormone therapies and human enhancements and the racial dimension of medicine, including medical racism. His books include *Testosterone Dreams: Rejuvenation, Aphrodisia, Doping, Dopers in Uniform: The Hidden World of Police on Steroids*, and *Black & Blue: The Origins and Consequences of Medical Racism*. He has taught an undergraduate race and medicine course nine times since 2001 and in 2017 taught a race and medicine elective at the University of Texas-Dell Medical School in Austin. He is professor of Germanic studies at the University of Texas at Austin.

Rachel Ingold is curator of the History of Medicine Collections in the David M. Rubenstein Rare Book & Manuscript Library at Duke University. Along with collecting materials related to the history of the health sciences (including global health), she has presented on the History of Medicine Collections at various conferences. Her work includes sponsoring digital projects, coordinating outreach efforts, and connecting users and researchers to primary sources—including providing instruction sessions for undergraduate students. She is the immediate past-president of the Archivists and Librarians for the History of Health Sciences.

Therese Jones is associate director of the Center for Bioethics and Humanities and director of the Arts and Humanities in Healthcare Program at the University of Colorado Anschutz Medical Campus. She is associate professor in the Department of Medicine. She has published and presented extensively on HIV/AIDS and the arts including *Sharing the Delirium: Second Generation AIDS Plays and Performances*; literature, film and medicine; and medical education. She is the editor of the *Journal of Medical Humanities* and lead editor for the *Health Humanities Reader*.

David Kline is a lecturer in religious studies at the University of Tennessee, Knoxville. He is the co-author of *Embodiment and Black Religion: Rethinking the Body in African American Religious Experience*.

Craig M. Klugman is professor of bioethics and health humanities in the Department of Health Sciences at DePaul University. He works on ethics at the end of life, public health ethics, and pedagogy and research methods in the health humanities. He is the editor of *Medical Ethics*, co-editor of *Ethical Issues in Rural Health* and *Research Methods in the Health Humanities*, producer of *Advance Directives*, and blog editor at bioethics.net.

Arno K. Kumagai is professor of medicine and vice chair for education, Department of Medicine at the University of Toronto. He also holds the F. M. Hill Chair in Humanism Education at Women's College Hospital, University of Toronto, where he has a clinical practice focused on working with individuals with type 1 diabetes mellitus. He has published extensively on the use of narratives in medical education, transformative learning, dialogical teaching, and teaching for equity and social justice and is the holder of numerous teaching awards in basic science teaching, humanism, educational innovation, and diversity.

Alex Lubet is Morse Alumni/Graduate & Professional Distinguished Teaching Professor of Music and an affiliate faculty member of the Center for Bioethics at the University of Minnesota. He is the author of *Music, Disability, and Society*, the first sole-authored monograph in the field of disability studies in music, and dozens of articles and chapters on disability issues within and beyond music. He is also a scholar of popular music and jazz, especially the music of Bob Dylan, whose journalistic pieces have appeared in such media outlets as *Newsweek, Salon.com, The Raw Story, San Francisco Chronicle, Associated Press, Houston Chronicle*, and *Seattle Post-Intelligencer*. He is also a composer, whose works have received over 500 performances on six continents, and a multi-instrumentalist who has concertized in North America, Europe, and Asia and recorded well-reviewed albums on the PARMA and pfMENTUM labels.

Melinda A. McGarrah Sharp is associate professor of practical theology and pastoral care at Columbia Theological Seminary in Decatur, Georgia. Her scholarship and teaching unfold at the intersections of pastoral theology, ethics, and postcolonial theory. Author of *Misunderstanding Stories: Toward a Postcolonial Pastoral Theology*, she has also contributed to multiple edited collections. She co-edits the *Journal of Pastoral Theology* and is a trained clinical ethicist.

Jarah Moesch, previously a postdoctoral scholar and associate director of design cultures and creativity at the University of Maryland, is currently a member of the Critical Design Lab at Vanderbilt University. Jarah is an artist-scholar whose work explores issues of justice through the design, production, and acquisition of embodied knowledges, specifically with the ways particular values are embedded within the design of systems and "industrial complexes," from healthcare and bioethics to ecologies on Earth and in outer space. Jarah uses these concerns to design new worlds. Jarah is the co-author of "Feminist Worlding: Media Ecologies Learning," in *Feminist Cyberspaces*, as well as essays "#transform (the underlying systems of digital) health" and "Questioning the Question" in the Field Guide Survey for *Media Commons*. Jarah's artwork has been shown in festivals and exhibitions across the United States and internationally.

Kirsten Ostherr is the Gladys Louise Fox Professor of English at Rice University in Houston, Texas, where she is a media scholar, health researcher, and technology analyst. She is founder and director of the medical humanities program and the Medical Futures Lab. She is the author of *Medical Visions: Producing the Patient Through Film, Television and Imaging Technologies* and *Cinematic Prophylaxis: Globalization and Contagion in the Discourse of World Health*. She is editor of *Applied Media Studies* and co-editor of *Science/Animation*, a special issue of the journal *Discourse*. Her research on trust and privacy in digital health ecosystems has been featured in *Slate*, the *Washington Post, Big Data & Society*, and *Catalyst*.

Susan Pacheco is associate professor of pediatrics in the Division of Pulmonary Medicine in the McGovern Medical School, University of Texas Health Science Center in Houston. She is an internationally recognized expert on the effects of climate change on children.

Nicole M. Piemonte is Assistant Dean for Medical Education and an assistant professor in the Department of Medical Education at Creighton University School of Medicine in Arizona. She received a Ph.D. in medical humanities from the University of Texas Medical Branch, where she studied continental philosophy, medical ethics, literature and medicine, and medical epistemology. Her teaching and research focus broadly on questions about illness, mortality, and compassion—and how the lived experiences of vulnerability and suffering can contribute to the cultivation of the (medical) self. She is the author of *Afflicted: How Vulnerability Can Heal Medical Education and Practice*.

Keisha Ray is assistant professor in the McGovern Center for Humanities and Ethics at University of Texas Health Science Center at Houston (UT Health). She works on topics in bioethics with a particular focus on biomedical enhancement and racial justice in healthcare. She has published articles in journals such as the *American Journal of Bioethics*, where she also regularly contributes blog posts to the online site. She has also published articles in the *American Journal of Bioethics—Neuroscience* and *Topoi: An International Review of Philosophy*. She has also contributed chapters to multiple anthologies.

Sarah Shannon is the Dean of the Montana State University College of Nursing. She taught healthcare and professional ethics to BSN nursing students for over twenty years at the University of Washington and was honored five times for her teaching excellence. She has published extensively on improving communication among healthcare teams, patients, and families around ethically-challenging topics including end-of-life decision-making in the intensive care setting, disclosure of healthcare errors, and conflict within the healthcare team, as well as on issue of professional practice and nursing ethics.

Jamie Shirley is a senior lecturer and the Director of Nursing Programs for the School of Nursing and Health Studies at the University of Washington Bothell. She teaches ethics, aesthetics, policy, and leadership in the graduate and undergraduate programs. Her work addresses issues of dependency, for people with illness and disabilities and for their caregivers, as well as legal guardianship and decision-making for persons without capacity. She is also a clinical ethics consultant for the UW Medicine system.

Kearsley A. Stewart is professor of the practice at Duke University, with joint appointments in the Duke Global Health Institute and Department of Cultural Anthropology. Stewart's current research interests include research ethics of HIV/AIDS clinical trials in Africa, global health pedagogy, and global health humanities. She is co-director of the Duke Health Humanities Lab; faculty associate with the Trent Center for Bioethics, Humanities and History of Medicine; and a member of the Duke University Library Council. Her work has appeared in *The Lancet, Academic Medicine, Global Public Health, Journal of Bioethical Inquiry, Africa Today, Journal of Empirical Research on Human Research Ethics*, and *Learning and Teaching: The International Journal of Higher Education in the Social Sciences*, among others.

Kelley K. Swain works at the crossroads of literature and science, writing science poetry and literature reviews and teaching medical humanities. She has written over fifty essays for *The Lancet* journals. She is the author of poetry collections *Darwin's Microscope, Opera di Cera*, and *Atlantic*; the memoir *The Naked Muse*; and the novel *Double the Stars*. In 2016, she was part of Visions of Nature, the first poetry residency at the Oxford University Museum of Natural History, the result of which was the anthology *Guests of Time*. Swain has edited two anthologies of science poetry, *Sonnets and Slide Rules* and *Pocket Horizon*.

Delese Wear is professor of family and community medicine at the Northeast Ohio Medical University. She is a co–course director of Human Values in Medicine, a longitudinal humanities course, along with a required capstone course for graduating medical students.

Joseph Zarconi is professor and chair of internal medicine and senior associate dean for health affairs at the Northeast Ohio Medical University College of Medicine in Rootstown, Ohio, where he also serves as co–course director for the reflective practice and clinical epilogue and capstone courses. He is also a practicing nephrologist and is active in the teaching of medical students and residents. He has presented at state, national, and international meetings and co-authored peer-reviewed journal articles and book chapters on topics relating to medical education, narrative medical practice, narrative ethics, humanism and professionalism, cultural consciousness, close reading, and social justice, as well as two books on narrative in healthcare. He is a member of the Northeast Ohio Medical University's Master Teacher Guild and has been recognized as a master teacher by the American College of Physicians.

Introduction

FOR IMPOSSIBLE DEMANDS

Olivia Banner

Health humanities educators are a diverse group of bricoleurs, in their teaching no less than in their scholarship. Coming from the humanities (English, art history, religious studies, the applied arts, film and media studies, philosophy, bioethics) and the social sciences (history, sociology, and anthropology), based in diverse locations across higher education (in the baccalaureate arts and sciences, in graduate programs, in medical schools, and in other health professions programs), scholars arrive to teach health humanities courses equipped with divergent disciplinary and field training and their distinct associated pedagogies; and they are often expected to put that training to distinctly different uses. This volume aims to illuminate those many different pedagogical approaches and applications and, in doing so, to advance a broader conversation bubbling among educators and scholars about how to redefine the field. Taking place in the informal spaces of mailing lists and professional conferences, these discussions have still not settled on any one term or definition for the field. An annual health humanities conference, a recent co-authored volume on health humanities, a co-edited reader on health humanities, and the International Health Humanities Network exist alongside a comprehensive introduction to medical humanities, two journals of medical humanities, and quite a few institutional programs that bear its name.[1] The Modern Language Association's special forum on the topic, Medical Humanities and Health Studies, splits the difference by using both the older name and a newer entity that lays claim to areas other than the humanities. Others have proposed and are using *critical medical humanities* to demarcate a specific approach to medical humanities that challenges some of its underlying models, for example, the medical model implied in the phrase.[2] Disability studies scholars and their allies are located among the latter group, although (and at the risk of being reductive) much of the orientation of disability studies is at odds with fields that prioritize *health* as a privileged term and *medicine* as an overarching framework, so some disability studies scholars disavow the term. Another scholar working in the area of critical media studies suggests a branching field that might be called *digital medical humanities*,[3] while another offers *biohumanities* to encompass and stimulate news ways of articulating the object under investigation—not the medicine of "medical humanities" or the clinic of "bioethics" but rather "textual representations and interpretations of biological, ecological, historical, and structural determinants of both the amelioration and the exacerbation of *suffering*."[4]

The editors of this volume ultimately settled on *health humanities*, and lingering for a moment on two questions that underpinned that choice will help set out both the ways in which this volume extends current field dynamics and how it concentrates particular forces. First, why *health humanities* over *medical humanities*? In their overview of the field, *Medical Humanities: An Introduction*, Thomas R. Cole, Nathan Carlin, and Ronald Carson define *medical humanities* as "an inter- and multidisciplinary field that explores contexts, experiences, and critical and conceptual issues in medicine and health care, while supporting professional identity formation."[5] This definition identifies two boundaried sites—medicine/healthcare and professionalization—that some definitions of *health humanities* claim to violate.[6] Paul Crawford and his co-authors, for example, articulate *health humanities* as a term that better encompasses the wide range of professional identities and nonprofessionals—those typically marginalized by the medical humanities such as patients, caregivers, and allied health professionals—that a humanities addressing health could include.[7] In their *Health Humanities Reader*, Therese Jones, Delese Wear, and Lester Friedman build on Crawford et al.'s definition and add that the term *health humanities* allows for a less medicine-centric academic enterprise. Like Jones, Wear, and Friedman's volume, *Teaching Health Humanities* addresses more than only medicine and healthcare; and some of its contributors teach students who will not become future healthcare professionals. As our volume similarly expands far beyond the scene of medicine and addresses educators working with many different kinds of students, we selected *health humanities* as the term most appropriate for encapsulating its contributions.

Second, for the purposes of this volume, how do we define *health humanities*? To be clear, there is not yet a canonical definition of *health humanities*; and we do not aim to advance a specific, field-defining formulation of it. Instead, just as the *Health Humanities Reader* sets out to illustrate what health humanities might be through the essays it includes, so too does this volume offer its chapters as illustrations of what its practitioners understand health humanities pedagogy to be. Having said that, we have brought contributors together with some operative assumptions about what health humanities is and could be. We work with these assumptions: health humanities is broad in nature (addressing topics outside medicine and healthcare and outside professional identity formation); inclusive (open to diverse perspectives, including those from outside traditional "medical humanities" training); open to, even privileging, disability studies and, by implication, a range of intersectional theories about health, illness, and axes of difference as constituted through structural hierarchies; and distinctly focuses on experience and analysis, in contrast to the instrumentalized form of medical humanities that can characterize its intersections with bioethics.

However our contributors locate themselves or whatever term they use to define their approach, they appear in this volume because their work illustrates how teaching can serve as a node by which to encourage a shift away from what Therese Jones has categorized as the ethical and instrumental imperatives of early iterations of medical humanities and toward social, political, and cultural imperatives.[8] Neither medical humanities nor its associated narrative medicine has ever shied away from acknowledging the social determinants of health or the social embeddedness of both patients and doctors, yet these have not always taken center stage in their scholarship or pedagogical praxis. Rather, the focus has been, as Rebecca Garden and Andrea Charise put it in their chapters, on the "god terms" of empathy, listening, moral imagination, and self-reflection. Recently, though, there has been heightened interest in centering the social, the political, even the economic in medical humanities work; and this volume seeks to build on these growing pains, with the specific aim of helping to foster new ways of thinking about pedagogical aims and methods. The appearance of many volumes focused on encapsulating the field(s) of health humanities and its array of topics, methods, and modes of expression—that is, its disciplinary and field reach as well as its articulation in both scholarly and artistic forms—speaks to the increasing visibility and significance of the field. A proposed future volume on methods in health humanities promises to deepen our understanding of this neglected topic in health humanities scholarship, and another proposed future volume on race and ethnicity in the global health humanities will exponentially increase this currently underdeveloped area of the field.[9] While many of these volumes either discuss teaching in broad terms or include component essays focused on teaching, none hone in on the contemporary scene of cross-fertilization across pedagogies as younger scholars enter the arena or as existing scholars graft fresh pedagogies from developments in their own fields.[10] This volume, then, was conceived as a way to nurture continued seeding of the field.

It was also conceived as a way to nurture our imaginations about what health humanities could do—that is, how it could evolve to address some of the most urgent crises of our times. In my experience teaching premed undergraduates, their capacity to imagine solutions to those crises or to imagine worlds alternate to our contemporary one seems underdeveloped: somehow, even though they had not even begun their true professional education, they already could not think beyond "there is only so much understanding of a person and his or her social context you can do in a 15-minute, let alone a 7-minute, exam." It is as if their imaginations have atrophied when confronted with the impossible Rubik's cube of our for-profit healthcare system. This fatalism, that healthcare and its practice are situated within a monumentally immovable edifice, seems, at times, to suffuse other areas of medical education, including the health humanities. It does seem that the time is right to develop that capacity to imagine alternatives, even if, as the adage goes, it is easier for most people to imagine the end of the world than the end of capitalism, which is the endpoint I had to ask my students to imagine so that they could imagine healthcare otherwise.[11] In their essay on climate change, David Kline, Thomas R. Cole, and Susan Pacheco offer a timeless slogan—"Be realistic. Demand the impossible"—to remind us that if ever there was a time to face down the barriers we have erected to more radical ways of thinking, now is it. In the case of climate change, that means helping students confront their own intellectual paralysis when faced with the terrifying enormity of global warming. But it might also mean revising some of our notions of the aims of health humanities and what it can achieve more generally.

Mapping the Chapters

The contributions in this volume are arranged to help guide the reader toward such imaginative tools. Briefly, the first section's essays cover familiar territory, mapping out where and how health humanities education currently occurs within educational institutions. Chapters in the second section address the why and the how of the politics of pedagogy, with contributions that explore how to create syllabi and pedagogical exercises that illuminate the politics, social determinants, and sociocultural factors of health. The third section's chapters reveal how health humanities educators take up a diverse range of media and cultural practices in focused and considerate manners, whether such media and practices serve as supplemental or illustrative course material or as the actual basis for courses that examine the mediation of media.

The first section, on where we are now, provides readers a window into the range of institutional locations where traditional health humanities education occurs. It does not aim to be exhaustive; rather, we purposefully selected disparate areas where such courses are institutionally embedded so that readers could get a sense of that difference and how different locations are being addressed through divergent approaches. To be clear, all of the essays in all three sections broaden that window's frame, but the first section's essays are concerned more with presenting traditional ways and spaces in which health humanities are taught. As the fields continue to evolve, it will certainly be useful as a historical marker of where the field was situated in this particular decade—even, perhaps, in a particular moment of political and social conjunctures whose impact on higher education, healthcare, and the classroom environment we cannot yet know. In their essays, contributors to the first section explain how they teach health humanities in baccalaureate undergraduate health humanities programs, nursing education, undergraduate medical school programs, theological education, and online bioethics.

For readers familiar with traditional course objectives in health humanities (those "god terms" of empathy, compassion, reflection, moral imagination) these essays help illuminate how such key principles are integrated for diverse curricular needs. In addition, most go beyond these first principles to argue for an education that recognizes that compassionate care requires understanding people's social context. Craig Klugman's chapter provides a history of how the health humanities moved into the baccalaureate setting and what its nonprofessionalizing context allows, freedoms often not available at the medical school level, when both students and accrediting auditors have specific aims that courses must fulfill. In their chapter, Nicole Piemonte and Arno Kumagai make the case that those first principles are applicable to socially engaged pedagogical objectives. For example, in their explanation of it, reflective writing is not only a method for deepening students' appreciation of the self and the other but also a way to address the frustrations students experience upon encountering social injustice in the medical system. Melinda McGarrah Sharp reveals how cultivating moral imagination aligns with principles of feminist intersectionality and other social liberationist thought, where moral imagination becomes a wedge into contemplating relations among marginalized individuals and the systems in which they live and die. In their chapter on nursing education, Jamie Shirley and Sarah Shannon illustrate how they encourage moral imaginative skills alongside critical analytic skills that will allow students to deal with moments of discomfort or to recognize their own errors. Significant in their essay is how these two skills interact with the feminization of the nursing profession. One of Shirley and Shannon's goals is to foster nurses' confidence in their own judgment so that they do not underestimate their own contribution to a team of healthcare providers. While they note that they must also ensure that their students do not become overconfident, it is intriguing that much of the emphasis in medical humanities has been on shaping (the masculinized profession of) physicians away from an egocentric stance in the healthcare setting. Shirley and Shannon remind us that this plays differently with a profession whose feminization has affected the authority its members are accorded. Amy Haddad's chapter, which explains the unique challenges of teaching in the online environment, illuminates how health humanities content integrated into a bioethics course deepens the grounds for bioethical decision-making, affording students the chance to draw on their emotions and imaginations, rather than relying solely on the logic-based skills typically used to justify bioethical decisions. Additionally, Haddad's use of the term *humanize* to refer to the process by which the online instructor must overcome the separation instituted by asynchronous, technologically enabled learning environments underlines the new era of "technologization" we have entered. If some of the original impetus for the birth of the medical humanities was a frustration with medicine's technologization in the 1970s, the health humanities today faces new methods through which technology affronts not only the healthcare experience but also education.

It is in the second section, in particular, that our contributors ask health humanities reader-educators to imagine their own practice differently. Each chapter centers one or more of the lacunae that have characterized medical humanities work: race, gender, sexuality, age, disability, and postcolonial/diasporic differences are all represented here. Race, as much recent work establishes, has been sorely neglected as a topic both in medical education as well as in the medical humanities; and the two chapters on the topic here articulate that neglect, the reasons for it, and some reparative pedagogical work that helps address it.[12] The section begins with work by John Hoberman enumerating the many ways in which health education reiterates the structural racism that permeates the practice of medicine, in particular by the absence of racial topics for required courses. In doing so, medical training contributes to continued error-prone diagnostic and therapeutic practices. Hoberman summarizes the course he taught at the University of Texas at Austin's Dell medical school, which aimed to educate medical students about these issues and that one can only hope will grow in enrollment size. Keisha Ray's contribution outlines how she incorporates teaching about race in her own courses. Ray's method draws on the rich critical race and feminist studies traditions of valuing testimony as evidence—a kind of *situated knowledge*, to use the feminist epistemology term, that individuals develop through their own experiences of their intersectional oppressions.[13] While Hoberman tends to emphasize sociological approaches that contextualize individual patient experiences within broader histories of their racialized category, Ray emphasizes the particularized knowledge derived from embodied experience. Her chapter additionally demonstrates how the testimony of patients of color can be combined with students' explorations of their own intersectional positions to foster their capacities to identify the multiple (and unique) identities each patient/person brings to the clinical context. For Ray, like other contributors in this section, the emphasis on "empathy" has outworn its value; and it is time to foster methods of teaching that institute practices of justice.

Like the two initial essays on race, which demonstrate how race has remained neglected in medical school education and, by implication, the medical humanities, the ones that follow take up categories of human differences that have been underaddressed in medical humanities (and medical education more broadly). Part of this lack of attention derives from the whiteness and Western-ness of health humanities itself, which Sayantani DasGupta's essay on diasporic and postcolonial models implicitly explores. DasGupta urges us to unpack the metaphor of the "home"—to consider that it is used to signal "comfort" and "familiarity" in Western contexts in which certain people are Othered, and thus never configured as "at home." In her teaching, DasGupta, following postcolonial and black feminist theorists, centers those who are marginalized, refusing to allow the white Western gaze to control the knowledge-space of her classroom. Instead, students explore stories authored by postcolonial and African American writers that trouble simplistic notions of home and where the concepts of illness and care on offer differ significantly from dominant cultural notions. Such works implicitly trouble the reigning paradigm that the healthcare professions should expand their services to "underserved populations," for such discourses do not stop to consider that marginalized communities may have already developed their own distinct modalities of care. In line with her work on narrative humility, DasGupta foregrounds that ultimately the experience of the Other is always unknowable and that, by acknowledging that fact, new understandings might arise. DasGupta's essay is especially important because it works to encourage readers to question their own notions of "home," including when it comes to thinking about global health. DasGupta pushes us to think whether we construct a Western gaze in our own classrooms. More than this, she describes how she collaboratively creates the topics for her courses, which she glosses as "a collaborative set of inquiries between faculty and student co-learners." This is not a question of answering to the neoliberal framing of the university as serving student-customers; it is a way of practicing pedagogical humility and realizing that the best way to discover and address our own gaps in knowledge is to ask our students to identify them and then help us formulate the proper response.

The essay co-authored by Michael Blackie, Delese Wear, and Joseph Zarconi similarly addresses ongoing lacunae in health humanities teaching around differences. Their piece discusses the difficulty in talking about class with students who come from backgrounds of economic privilege and/or who lack the vocabulary to enter conversations about class. They enumerate key errors in thinking that characterize how students and health education frame poverty and class, then elaborate a number of exercises to help students move beyond such limited frameworks. As they note, some of these limitations arise from the focus on the single-story method, where an individual story morphs into a stereotype that then prohibits identifying the complexity of actual human beings. This might seem to suggest that the humanities practice of focusing on one story would be a dangerous continuation of this method; however, rather than discard it, they use the film *Precious* (dir. Lee Daniels, 2009) to demonstrate how a single representation of an African American girl living in poverty can illuminate for students intersections of oppression and, in particular, the structural determinants of wealth and health. Importantly, their chapter does not address class alone but draws out an intersectional approach that also considers race, gender, sexuality, and ability. In doing so, it exemplifies the significance of intersectionality for health humanities teaching.

Andrea Charise's chapter similarly touches on intersectional issues, in this case by examining age in relation to class and race. Her university has a demographic composition typical of large urban universities (i.e., working and lower-middle class, racially and ethnically diverse), so her students' experiences of aging are vastly different from those of the (white, middle-class) people thus far centered in age studies. When she assigned a text conventionally used in age studies classes (*King Lear*), Charise was surprised to find students consuming the text alongside other mediated interpretations of it (e.g., YouTube videos of theatrical and other interpretations of the play). By observing their media habits, Charise discovered she could enable a learning experience in which students remixed age studies and its texts, in doing so integrating—even centering—their non-white, non-middle-class cultural references and texts.

Rebecca Garden too discusses this sort of collaborative design in her chapter on the accessible health humanities course. It is an all too familiar fact that the built environments of many universities and healthcare institutions are not accessible, but perhaps less recognized is that learning environments too are also not accessible. Extending work by disability studies scholars, Garden explains what it takes to fashion accessibility into a course—what disability activists call "baked in, rather than added on" access.[14] She includes extremely detailed notes about each component of the pedagogical environment and how to ensure that it is accessible not only to students but also, just as importantly, to community members who visit the class. Recognizing the signal importance of pushing this information out to other educators, Garden includes an appendix of access basics that maps out how to construct an accessible environment. In addition, Garden articulates the theoretical connections between health humanities and disability studies and how disability studies serves the aims of a social justice practice that targets the structural determinants of health. A disability studies framework that distinguishes between the social and medical models of disability clearly illuminates how *the social* affects bodies and minds. In this, disability studies is a prime, possibly master theoretical framework by which to approach what sociologists and the healthcare professions term the *social determinants of health*. Garden's explanation of its theoretical import should provoke greater reflection on how teaching the social versus medical model of disability might lend to structural competency efforts as well.

David Kline, Thomas R. Cole, and Susan Pacheco's chapter on climate change takes to its logical endpoint what needs to be addressed if we are to fully understand those determinants: the effects of climate change. The intensification of weather extremes is exacerbating already existing social and health inequalities (one need only note Hurricane Katrina as a visible recent instance), and ignoring this issue does not prepare medical students to understand the scope of health in a warming world that they will enter. In fact, it is perhaps by addressing climate change, the enormity of which often paralyzes students, that health humanities educators can best expand the scale of how students conceive of "health"—not as something that happens to individuals but as something occurring at the levels of communities, populations, even continents.

The question of scale carries over into Lisa Diedrich's chapter. In her classes, Diedrich introduces theoretical models that can help students understand the relationship between the micro and macro, the individual and the social, the local and the global. For example, the concept of structural violence helps elucidate those scalar relationships in a global health course; in gender and health courses, the feminist concept of intersectionality allows students to consider how law, policy, and culture are imbricated in shaping how those who are vulnerable experience health and illness. Teaching in a women's studies department and with a women's studies background, thus well versed in what interdisciplinary study can illuminate, Diedrich provides a clear justification for why feminist theory itself is necessary for illuminating the politics of health; she also reveals key nodes through which those less versed in the theory might consider incorporating it into their own courses.

The third section serves many purposes. One is to give readers insight into how to incorporate new media into their existing courses. Using media in teaching has a long history in health humanities education as educators incorporate a film, a television episode, and a novel here and there in order to elucidate certain themes. The chapters that focus specifically on media illuminate newer forms of media that have received less attention. For example, Nathan Carlin explains how he incorporates the new media format of the radio podcast into his ethics class, while Jarah Moesch describes an entire course built around examining the medical record and information technologies. In their essay on using archives in a global health humanities classroom, Kearsley Stewart and her co-authors present an assignment that asks students to remix and cut up material from their library's large archive of gray literature about HIV/AIDs. Alex Lubet, who teaches at the intersections of disability studies, music studies, and bioethics, presents his methods for revealing the disjunctures and overlaps between bioethics and disability studies. In his unique class, he uses examples drawn from music history and cultural representations of music and musicians to explore course concepts, and he frames the learning environment that happens in his course as analogous to what happens in the music composition process.

Two contributions on visual art, a media format with a rich history in medical humanities, help illuminate distinctive ways in which the medium is incorporated today. Marcia Brennan's essay foregrounds how she implements aesthetic appreciation for palliative care patients. With Brennan's guidance, these patients create material artifacts that their survivors can keep as a memory of this transient time. It would not diminish the significance of Brennan's work to note that such application can travel into other spaces of care, including the classroom. Therese Jones's chapter describes how she integrates visual culture health activism into her courses in order to propel students not only to "see" more rigorously but also to develop their sense of how to witness as they look, stare, view, and otherwise exercise their optic skills. By having students view visual health activist texts as well as participate in creating such projects, Jones fosters her students' capacity to imagine themselves involved in both witnessing and co-constructing dialogues about the experience of the healthcare system, from the viewpoint of patients as well as practitioners.

The second aim is one that the editors (especially Banner) hope to see more work on. As I, Kirsten Ostherr, and others have argued, health humanities need not stay on the sidelines as digital health technologies penetrate the edifice of medical practice.[15] Instead, an invigorated health humanities, buttressed by the understanding that media and technology, like health, have politics, should be taking these new media forms into the fold. Ostherr's contribution illuminates how to teach in a participatory classroom that mingles practice with theory to guide interventions into communicative media design. Drawing on models developed by art + science design thinkers, Ostherr creates a course organized around solving design problems that currently exist within healthcare settings. But students do not design in an abstract space of theory; rather, they construct solutions guided by media theory and, most significantly, the people their designs will ultimately affect, namely patients and caregivers. Although Ostherr's course does not linger on the typical medical humanities "god terms" of empathy and witnessing, it does emphasize a model of what Ostherr calls "reciprocity": a responding to the needs of patients. In this, it refuses a paternalistic model in which students would presume to know more than patients—instead, it inculcates a responsibility to patients themselves.

Moesch's contribution exemplifies how digital culture scholars enlist their training in the politics of media and technology to show students that such politics affect medicine's ability to address diversity and to encourage students to imagine alternative possible systems. Moesch's chapter could just as well have been included in the volume's second section, so clearly does it demonstrate how ideologies of gender and sexuality affect technology development, which affects people's health and healthcare. Even more so, though, these chapters reveal the extent to which digital health tools are imbued with neoliberal imperatives and the ways in which a robust health humanities could foster students' capacities to identify those logics. Moesch's teaching, for example, illuminates that proprietary models of health information technologies sustain how insurance companies determine what gender and sex are and can be within healthcare contexts. She then asks students to imagine reorganizing the electronic medical record to allow for greater diversity. The annotated syllabus she includes here should help educators without experience in critical media studies, who might see it as too unfamiliar to incorporate in their own teaching, feel more comfortable with it, for it shares with other humanities fields the core interpretive practice of close reading.

Pedagogy in Impossible Times

Throughout this book, even when contributors may dip into the neoliberal language of "outcomes" and "effectiveness," the general push to contour teaching to fit into quantification and measurement models is exposed as inimical to the real work of teaching.[16] Diedrich, for example, takes an issue that arises out of the neoliberal context of increased demands on our time and often plagues health educators as they plan their course syllabi or daily lessons—"we don't have time" to explore questions that accreditation practices have deemed superfluous or to imagine alternate worlds—and flips it on its head: she suggests that we could imagine ourselves as having enough time and discovering what that allows us to newly explore. She provocatively supplies only a brief suggestion of one possible exploratory route here—that health humanities students might enter women's and sexuality studies education, rather than the typical direction of educators from women's and sexuality studies entering health humanities contexts.

Diedrich is gesturing to the complications that are arising as undergraduate health humanities programs gain in stature across the United States, an increase documented in Sarah Berry, Erin Lamb, and Therese Jones's recent report on the increase in health humanities majors and minors. As they note in their report, "At a time when Liberal Arts education, and humanities programs in particular, are under fire in many public quarters, programs in the Health Humanities are experiencing dramatic growth. Since the turn of the century alone (from 2000–2016) the number of Health Humanities programs has more than quadrupled, increasing from 14 to 58, with another 7 known programs currently in development."[17] This striking correlation has led some to worry about causation—whether the always-under-attack humanities fields are being engulfed by majors that are pre-vocational, the humanities workforce having to justify its existence by recourse to instrumentalist arguments such as "the humanities can help our students get into good medical schools," "a humanities background protects against physician burnout," and so forth. In his essay, Klugman also remarks on this sort of jousting between the bench sciences and the health humanities minor, where, possibly due to the ways in which universities today require numbers to justify continued funding of departments, departments may even actively try to coerce students away from the temptation of health humanities courses, which seduce students to play in ludic culture and, possibly, change their majors (or add a minor). And Piemonte and Kumagai argue that the health humanities should simply refuse such reductive schema of calculative assessment, that the work they do is incommensurable with the epistemological framework of evidence-based learning—in fact, the work they do actively undermines that epistemological framework. Certainly, the testimonial model offered by Ray similarly refutes that epistemology.

When Diedrich makes the case for the stimulating intersections between illness politics and feminist theory both in thought and in teaching, she helps us remember that there are other spaces of intellectual exploration and knowledge to which we should push our students, not for their future in healthcare but for their overall education. In other words, the humanities (and, in the case of interdisciplinary fields such as women's studies, all the arts and sciences) have intrinsic value in and of themselves, as methods that help people learn how to think about their world, not just to prepare for their professional lives. This is surely something of which health humanities educators are perfectly aware. It seems, though, that in this current conjuncture, when both the educational and the medical institutions that are under assault take recourse in quantification, technologies of measurement, and measures of those institutions' "value," health humanities educators could become a little more realistic and demand the impossible.

Notes

1. Therese Jones, Delese Wear, and Lester D. Friedman, eds., *Health Humanities Reader* (New Brunswick, NJ: Rutgers University Press, 2014); Paul Crawford et al., *Health Humanities* (London: Palgrave Macmillan, 2015); Thomas R. Cole, Nathan S. Carlin, and Ronald A. Carson, *Medical Humanities: An Introduction* (Cambridge: Cambridge University Press, 2014). The two journals are the US *Journal of Medical Humanities* and the UK-based *Medical Humanities*.

2. Alan Bleakley, "Towards a 'Critical Medical Humanities,'" in *Medicine, Health, and the Arts: Approaches to Medical Humanities*, ed. Victoria Bates, Alan Bleakley, and Sam Goodman (Abingdon, UK: Routledge, 2014), 17–26; Sarah Atkinson et al., "'The Medical' and 'Health' in a Critical Medical Humanities," *Journal of Medical Humanities* 36, no. 1 (2015): 71–81; William Viney, Felicity Callard, and Angela Woods, "Critical Medical Humanities: Embracing Entanglement, Taking Risks," *Medical Humanities* 41, no. 1 (2015): 2–7; Lisa Diedrich, *Indirect Action: Schizophrenia, Epilepsy, AIDS, and the Course of Health Activism* (Minneapolis: University of Minnesota Press, 2016); Ann Whitehead and Angela Woods, eds., *The Edinburgh Companion to the Critical Medical Humanities* (Edinburgh: Edinburgh University Press, 2016); Olivia Banner, *Communicative Biocapitalism: The Voice of the Patient in Digital Health and the Health Humanities* (Ann Arbor: University of Michigan Press, 2017).

3. Kirsten Ostherr, *Medical Visions: Producing the Patient through Film, Television, and Imaging Technologies* (Oxford: Oxford University Press, 2013).

4. Catherine Belling, "Introduction: From Bioethics and Humanities to Biohumanities?" *Literature and Medicine* 34, no. 1 (Spring 2016): 5.

5. Cole, Carlin, and Carson, *Medical Humanities*, 12.

6. Although, to be precise, Cole, Carlin, and Carson's definition is expanded on in their volume as well. See ibid., 8–15.

7. Jones, Wear, and Friedman, *Health Humanities*, 6, citing Paul Crawford et al., "Health Humanities: The Future of Medical Humanities?" *Mental Health Review Journal* 15, no. 3 (2010): 4.

8. Therese Jones, "'Oh! The Humanit(ies)!': Dissent, Democracy, and Danger," in *Medicine, Health, and the Arts: Approaches to the Medical Humanities*, ed. Victoria Bates, Alan Bleakley, and Sam Goodman (Abingdon, UK: Routledge, 2014), 27–38.

9. Erin Lamb and Craig Klugman, *Methods of the Health Humanities* (Oxford: Oxford University Press, forthcoming).

10. There are, however, other volumes in progress that will similarly expand our understanding, for example, Esther Jones, ed., *Health Humanities in Global Context: Race and Ethnicity across the World.*

11. The exact quotation comes from Frederic Jameson, "Future City," *New Left Review* 21 (May 2003): 76.

12. Work enumerating its absence in the medical humanities includes, among others, John Hoberman, *Black and Blue: The Origins and Consequences of Medical Racism* (Berkeley: University of California Press, 2012); Olivia Banner, "Structural Racism and Practices of Reading in the Medical Humanities," *Literature and Medicine* 34, no. 1 (2016): 25–52.

13. For "situated knowledge," see Sandra Harding, "'Strong Objectivity' and Socially Situated Knowledge," in *Whose Science? Whose Knowledge?* (New York: Cornell University Press, 1991), 138–63; see also Donna Haraway, "Situated Knowledges: The Science Question in Feminism and the Privilege of Partial Perspective," *Feminist Studies* 14, no. 3 (1988): 575–99; Patricia Hill Collins, "Learning from the Outside Within: The Sociological Significance of Black Feminist Thought," in *The Feminist Standpoint Theory Reader: Intellectual and Political Controversies*, ed. Sandra Harding (New York: Routledge, 2004), 103–26; bell hooks, "Choosing the Margins as a Space of Radical Openness," in *The Feminist Standpoint Theory Reader: Intellectual and Political Controversies*, ed. Sandra Harding (New York: Routledge, 2004), 153–60; Chela Sandoval, "U.S. Third World Feminism: The Theory and Method of Differential Oppositional Consciousness," in *The Feminist Standpoint Theory Reader*, 195–210. For "intersectionality," see Kimberlé Crenshaw, "Mapping the Margins: Intersectionality, Identity Politics, and Violence against Women of Color," *Stanford Law Review* 43, no. 6 (1991): 1241–99; Patricia Hill Collins, *Black Feminist Thought: Knowledge, Consciousness, and the Politics of Empowerment*, 2nd ed. (New York: Routledge, 2000).

14. See especially Liat Ben-Moshe et al., eds., *Building Pedagogical Curb Cuts: Incorporating Disability into the University Classroom and Curriculum* (New York: Syracuse University Press, 2007); Margaret Price, *Mad at School: Rhetorics of Mental Disability and Academic Life* (Ann Arbor: University of Michigan Press, 2007).

15. See Ostherr, *Medical Visions*; Banner, *Communicative Biocapitalism.*

16. This follows other work criticizing how the culture of quantification diminishes the medical humanities, including, among others, Rafael Campo, "'The Medical Humanities,' for Lack of a Better Term," *JAMA* 294, no. 9 (2005): 1009–11; Catherine Belling, "Sharper Instruments: On Defending the Humanities in Undergraduate Medical Education," *Academic Medicine* 85, no. 6 (2010): 938–40.

17. Sarah L. Berry, Erin Gentry Lamb, and Therese Jones, *Health Humanities Baccalaureate Programs in the United States* (Hiram, OH: Center for Literature and Medicine, Hiram College, 2016), http://www.hiram.edu/wp-content/uploads/2016/11/HHBP_12_2_16.pdf.

Works Cited

Atkinson, Sarah, Bethan Evans, Angela Woods, and Robin Kearns. "'The Medical' and 'Health' in a Critical Medical Humanities." *Journal of Medical Humanities* 36, no. 1 (2015): 71–81.

Banner, Olivia. *Communicative Biocapitalism: The Voice of the Patient in Digital Health and the Health Humanities*. Ann Arbor: University of Michigan Press, 2017.

Banner, Olivia. "Structural Racism and Practices of Reading in the Medical Humanities." *Literature and Medicine* 34, no. 1 (2016): 25–52.

Belling, Catherine. "Introduction: From Bioethics and Humanities to Biohumanities?" *Literature and Medicine* 34, no. 1 (Spring 2016): 1–6.

Belling, Catherine. "Sharper Instruments: On Defending the Humanities in Undergraduate Medical Education." *Academic Medicine* 85, no. 6 (2010): 938–40.

Ben-Moshe, Liat, Rebecca Cory, Mia Feldbaum, and Ken Sagendorf, eds. *Building Pedagogical Curb Cuts: Incorporating Disability into the University Classroom and Curriculum*. New York: Syracuse University Press, 2007.

Berry, Sarah L., Erin Gentry Lamb, and Therese Jones. *Health Humanities Baccalaureate Programs in the United States*. Hiram, OH: Center for Literature and Medicine, Hiram College, 2016. http://www.hiram.edu/wp-content/uploads/2016/11/HHBP_12_2_16.pdf.

Bleakley, Alan. "Towards a 'Critical Medical Humanities.'" In *Medicine, Health, and the Arts: Approaches to Medical Humanities*, edited by Victoria Bates, Alan Bleakley, and Sam Goodman, 17–26. Abingdon, UK: Routledge, 2014.

Campo, Rafael. "'The Medical Humanities,' for Lack of a Better Term." *JAMA* 294, no. 9 (2005): 1009–11.

Cole, Thomas R., Nathan S. Carlin, and Ronald A. Carson. *Medical Humanities: An Introduction*. Cambridge: Cambridge University Press, 2014.

Collins, Patricia Hill. *Black Feminist Thought: Knowledge, Consciousness, and the Politics of Empowerment*. 2nd ed. New York: Routledge, 2000.

Collins, Patricia Hill. "Learning from the Outside Within: The Sociological Significance of Black Feminist Thought." In *The Feminist Standpoint Theory Reader: Intellectual and Political Controversies*, edited by Sandra Harding, 103–26. New York: Routledge, 2004.

Crawford, Paul, Brian Brown, Charley Baker, Victoria Tischler, and Brian Abrams. *Health Humanities*. London: Palgrave Macmillan, 2015.

Crawford, Paul, Brian Brown, Victoria Tischler, and Charley Baker. "Health Humanities: The Future of Medical Humanities?" *Mental Health Review Journal* 15, no. 3 (2010): 4–10.

Crenshaw, Kimberlé. "Mapping the Margins: Intersectionality, Identity Politics, and Violence against Women of Color." *Stanford Law Review* 43, no. 6 (1991): 1241–99.

Diedrich, Lisa. *Indirect Action: Schizophrenia, Epilepsy, AIDS, and the Course of Health Activism*. Minneapolis: University of Minnesota Press, 2016.

Haraway, Donna. "Situated Knowledges: The Science Question in Feminism and the Privilege of Partial Perspective." *Feminist Studies* 14, no. 3 (1988): 575–99.

Harding, Sandra. "'Strong Objectivity' and Socially Situated Knowledge." In *Whose Science? Whose Knowledge?*, 138–63. New York: Cornell University Press, 1991.

Hoberman, John. *Black and Blue: The Origins and Consequences of Medical Racism*. Berkeley: University of California Press, 2012.

hooks, bell. "Choosing the Margins as a Space of Radical Openness." In *The Feminist Standpoint Theory Reader: Intellectual and Political Controversies*, edited by Sandra Harding, 153–60. New York: Routledge, 2004.

Jameson, Frederic. "Future City." *New Left Review* 21 (May 2003): 76.

Jones, Esther, ed. *Health Humanities in Global Context: Race and Ethnicity across the World.* New York: Palgrave Macmillan, forthcoming.

Jones, Therese. "'Oh! The Humanit(ies)!': Dissent, Democracy, and Danger." In *Medicine, Health, and the Arts: Approaches to the Medical Humanities*, edited by Victoria Bates, Alan Bleakley, and Sam Goodman, 27–38. Abingdon, UK: Routledge, 2014.

Jones, Therese, Delese Wear, and Lester D. Friedman, eds. *Health Humanities Reader.* New Brunswick, NJ: Rutgers University Press, 2014.

Lamb, Erin, and Craig Klugman. *Methods of the Health Humanities*. Oxford: Oxford University Press, forthcoming.

Ostherr, Kirsten. *Medical Visions: Producing the Patient through Film, Television, and Imaging Technologies*. Oxford: Oxford University Press, 2013.

Price, Margaret. *Mad at School: Rhetorics of Mental Disability and Academic Life*. Ann Arbor: University of Michigan Press, 2007.

Sandoval, Chela. "U.S. Third World Feminism: The Theory and Method of Differential Oppositional Consciousness." In *The Feminist Standpoint Theory Reader: Intellectual and Political Controversies*, edited by Sandra Harding, 195–210. New York: Routledge, 2004.

Viney, William, Felicity Callard, and Angela Woods. "Critical Medical Humanities: Embracing Entanglement, Taking Risks." *Medical Humanities* 41, no. 1 (2015): 2–7.

Whitehead, Ann, and Angela Woods, eds. *The Edinburgh Companion to the Critical Medical Humanities*. Edinburgh: Edinburgh University Press, 2016.

PART I

Places of Pedagogy

1

Undergraduate Education

Craig M. Klugman

Introduction

Thirty students wander among desks in a bright classroom. On the desks are pieces of art accompanied by short essays explaining the significance of each piece. On one table lays a black-and-white photograph showing a disheveled, older man sitting on a park bench. The essay explains that the student took the picture after seeing the subject drop his inhaler. She helped him to find it and then started talking to him about his chronic obstructive pulmonary disease and his experiences with the healthcare system. Another display shows a home-made graphic novel, detailing a student's ongoing experiences trying to find a diagnosis for her boyfriend's mysterious illness. In a third, a collage shows a computed tomography scan superimposed on top of medical articles about the imaging method and hospital bills for the procedure. The accompanying essay describes the collage as representing the cost of cutting-edge technology. This is Gallery—the final exam in a baccalaureate health humanities class. The students' assignment is to create an original piece of art based on a theme from the course and write a short essay that explains the work. Although many of these scientific students complain about their lack of creativity, they produce impressive works of thoughtful art.

In this chapter, I will explore how the health humanities moved into the baccalaureate environment and show that this presence is growing rapidly. The undergraduate health humanities experience is different from that in a medical school because the baccalaureate student has more time, more curricular space, and fewer preconceived notions about "what is important." The undergraduate student body is a larger population than those of graduate and professional schools. Baccalaureate students are more diverse in terms of sex, race/ethnicity, and career path. While in a medical school the majority of students will become doctors, in an undergraduate setting students may be headed for medical, nursing, public health, physical therapy, or other allied health careers or will not work in health at all. Alongside these advantages are certain challenges for approaching this work with an undergraduate population that I explore. These differences become evident in long-term assignments such as Gallery and a narrative ethnography project.

In medical humanities, the term *undergraduate* is often used to refer to the years in medical school. However, here I use the term *undergraduate* to refer to the years spent pursuing a baccalaureate degree.

A Brief History of Undergraduate Health Humanities

In 1910, Abraham Flexner refined medical education into the scientism we know today when he released his report *Medical Education in the United States and Canada*.[1] Flexner proposed that medical training be based on the scientific model and that students come to medical school with a strong background in the sciences. The sciences ended up replacing humanities, arts, and social science coursework. Regretfully, in 1925, Flexner wrote to his brother that he had assumed students would enter medicine with a liberal arts background rich in humanities when he wrote his report.[2] Post–Flexner report students lacked this essential exposure.

In response to the lack of humanities learning in medical students, in 1967 the Pennsylvania College of Medicine began a quiet revolution by introducing medical humanities into its medical curriculum. Over the next several decades many medical schools adopted similar programs that incorporated literature, history, narrative, law, ethics, and cultural studies into the four-year medical school experience. At the same time preparation for medical school had not changed since Flexner released his report: students in the 2000s still prepared for medical school by taking a science-intensive course of baccalaureate study, often eschewing the humanities, arts, and social sciences for advanced biology, genetics, physics, and chemistry.

This emphasis is reflected in the Medical College Admission Test (MCAT), which is the gatekeeper to studying medicine in the United States and Canada. The test first appeared under this name in 1948 but is found in earlier incarnations as far back as 1928. These early tests required knowledge of "modern society" such as history, economics, and sociology. Since 1977 the test focused more on science and quantitative reasoning, having deleted the society section. To prepare for this test, students were encouraged to major in biology, chemistry, and biochemistry.[3] However, change appeared in 2011 when the Association of American Medical Colleges announced that as of 2015 the exam would reduce the percent of science tested and add sections on human behavior/culture and on logical analysis/reasoning.[4] In addition to science, students are now encouraged to take courses in psychology, sociology, and philosophy/ethics.

Outside of the United States, medical school entrance exams focus on reasoning skills rather than scientific knowledge. For example, the UK

Clinical Aptitude Test looks at verbal reasoning, decision-making, quantitative reasoning, abstract reasoning, and situational judgment. The Australian Undergraduate Medicine and Health Sciences Admissions Test focuses on logical reasoning and problem-solving, interpersonal understanding, and pattern identification. However, in India, the National Eligibility cum Entrance Test focuses solely on knowledge of physics, chemistry, and biology.[5] At the time of writing, there has not been a strong movement toward baccalaureate health humanities in these countries.

In 1978, an article in the *New England Journal of Medicine* questioned the scientific approach to premedical education and suggested that a broader curriculum based in the humanities would be more appropriate.[6] In the 1980s, Davidson College in North Carolina began its Center for Medical Humanities (now the Department of Health and Human Values), and in 1990 Hiram College began the Center for Literature and Medicine, both of which offered classes and formal curricula that incorporated more humanities into premedical education and more medicine into traditional humanities teaching. In the United States, the new MCAT increased the popularity of undergraduate health humanities programs and is changing how baccalaureate institutions prepare their students for medical school. Although biology and chemistry are still popular majors for premed students, as of 2018 sixty-eight health humanities programs exist in the United States and the first minor in Canada has started enrolling students.[7] At the baccalaureate level, health humanities can take the form of majors, minors, concentrations, or certificates. This count does not include student clubs, which provide another opportunity for engagement. While more applicants to medical school major in biology, the success rate of applicants from the humanities is higher.[8]

Why Health Humanities in Baccalaureate Education

HEALTH HUMANITIES VERSUS MEDICAL HUMANITIES

The term *health humanities* is most often used in the undergraduate (baccalaureate) arena instead of medical humanities. The shift in term is more encompassing and representative of the shift from disciplinary to multi- and interdisciplinary ways of knowing and practicing. The field of health humanities acknowledges that health is composed of several social determinants including economic stability, education, social and community context, neighborhood and built environment, and medical care. Medicine is only one aspect of "health."[9] Many students who declare themselves interested in medical school will never apply to medical school or will choose to go into nursing, dentistry, public health, or other allied health professions. Many students who might be interested in classes labeled "medical humanities" may turn away, thinking that such courses are only for people interested in medical careers.

In a practical sense, gaining approval for a *medical humanities* curriculum at an undergraduate institution can be challenging. At my own school, we received such feedback as "with that name, would students in such a curriculum feel like a failure if they did not get into medical school" and "it seems like this would be good preparation for nursing students, but the term *medical* will keep those students away." Thus, the use of *health* instead of *medicine* is more welcoming and encompassing of the many professions and perspectives that students may study.

WIDER AUDIENCE

A medical humanities program in a medical school reaches a very narrow audience. A large medical school may have one thousand students over all four years. If the medical school is part of a stand-alone health science center, then there may be an audience of two thousand students. In a baccalaureate institution, the potential audience could be in the tens of thousands. My own university has sixteen thousand undergraduate students, and the health sciences major (the home for the health humanities) has 850 students. Students from outside of the home major may also take health humanities classes out of interest or because they are requirements in other majors, minors, and certificates.

Even if a student in an undergraduate health humanities course decides not to go into any health profession, that student still benefits from exposure to this field. Every student will someday be a patient or a caregiver for a patient. Their exposure to the health humanities offers them tools for making sense of the illness experience, communicating with healthcare professionals, and finding others going through similar experiences (whether through support groups or reading a book written by someone who had the same illness). The health humanities are not solely for people who practice medicine and health professions. They have a great deal to teach those who are sick or someday will be sick. In the baccalaureate institution, all students have access.

GREATER DIVERSITY

Not only can undergraduate health humanities reach a greater number of students, but there is also a greater diversity in the types of students. For example, consider the distribution of students based on sex and race/ethnicity between undergraduate and medical schools in the United States (Table 1.1).

MORE TIME AND SPACE IN THE CURRICULUM

In the undergraduate setting, students have more time and space in their course of study to engage in health humanities. Students in an undergraduate program tend to have class twelve to eighteen hours per week (depending on how many

TABLE 1.1

Comparison of Diversity in Students at US Baccalaureate and Medical Schools*

	Baccalaureate	Medical Schools
Total population	20,207,460	20,055
Sex		
Male	43.5%	52.8%
Female	56.5%	47.2%
Race/ethnicity		
White	55.6%	51.7%
Black	39.8%	6.4%
Hispanic	13.8%	8.4%
Asian	6%	20.1%
Pacific Islander/Hawaiian	0.2%	0.1%
American Indian	3%	0.7%
Resident nonalien	4.5%	1.3%

*May not add up to 100% because of nonresponses and "other" categories.[18]

credits they are taking) over four years. In medical school, only about 70% of schools require humanities education, and those offer a median of twenty-nine hours of exposure.[10] Even if humanities are available, most medical students pack their classroom work into the first two years (first eighteen months in many newer curricula), with some short selectives/electives in the third and fourth years. The baccalaureate student has more time and more space in the academic program to devote to a class or formal program in health humanities. In addition, an undergraduate course will meet for thirty-three hours (quarters) to forty-five hours (semester) per academic term. On top of that, students are expected to spend two to three hours working outside of class for every hour in class. Thus, in a single undergraduate course, students spend more time studying health humanities than most students do over four years of medical school.

In an undergraduate institution, the health humanities course counts the same as any other course as far as number of credits and time spent in the classroom (with the exception of lab courses). Every class is assigned a separate grade that counts equally toward the grade point average. In most medical schools, it is rare for health humanities to be a separate grade and, if it is, to receive the same weight. An undergraduate health humanities course does not have to fight for limited curricular time or for space on a comprehensive exam.

UNFORMED PROFESSIONAL IDENTITIES

The undergraduate student walking into a university does not necessarily know what is emphasized and de-emphasized in medical training. The student has not yet experienced the hidden curriculum of medicine or taken standardized tests that predominantly emphasize science over humanities. Having taught at two medical schools, I found that there were some students who gravitated to the humanities but that the vast majority found them to be "a break from real studying" or "irrelevant to being a doctor," as several students wrote on ethics/humanities module evaluations. The undergraduate student, for the most part, has no such assumptions. This younger student asks, What do I need to know to be a professional? Thus, students at this stage of learning are more open to and accepting of humanities work and more clearly see its relevance. A student may not understand how the Krebs cycle will assist in healing patients, but he or she can instantly see why viewing a play about a person dying of cancer will help him or her relate to future patients, or even to a family member, suffering from the same disease. The health humanities are universal and provide a meaningful base on which students can build a professional identity.[11]

SUCCESS IN MEDICAL EDUCATION

The majority of applicants to medical school do major in the biological sciences. In part, premed advisors often encourage students to pursue biology-related degrees since such degrees allow a student to count the premed requirements toward a degree program and because they are trained to offer this advice. But since the mid-1990s, data on student performance in medical school based on their baccalaureate major have shown that humanities students do as well as those with any other major.[12] In the United States, humanities students generally have higher MCAT scores than those with other majors, and a 1983 article found that humanities majors were more likely to choose primary care specialties.[13]

Lessons for the Undergraduate Instructor

For the health humanities scholar coming out of a medical school environment (whether for graduate training or a previous faculty position), the baccalaureate environment can be alien. The students are younger and less mature. They often want advice on such varied issues as choosing a career and how to get along with a disliked roommate. They are exploring being adults and making many of their own decisions for the first time. While some approaches, lectures, and assignments from medical and graduate school may translate to the undergraduate setting, most will require significant reworking. Therefore, I offer these nine suggestions for working with an undergraduate population. Later in this chapter, I will connect these general lessons to specific teaching strategies.

1. "*You know nothing Jon Snow.*" Undergraduate students lack background knowledge and skills that one might assume in a medical student who has already completed four years of college. For example,

in my first semester teaching after receiving my doctorate, I assigned baccalaureate students an ethical analysis essay about any issue in health. What I received looked nothing like what I expected or could understand. I realized that the students had no idea what an analysis is, never mind what ethics is. The next quarter I split the assignment into several parts: topic, introductory paragraph, annotated bibliography, detailed outline, and final paper. For each section, I distributed detailed instructions and examples of successful essays. I also gave each individual student detailed feedback as he or she turned in each of the subassignments. Instead of letting them choose any health-related topic, I gave them a list of six topics from which to pick. The result was that they learned all of the skills that go into writing an analysis paper and created a better product.

2. *Talk about all health professions, not just medicine.* Chances are that more undergraduate students will go into nursing, allied health professions, and public health than will go into medicine. This makes it important to be inclusive in teaching and discussion. It took about three years before all of my PowerPoint slides changed from "doctor" and "medicine" to "healthcare provider" and "healthcare."
3. *Relate knowledge and skills through examples that students understand.* Undergraduate students are younger and less experienced than graduate students. They are exploring their world and the artistic canons of culture for the first time. Many references we use in graduate programs and when talking to our peers will be lost on these students. For example, recently, I was teaching about Kant and used the classic thought experiment, "Your best friend is on the run and hiding in your basement. She begs you to tell no one that she is there. A KGB agent knocks on your door and asks where your friend is. What do you do?" Before we discussed the Kantian imperative that you must always tell the truth, I asked the students if they had any questions. One hand went up, and the student asked, "Yeah, what's the KGB?" I realized that these students had been four years old when the KGB was disbanded, so I had to find a more contemporary reference for them.
4. *Exams do not have to be multiple-choice.* In the medical schools where I worked, there was an emphasis on preparing students to succeed on the US Medical Licensing Examination Step exams. Toward that end we had to write final exam questions in the Step format that had to be approved by a test question committee. Besides, even if I could have assigned an essay, grading 225 essays was beyond my available time. In an undergraduate institution, the instructor decides the format of the question and what material to test. Now I can assign short essays in exams, alongside a few multiple-choice questions (so that they can get a taste of that experience) and even have students write a longer paper

over the term. With only thirty students in my classes, I have more time and space for grading their writing.

5. *Set the examples for how they will relate to people in the future.* The first time I received an email from a student that began with "Hey Craig," I knew that I had to set an example for courteous communication and interaction with students that would serve them well throughout life. Rather than getting frustrated at their attempts toward familiarity, I keep a series of stock answers to use in the teachable moment. To that student, I answered the question and then stated, "I just wanted to let you know, to help you in your future interactions, that unless someone has invited you to call them by their first name, in general a person with more education or a higher position than you should be addressed by an honorific and the last name." I then signed the note "Dr. K." Sure enough, the student apologized and expressed appreciation because no one had told her the proper way to address a professor before.
6. *Grammar counts*. Often, when I did assign short essays in a medical school, I was advised not to worry about grammar or spelling because medical students did not need to know how to write and most likely had not had a writing class in a long time. In a baccalaureate course, I can set the future stage by having grammar and spelling as a component of every assignment. Plus, the university has a writing center, so if I find that a student needs to work on his or her writing, I refer the student to the writing center for assistance.
7. *Classroom time should be spent in active learning.* "Flipped classroom" and "student-directed learning" are among several popular pedagogies in undergraduate teaching. In both of these examples, the assumption is that knowledge is readily available to students through books and the Internet. In face-to-face interactions, one teaches and students practice active skills such as how to find good sources of information. This has led to the growth of "hybrid courses," where reading, online lectures, and exercises are completed at home on the student's time before arriving to the classroom.[14] Whereas a traditional class would meet twice a week for seventy-five to ninety minutes each time, in a hybrid class students meet once a week for seventy-five to ninety minutes, and the other "class period" time is spent on self-study using online materials provided by the instructor. Passive learning such as listening to a lecture occurs online, at home (or in the library). Since the limited resource in a course is classroom time, the instructor is encouraged to spend that time on active learning such as discussion, group work, and more detailed exercises. In these pedagogies, the instructor is not a topic expert so much as a learning facilitator.
8. *Hold students accountable.* I do not assign a task and assume students will complete it. College students do activities for a reward, not for

their own personal learning. They only complete those things which the instructor will read and grade. If there is not an assessment, then they will put in less time and might even skip the activity.[15] For example, few students will read a book to be discussed in class. At the beginning of the class session I give a reading quiz to make sure that students are familiar with the work, and then we can have a discussion. Knowing that there is a graded quiz, more students complete the reading. In the Gallery exercise, accountability means that students conduct peer scoring of art. Even this simple element encourages students to pay greater attention to their classmates' projects.

9. *More time does not equal more topics.* Although classes are longer and there are opportunities for assignments that extend over months, the fact that students may lack critical thinking skills means that instructors end up teaching less content and more skills. For example, in reading *The Nichomachean Ethics*, I have students bring one chapter to class. I break them up into eight groups, and each group is assigned a section of the text. The goal of that group is to write one or two sentences to explain what Aristotle is saying. During a fifteen-minute work period, I visit each group to listen and to offer some direction for their interpretation. Then each group writes its sentence on the board. In eight sentences, the class has interpreted the chapter in words that make sense to them and are accurate to the original text. Students find it difficult to read an original text, but when they are shown how to break it apart and how to engage the text, they learn the skills and can read the next chapter with greater ease and understanding. Plus, they learn to discuss meaning and interpretation with their peers. The additional course time does not mean that you will cover topics in further depth or pack more topics in (you can do that by offering multiple courses) but rather that you can go slower and work with students to develop their skills.

PUTTING THE SKILLS TOGETHER

In my health humanities course, students are assigned to write a narrative ethnography, a practice that encompasses several skills over the ten weeks of the quarter. The goal is for students to be able to interview people, write their story, and analyze the story they have written. In the second week of a ten-week course, students participate in a narrative medicine exercise based on one developed by Rita Charon of the narrative medicine program at Columbia University. Students break into pairs. One person is the teller, and the other is the listener. In the first stage, the teller spends five minutes telling a true story based upon a prompt offered by the instructor. For the next five minutes, the listener writes down the story he or she heard, and the teller writes down what it was like to tell the story. They then switch roles. At this point the class comes together, and pairs are asked to volunteer to read one set of stories. Thus, the listener will read what he or she wrote of the story he or she heard. He or she may not add anything to the story, only read what is handwritten on the page. The class then performs a literary analysis of the story prompted by the instructor. For example, the class is asked, Who are the characters? What is the plot? Where is the setting? Describe themes and symbols. The original teller is asked how much of the oral story the listener captured and then shares his or her essay about telling the story.

In the second stage, students are assigned a published pathography due in the fourth week of the term. I provide students a list of written works, films, and graphic novels from which they may choose. The student then writes his or her analysis of the work based on guiding questions. As an instructor, I grade the assignment with detailed comments and suggestions and return it to the student.

The third and final stage has students interview a person suffering from an illness and write his or her story. This paper is submitted in the ninth week of the quarter. As the instructions detail, the goal is to discern the patient's illness narrative or the patient's perspective of living with the illness. I do not assign patients to the students as part of the assignment. It is for them to find people who suffer an illness. I instruct students in being courteous and professional in speaking with their subjects, including asking for their permission and explaining that this is a class assignment that will be shared with the members of the course. A few students have reported that their first-choice interviewee said no to the conversation and that they had to find a second subject. Many interview friends or family members, but a few will interview people they encounter in their lives such as a custodian, an administrative assistant, or even a person they meet on the bus. Some of the illnesses are serious, and some are trivial, though they might be serious to those experiencing them. One of the goals is for the students to realize that many people experience illness and suffering all around and that without asking, you might never know.

The student then writes the patient's story. Often, students choose a third-person point of view, but some have chosen the first person. The last section of the paper is to analyze their own writing, looking at perspective, voice, character, plot, theme, symbol, setting, and more, just as they did in class and in the pathography. Each of these stages is listed as a separate assignment and receives a different grade, but the earlier activities build upon one another to allow the student to conduct the detailed and complex final paper.

The following progression of assignments demonstrates the seven lessons I have laid out.

1. *You know nothing.* Students start without knowing about illness narratives and health humanities deep reading. By the end they are able to do so on their own. They practice the skills and partake in discussion to learn about illness narratives, pathographies, and narrative medicine.

2. *Illness is about more than medicine.* Students are not taught to ask patients what doctors they have seen but rather what treatment and help they have sought. The emphasis is on the idea that caring happens in a host of ways by a variety of professions and non-professionals.
3. *Relate knowledge and skills through examples that students understand.* Not only do they learn about the ideas of Arthur Kleinman, Rita Charon, and Kathryn Montgomery on illness narratives, but also through specific examples (themselves, a text, and an interview) the concept is brought to life.[16]
4. *Exams do not have to be multiple-choice.* This work is not short answer and has no right or wrong responses.
5. *Set examples for future interactions.* The instructions teach students about proper behavior and address.
6. *Grammar counts.* Grammar is part of the grade.
7. *Active learning.* The first exercise is an active, in-class activity that can only be done with others. Reading and writing then occur on the students' own time. If they have questions, the instructor is an email or phone call away.
8. *Hold students accountable.* At each stage students learn and demonstrate graded skills. The in-class exercise counts toward a course attendance and participation grade. The text analysis and narrative analysis are graded according to a rubric that I share with students ahead of time. The instructor must read all writing, assign a grade using the rubric, and make copious comments on the student's work.
9. *You may have more time, but you may end up teaching less.* In a ten-week quarter, the three parts of this assignment consume a considerable amount of time. I would love to have them do other assignments and demonstrate other skills, but doing so would be a superficial study and diminish all learning in a short period of time. Thus, we focus on fewer skills but learn them in greater depth.

This approach requires a great deal of time and energy from both the instructor and the student. As an instructor, I have to design the detailed instructions and examples, spend time and effort on careful formative grading, and respond to frequent student questions. The end result, however, is a student with an expanded knowledge base and an important health humanities skill.

Gaining Institutional Acceptance

When I arrived at DePaul, I created and submitted for approval a health humanities course. The college of science's curriculum committee was unsure of how it deepened students' knowledge of science but as an elective the committee was willing to let it pass. I then applied to have this course count for the "arts and literature" learning domain in the general education requirements. The course was rejected, with a long list of suggestions and reasons. A year later I revised and resubmitted and was rejected outright. This time there were few comments, but the message was that this domain was the province of the humanities departments. A second message was that the health humanities was not a methodological way of knowing in itself but rather a superficial examination of the humanities in instrumental service to health. I did not apply a third time.

In the undergraduate environment, the health humanities can be threatening. As a stand-alone course, it threatens those in the traditional humanities who feel that students in the sciences and health will not venture out to learn from them but stay closer to their science. Considering that there has been a dramatic drop in the number of humanities majors and the percent of all faculty teaching in humanities, this is a real concern.[17] As part of a major or minor program, health humanities is a threat to the traditional premed majors. At my institution, the bench biologists and chemists who are used to teaching these students believe that their hard science curriculum is the best preparation for medical school, even though few (if any) of them have ever taught in a medical school. The biology department is often trying to find out how many of its students were accepted into medical school versus the number in the health sciences program. Another fear of the traditional sciences is that interdisciplinary health and health humanities programs will "steal" their students. What is even worse from their perspective is that while they lose numbers of majors, their teaching workload remains the same since the health humanities students will still be taking the same biology and chemistry premed science courses. In some cases, I was told that our students were not as competitive as the biology majors in those classes. Several bench science courses saw their prerequisites increased so that one could not take the class without being a science major. The result is that interdisciplinary health had to create and offer its own science classes, which ultimately were more popular than the pure science options because we connected the science to the humanities and social sciences.

Undergraduate health humanities is about interdisciplinary learning. The goal is to help students bring together the humanities, arts, social sciences, and sciences to gain a larger, 360-degree view of health. The health humanities prime students to think about illness as not just a malfunction of the body or an invading pathogen but also a change in a life and a process that takes place within a community, a set of health policies, and a particular economic environment. Students learn to view health issues from perspectives that inform one another. My hope is that when these students move on to health careers, to being patients, and to being caregivers to loved ones, they remember this bigger picture.

PEDAGOGY EXERCISE SECTION

Assignment Handouts

GALLERY

Throughout the course we have been engaging with texts of all kinds, from visual art to film to narrative. Now it is your turn to appreciate the process of creating such works. For your final assignment, you are to create an original work of narrative art that represents a theme from the course. You may choose something inspiring from the book you individually chose and read for the course or from any other aspect of the course. Your piece should have a definite theme.

You can create any artistic piece such as a painting, sculpture, photograph, short story, poem, fabric art, play, music, video, or dance, to name a few forms. Any form of creative expression is acceptable.

This assignment has several components.

1. Your creative expression. Do not leave this to the last minute. It is much harder to put together a truly effective and thoughtful creative piece than you may think.
2. A short essay of at least 500 words that discusses your work from a narrative perspective and explains:
   a. Why did you chose this particular medium?
   b. What should the viewer/reader look for in your work?
   c. What was your inspiration for the piece?
   d. What themes are reflected in the work?
3. A presentation for the final class meeting. This "Gallery" will be an opportunity for the entire class to see our creations. If you require any special display space, please let the instructor know. For example, you may want an easel to show your artwork, a sound system to play a song, an area to perform a dance, etc.

GRADING RUBRIC

CRITERION	POSSIBLE POINTS
Production of a thoughtful creative expression	40
Critical essay of minimum 500 words that discusses the work	26
Public presentation to the course at Gallery session	20
Peer grading	14
Total	100

GALLERY PEER GRADING SHEET

Your task is to give a peer review grade for each of our classmates' creative efforts. Place a checkmark or an X in the score that is closest to your assessment. Use the following guide in making your assessment:

2—Piece of art is creative, clearly reflects a theme from the course, and is artistically pleasing; and it appears that the artist put in a great deal of effort. Essay is well written and masterfully describes the art piece.

1—Piece of art is interesting, reflects a theme from the course, and has been completed; and it appears that the artist put some time into the effort. Essay is cogent and describes the art piece.

0—No art is produced, or the piece of art reflects a minimum of effort or does not relate to a course theme. Essay is missing or difficult to read and does not ably describe the art piece.

ARTIST NAME	SCORING (PUT AN X IN APPROPRIATE BOX)		
	2—EXCELLENT	1—GOOD	0—UNACCEPTABLE

ILLNESS NARRATIVE ETHNOGRAPHY ASSIGNMENT

You are to submit a minimum 1,500-word essay that describes a person's experience of illness and what it meant to him or her. In order to accomplish this task you must do the following:

1. Interview a person who has been a patient for an illness. Ideally, this is a person whose story you do not know well. You should ask the person in advance and schedule a time to talk. Be sure to let the person know what the interview is for, what it is about, and approximately how long it will take. Ask permission to take notes (please note that audio or visual recording requires a separate written, signed consent that must be approved by the university). Be sure to follow up with a thank you note and, when written, send the patient a copy of your essay.
2. Write a 1,500-word essay. About 1000 words (66%) should tell the patient's story. Make sure you answer the following questions:
   a. Provide some context for the interview:
      i. Who did you interview, and why this person?
      ii. Who is this person?

   b. What does the patient think caused the problem?*
   c. Why does the patient think it started when it did?*
   d. What does the patient think the illness does to him or her? How does it work?*
   e. How severe is the sickness?*
   f. What kind of treatment did the patient think he or she should have received and what did he or she receive?*
   g. What are the results the patient expected from the treatment? Was it successful?*
   h. What are the chief problems the sickness caused for the patient?*
   i. What does the patient fear most about the sickness?*
   j. With whom has the patient shared the story before?
3. The rest of the essay (about 500 words) should be an analysis of the illness narrative.
   a. What is the plot of the story?
   b. Who are the characters?
   c. What are the symbols, and what do they mean?
   d. What are the themes in the story?
   e. What is the patient's desired goal (cure, treatment, end to suffering, recompense, etc.)?
   f. From what perspective is the story told (first person, second person, third person)?
   g. What is the setting of the story?
   h. What do you think the story means?

GRADING RUBRIC

CRITERION	POSSIBLE POINTS
Well written (followed rules of spelling and grammar)	13
Provided context for interviewee	13
Critical description of patient's explanatory model of illness (area 2)	40
Critical narrative analysis (area 3)	34
Total	100

* From Arthur Kleinman's Explanatory Model of Illness.

Notes

1. Abraham Flexner, *Medical Education in the United States and Canada: A Report to the Carnegie Foundation for the Advancement of Teaching*, The Flexner Report, Bulletin 4 (Boston: Updyke, 1910).

2. D. J. Doukas, L. B. Mccullough, and S. Wear, "Reforming Medical Education in Ethics and Humanities by Finding Common Ground with Abraham Flexner," *Academic Medicine* 85, no. 2 (2010): 318–23.

3. W. C. Mcgaghie, "Assessing Readiness for Medical Education: Evolution of the Medical College Admission Test," *JAMA* 288, no. 9 (2002): 1085–90.

4. Association of American Medical Colleges, "AAMC Releases Preliminary Recommendations for New Mcat Exam," modified 2011, accessed September 1, 2016, Association of American Medical Colleges "What You Need to Know About the New MCAT Exam," accessed August 13, 2018, https://students-residents.aamc.org/video/what-you-need-know-about-new-mcat-exam/.

5. UKCAT Consorium, "UKCAT Test Format," modified 2017, accessed October 31, 2017, https://www.ukcat.ac.uk/ukcat-test/ukcat-test-format/; Australian Council for Educational Research, "UMAT: Undergraduate Medicine and Health Sciences Admission Test. Preparation Strategy," modified 2017, accessed October 31, 2017, https://umat.acer.edu.au/prepare/preparation-strategy; Central Board of Secondary Education, "National Eligibiulity Cum Entrance Test," modified 2017, accessed October 31, 2017, http://cbseneet.nic.in/cbseneet/Welcome.aspx.

6. L. Thomas, "Notes of a Biology-Watcher. How to Fix the Premedical Curriculum," *New England Journal of Medicine* 298, no. 21 (1978): 1180–81.

7. Sarah L. Berry, Erin Gentry Lamb, and Therese Jones, "Health Humanities Baccalaureate Programs in the United States," Hiram College, 2017, accessed October 31, 2017, http://www.hiram.edu/academics/center-of-distinction/center-for-literature-medicine/baccalaureate-health-humanities-programs-in-the-u-s/. Also personal communication with Erin Lamb, October 31, 2017.

8. Association of American Medical Colleges, "Table A-17: MCAT and GPAs for Applicants and Matriculants to U.S. Medical Schools by Primary Undergraduate Major, 2016–2017," modified 2017, accessed October 31, 2017, https://www.aamc.org/download/321496/data/factstablea17.pdf.

9. T. Jones et al., "The Almost Right Word: The Move from Medical to Health Humanities," *Academic Medicine* 92, no. 7 (2017): 932–35; US Department of Health & Human Services, "Social Determinants of Health," modified 2017, accessed October 31, 2017, https://www.healthypeople.gov/2020/topics-objectives/topic/social-determinants-of-health. The name shift is even found in the naming/renaming of national and international academic societies: International Health Humanities Network (UK), Canadian Association for Health Humanities, and Health Humanities Consortium (US).

10. Craig M. Klugman, "Medical Humanities Teaching in North American Allopathic and Osteopathic Medical Schools," *Journal Medical Humanities* (2018), doi:10.1007/s10912-017-9491-z.

11. C. M. Klugman, "How Health Humanities Will Save the Life of the Humanities," *Journal of Medical Humanities* 38, no. 4 (2017): 419–30.

12. Michael R. Grey et al., "How Do Australian Doctors with Different Pre-Medical Backgrounds Perform as Interns?" *Education of Health* 14, no. 1 (2001): 87–96; D. Muller and N. Kase, "Challenging Traditional Premedical Requirements as Predictors of Success in Medical School: The Mount Sinai School of Medicine Humanities and Medicine Program," *Academic Medicine* 85, no. 8 (2010): 1378–83; Andrea Wershof et al., "Evaluating the Impact of the Humanities in Medical Education," *Mount Sinai Journal of Medicine* 76, no. 4 (2009): 372–80; S. R. Smith, "Effect of Undergraduate College Major on Performance in Medical School," *Academic Medicine* 73, no. 9 (1998): 1006–1008.

13. C. Zeleznik, M. Hojat, and J. Veloski, "Baccalaureate Preparation for Medical School: Does Type of Degree Make a Difference?" *Journal of Medical Education* 58, no. 1 (1983): 26–33; Association of American Medical Colleges, "Table A-17."

14. Maureen J. Lage, Glenn J. Platt, and Michael Treglia, "Inverting the Classroom: A Gateway to Creating an Inclusive Learning Environment," *Journal of Economic Education* 31, no. 1 (2000): 30–43.

15. Jeffrey S. Nevid and Katie Mahon, "Mastery Quizzing as a Signaling Device to Cue Attention to Lecture Material," *Teaching of Psychology* 26, no. 1 (2009): 29–32.

16. Rita Charon, *Narrative Medicine: Honoring the Stories of Illness* (New York: Oxford University Press, 2006); Arthur Kleinman, *The Illness Narratives: Suffering, Healing & the Human Condition* (New York: Basic Books, 1988); Kathryn Montgomery, *Doctors' Stories: The Narrative Structure of Medical Knowledge* (Princeton, NJ: Princeton University Press, 1993).

17. Humanities Indicators, "Number of Faculty Members in Humanities and Other Fields," modified June 2016, accessed Octber 31, 2017, https://www.humanitiesindicators.org/content/indicatorDoc.aspx?i=71; Humanities Indicators, "Bachelor's Degrees in the Humanities," modified May 2017, accessed June 17, 2017, https://humanitiesindicators.org/content/indicatordoc.aspx?i=34.

18. Based on Association of American Medical Colleges, "Table A-9: Matriculants to U.S. Medical Schools by Race, Selected Combinations of Race/Ethnicity and Sex, 2013–2014 through 2016–2017," modified 2017, accessed October 31, 2017 https://www.aamc.org/download/321474/data/factstablea9.pdf; and National Center for Education Statistics, "Table 306.10. Total Fall Enrollment in Degree-Granting Postsecondary Institutions, by Level of Enrollment, Sex, Attendance Status, and Race/Ethnicity of Student: Selected Years, 1976 through 2015," prepared October 2016, accessed October 31, 2017, https://nces.ed.gov/programs/digest/d16/tables/dt16_306.10.asp.

Works Cited

Association of American Medical Colleges "What You Need to Know About the New MCAT Exam," accessed August 13, 2018, https://students-residents.aamc.org/video/what-you-need-know-about-new-mcat-exam/.

———. "Table A-9: Matriculants to U.S. Medical Schools by Race, Selected Combinations of Race/Ethnicity and Sex, 2013–2014 through 2016–2017." Modified 2017. Accessed October 31, 2017. https://www.aamc.org/download/321474/data/factstablea9.pdf.

———. "Table A-17: MCAT and GPAs for Applicants and Matriculants to U.S. Medical Schools by Primary Undergraduate Major, 2016–2017." Modified 2017. Accessed October 31, 2017. https://www.aamc.org/download/321496/data/factstablea17.pdf.

Australian Council for Educational Research. "UMAT: Undergraduate Medicine and Health Sciences Admission Test. Preparation Strategy." Modified 2017. Accessed October 31, 2017. https://umat.acer.edu.au/prepare/preparation-strategy.

Berry, Sarah L., Erin Gentry Lamb, and Therese Jones. "Health Humanities Baccalaureate Programs in the United States." Hiram College, 2017. Accessed October 31, 2017. http://www.hiram.edu/academics/center-of-distinction/center-for-literature-medicine/baccalaureate-health-humanities-programs-in-the-u-s/.

Central Board of Secondary Education. "National Eligibility Cum Entrance Test." Modified 2017. Accessed October 31, 2017. http://cbseneet.nic.in/cbseneet/Welcome.aspx.

Charon, Rita. *Narrative Medicine: Honoring the Stories of Illness.* New York: Oxford University Press, 2006.

Doukas, D. J., L. B. McCullough, and S. Wear. "Reforming Medical Education in Ethics and Humanities by Finding Common Ground with Abraham Flexner." *Academic Medicine* 85, no. 2 (2010): 318–23.

Flexner, Abraham. *Medical Education in the United States and Canada: A Report to the Carnegie Foundation for the Advancement of Teaching*. The Flexner Report, Bulletin 4. Boston: Updyke, 1910.

Grey, Michael R., Sallie-Anne Pearson, Isobel E. Rolfe, Francis. J. Kay, David A. Powis. "How Do Australian Doctors with Different Pre-medical Backgrounds Perform as Interns." *Education for Health Change in Learning and Practice* 14, no. 1 (2001): 87–96.

Humanities Indicators. "Bachelor's Degrees in the Humanities." Modified May 2017. Accessed June 17, 2017. https://humanitiesindicators.org/content/indicatordoc.aspx?i=34.

———. "Number of Faculty Members in Humanities and Other Fields." Modified June 2016. Accessed Octber 31, 2017. https://www.humanitiesindicators.org/content/indicatorDoc.aspx?i=71.

Jones, T., M. Blackie, R. Garden, and D. Wear. "The Almost Right Word: The Move from Medical to Health Humanities." *Academic Medicine* 92, no. 7 (2017): 932–35.

Kleinman, Arthur. *The Illness Narratives: Suffering, Healing & the Human Condition.* New York: Basic Books, 1988.

Klugman, C. M. "How Health Humanities Will Save the Life of the Humanities." *Journal of Medical Humanities* 38, no. 4 (2017): 419–30.

Klugman, Craig M. "Medical Humanities Teaching in North American Allopathic and Osteopathic Medical Schools." *Journal Medical Humanities* (2018). doi:10.1007/s10912-017-9491-z.

Lage, Maureen J., Glenn J. Platt, and Michael Treglia. "Inverting the Classroom: A Gateway to Creating an Inclusive Learning Environment." *Journal of Economic Education* 31, no. 1 (2000): 30–43.

McGaghie, W. C. "Assessing Readiness for Medical Education: Evolution of the Medical College Admission Test." *JAMA* 288, no. 9 (2002): 1085–90.

Montgomery, Kathryn. *Doctors' Stories: The Narrative Structure of Medical Knowledge.* Princeton, NJ: Princeton University Press, 1993.

Muller, D., and N. Kase. "Challenging Traditional Premedical Requirements as Predictors of Success in Medical School: The Mount Sinai School of Medicine Humanities and Medicine Program." *Academic Medicine* 85, no. 8 (2010): 1378–83.

National Center for Education Statistics. "Table 306.10. Total Fall Enrollment in Degree-Granting Postsecondary Institutions, by Level of Enrollment, Sex, Attendance Status, and Race/Ethnicity of Student: Selected Years, 1976 through 2015." Prepared October 2016. Accessed October 31, 2017. https://nces.ed.gov/programs/digest/d16/tables/dt16_306.10.asp.

Nevid, Jeffrey S., and Katie Mahon. "Mastery Quizzing as a Signaling Device to Cue Attention to Lecture Material." *Teaching of Psychology* 26, no. 1 (2009): 29–32.

Schwartz, Andrea Wershof, J. S. Abramson, I. Wojnowich, R. Accordino, E. J. Ronan, and M. R. Rifkin. "Evaluating the Impact of the Humanities in Medical Education." *Mount Sinai Journal of Medicine* 76, no. 4 (2009): 372–80.

Smith, S. R. "Effect of Undergraduate College Major on Performance in Medical School." *Academic Medicine* 73, no. 9 (1998): 1006–1008.

Thomas, L. "Notes of a Biology-Watcher. How to Fix the Premedical Curriculum." *New England Journal of Medicine* 298, no. 21 (1978): 1180–81.

UKCAT Consorium. "UKCAT Test Format." Modified 2017. Accessed October 31, 2017. https://www.ukcat.ac.uk/ukcat-test/ukcat-test-format/.

US Department of Health & Human Services. "Social Determinants of Health." Modified 2017. Accessed October 31, 2017. https://www.healthypeople.gov/2020/topics-objectives/topic/social-determinants-of-health.

Zeleznik, C., M. Hojat, and J. Veloski. "Baccalaureate Preparation for Medical School: Does Type of Degree Make a Difference?" *Journal of Medical Education* 58, no. 1 (1983): 26–33.

2

Teaching for Humanism

ENGAGING HUMANITIES TO FOSTER CRITICAL DIALOGUES IN MEDICAL EDUCATION

Nicole M. Piemonte and Arno K. Kumagai

Introduction

The inclusion of the humanities in medical education—though increasingly popular in recent years—is not a new initiative. In the 1960s, philosophers, theologians, and practitioners began to draw attention to the fact that the medical care of the time failed to address the lived experience of patients and expressed concerns about "the way medical students of the rising generation were being trained and, in particular, what was lacking in their education."[1] Daniel Fox, who offers a historical account of the political origins of the medical humanities, observes that groups concerned with medical education during this time primarily focused on three issues: depersonalization in medicine, the centrality of molecular biology in medical education, and the teaching of "mechanistic medicine."[2] Though the term *medical humanities* was not used at the time (and did not become widely used until the 1980s and 1990s), prominent figures in medicine, such as famed physician and bioethicist Edmund Pellegrino, advocated for the introduction of the humanities into medical education.[3] And in 1967, the Penn State College of Medicine Department of Humanities became the first such department in a medical school in the United States.

Forty years have come and gone since the medical humanities—now often referred to as the "health humanities" to emphasize inclusiveness—came on the scene, and the number of initiatives in medical education has grown significantly. In fact, it is difficult to determine exactly how many departments, tracks, certificate programs, concentrations, and courses exist in 141 allopathic medical schools in the United States and Canada. However, a recent unpublished survey suggests that approximately 71% of these schools have required medical humanities curricula, 92% offer electives, and 23% have a pathway or concentration.[4] The medical humanities are also quite popular in the United Kingdom, where most medical programs offer courses in one or more humanities subjects at some point during students' education.[5]

Despite their increasing presence, it is hard to discern the specific content of and pedagogical theory driving such initiatives as there exists no standard curriculum and initiatives vary widely across schools and programs. For those of us who have been engaged in the field for a while, however, there is general agreement that the point of the humanities in medical education is not simply to make more compassionate and empathic doctors. Cultivating compassion and empathy is important, to be sure—yet, for most of us who are committed to advocating for social justice, ameliorating healthcare disparities, and creating a healthcare system that serves the deepest needs of those who participate in it, cultivating critical perspectives among our students, alongside promoting compassion, is paramount. Indeed, we believe that true compassion for others encompasses—and perhaps even catalyzes—a desire to (at least) acknowledge the systems of power and oppression that cause physical and existential suffering among patients, their loved ones, and ourselves. In gathering together the wisdom and insight of many disciplines—including literature, philosophy, religion, history, art, bioethics, visual studies, gender studies, and the social sciences—teaching the humanities in medical school can foster a richer understanding of the human experience of illness, health, dis/ability, identity, gender, embodiment, healthcare, and so on.[6] The humanities underscore the fact that medicine is laden with existential questions about the meaning of life and death and that practicing medicine requires more than scientific knowledge and technical acumen.

Our approach to teaching the humanities in medical education is grounded in fostering an understanding of the lived experiences of others that disrupts taken-for-granted assumptions and perspectives—usually through stories, film, drama, and the arts—as well as encouraging critical consciousness through reflection on the self, others, and the world.[7] We do so with a particular emphasis on the development of a professional identity and ethical being-in-the-world of the students whom we teach. This chapter, therefore, is devoted to an exploration of the aims of engaging the humanities in medical education and a discussion of specific pedagogical approaches in educating physicians for humanistic practice. In particular, the roles of stories, dialogue, and reflection on the moral, existential, and interpersonal dimensions of medicine are considered; and examples of specific educational practices from the authors' own experiences are used to illustrate how educational and social theory may be used to design learning activities that foster an orientation toward a practice of medicine that embodies excellence, compassion, and justice.

Why the Humanities?

Since the 1960s, when professionals—including (and perhaps especially) doctors—suddenly found themselves facing unprecedented scrutiny, there has been a general consensus that the persistent conflicts of goals, values, and interests, as well as the complexity, instability, and uncertainty intrinsic to medical practice, cannot be resolved by applying narrow, specialized knowledge.[8] The world of medicine is a kind of microcosm of life, a concentration of the all-too-human elements of being alive: birth, death, illness, suffering, isolation, fear, love, uncertainty. Nearly every person who cares for the sick crosses the threshold into the space where human mortality and finitude—and the feelings of helplessness associated with them—come to the fore. As such, practicing medicine requires both scientific knowledge and a different kind of knowing and learning, one that involves more than an acquisition of facts and skills via lectures and textbooks, one that works to develop an *orientation* toward self and others, which occurs tacitly through dialogue, personal experience, and reflection.[9]

However, the general lack of emphasis on the existential elements of medical practice that remains with us today is concerning since, as sociologist Fredric Hafferty points out, medical education is more than training—it is a *socialization process*, one that has the power to influence and shape students' values and beliefs.[10] As spaces of personal transformation, medical schools and residency programs "are formidable—and formative—settings that structure and shape how future physicians will think, act, and identify themselves with core occupational values."[11] In other words, a student does not merely adopt new attitudes and behaviors during this time that are "added on" to an already formed self; instead, socialization or resocialization involves some aspects of students' selves being "*replaced* by new ways of thinking, acting, and valuing. . . . a dual process of moving into the new and moving away from the old."[12] This is a process, Hafferty claims, "for better and/or for worse—to change hearts *and* minds."[13]

Even so, medical students are rarely told explicitly that the education they are undertaking will have as much to do with their character as it does with their intellect.[14] Personal transformation is largely left unaddressed at the level of the formal curriculum and is instead "taught" via the *hidden curriculum*—that is to say, through the messages students receive and the experiences they have with patients, peers, and mentors that powerfully communicate what it means to be a doctor. This is particularly problematic, given that the hidden curriculum is predominantly shaped by the epistemology of modern medicine—what doctors know and how they come to know it. Within medicine, the "knowable" is namely the observable and measurable (usually empirical, scientific facts), and how one comes to know those facts is through one's observations or through measurements, lab tests, microscopy, imaging, and so forth. Traditional accounts of medicine are dominated by a discursive system grounded in an epistemological theory of the body as an anatomical/physiological/biochemical structure that is best known and understood through the methods of science and through the impartial observations of the physician.[15]

On its face, the assumption that medicine is a scientific endeavor may appear reasonable, considering that clinicians often rely on important technology and scientific modalities to "reveal" the workings of the biological body. However, Kathryn Montgomery argues that this epistemology, which emphasizes objectivity and neutrality as a means of practicing "good science," ignores the fact that clinical practice is inherently uncertain and reliant on experiential knowledge.[16] Moreover, epistemologies carry with them a certain kind of ethos, shaping ideas of the specific dispositions and values that will allow one to properly secure knowledge.[17] In becoming or embodying this particular scientific self, knowing and knower are melded together, and the knower becomes one who must resist the temptations of imagination and subjectivity. As a result, some students may come to see the adoption of an objective stance toward a patient and his or her illness as good, noble, or right—despite the fact that scientific objectivity can occlude the very human elements of illness and medicine, resulting in narrow and insufficient care of the suffering other. A student, for example, might believe that the most important elements of his or her training are the diagnosis and (biological) treatment of pathology, rather than an ability to understand what it is like to live with and manage a chronic condition like diabetes, arthritis, or cystic fibrosis every day. This is not to say that an objective and accurate assessment of biological disease is not critical (it is) but, rather, that it cannot account for the complete picture of patient care. Nor is this to say that learning to think critically and responding appropriately to human suffering are somehow opposed to being trained in the sciences. There are, of course, many medical students who endure the rigors of such an education while holding fast to an authentic sensitivity to the depths of human suffering and are keen to point out some of the shortcomings of modern medicine or reductionist scientific research. Nevertheless, in general, medical education is not known for fostering commitments to change the social and economic forces that shape health and illness, for deepening students' ability to genuinely empathize with others, or for encouraging conversations about the existential struggles that severe illness can trigger.

Despite the fact that much ink has been spilled emphasizing that medicine is a *science-using* practice that involves "subjective" skills like clinical intuition, practical experience, and the ability to relate to and engage with other people, notions about the need for objectivity and a narrow focus on biological disease continue to abound in medical education.[18] And while a training defined by such notions often prepares students well for the important tasks of diagnosing and treating biological breakdowns, it fails to prepare them for the care of patients who suffer in ways beyond biological dysfunction, patients whose worlds are turned upside down by unjustified tragedy or unspeakable loss. The pedagogical structure of medical education, which is created by and perpetuates an epistemology that deems human suffering as secondary or even extraneous, cries out for a different way of knowing the world—and this knowing is fostered, in part, through an engagement with the humanities, including stories of suffering and resiliency depicted through narrative, literature, poetry, theater, music, and art that grapple with enduring questions about what it means to be human.

What Does This Education Look Like?

Although biomedical theory and technical skill are critical in medicine, the humanities, which draw us back to the non- or pre-theoretical *experience* of medicine, remind us to consider the "for-the-sake-of-which" or end (*telos*) of medicine. German philosopher Martin Heidegger reminds us that "there are two kinds of thinking, each justified and needed in its own way"—calculative thinking and meditative thinking.[19] Although calculative thinking, which is largely analytical and set over and against the world and its objects in order to discover "correct" answers, has its place in medicine and medical education, a pedagogical culture that supports the personal and moral development of students must be infused with *meditative thinking*, a slower thinking defined by an openness to mystery, uncertainty, and humility in the face of the other who is ill or suffering. Such a culture may help reveal that calculative and meditative thinking are complexly intertwined in medicine since any observation or understanding of a patient's *dis-ease* is always an interpretation that requires attention to the patient's story—a realization that can help dissolve the dichotomy between "hard" and "soft" knowledge, between clinical objectivity and empathy, and between biomedicine and the humanities.

Incorporating the humanities into medical education—in an intentional, integrated, and sustained way—is what brings meditative thinking back to medicine and students back to themselves and to others. Although approaches to teaching the humanities in this context vary in content and in form, they are united in their ability to capture, engage, and educate the *moral imagination.* Ronald Carson describes the moral imagination as the emotional and intellectual capacity that allows one to imagine *something* of what it might be like to be in the situation of someone else.[20] Carson explains,

> One of our principal tasks as teachers in the medical humanities is to take our students where we find them, with their own mother tongues of morality, and—with the help of texts and ways of thinking drawn from our disciplines—to help them clarify their moral outlooks, become aware and

> respectful of other intelligences and sensibilities, and become fluent in their moral thinking. (26)

In offering students new ways of seeing the world and cultivating their moral imaginations through literature, poetry, and narrative accounts, for example, that express the human experience of medicine and illness, students might begin to recognize their own potential for or experience of suffering. Imagination and wonder have the power to transfigure them out of their typical ways of thinking and perceiving, taking them someplace else—even toward an understanding of what it might be like to be in the situation of someone who is in need of care.[21] Educating the moral imagination can help one grow into the kind of doctor patients need—one who, as Carson says, "knows how to listen for the storyline and hear the heartbeat of [patients'] lives."[22]

Questions remain, however, about whether and how one can educate the moral imagination or cultivate the kind of humility that is necessary to engage it. Carson argues that this can indeed be taught—not didactically but indirectly. That is to say, by emphasizing the way one learns from art, literature, and poetry—an exposure to stories of suffering and resiliency.[23] This way of teaching can feel foreign and uncomfortable to some medical students, especially to those who see such teaching as irrelevant to the task at hand—namely, learning "scientific" medicine. And yet, it is possible to uncover and cultivate students' moral imaginations—if we conceive of the educational project of medical school as something other than didactic instruction. Education, from the Latin *educere*, meaning "to lead" or "draw out," is not about inculcation or indoctrination but rather what Heidegger would call "leaping ahead" of students in order to draw out the whole selves they are becoming in their life of service to others. Especially since it is teeming with encounters with human vulnerability, medical school is, in many ways, the ultimate place for the liberal education of the whole self to occur. Cultivating clinical and moral discernment occurs through supporting students' personal development by engaging their own critical capacities and by recognizing and accepting that they will make mistakes as they discover, for themselves, what it means to be a good doctor.

Incorporating art and narrative into medical training in order to help students discover truth for themselves seems to many educators intuitively desirable. But why is this so? What is it about artistic or narrative representations that allow for a deeper understanding of medicine, illness, or suffering? As Cole, Carlin, and Carson point out, the arts can offer answers to "experience-near" questions—that is, questions about the personal and particular: What is it like to be a disillusioned medical student or a stressed-out resident? What is it like to live with a chronic illness?[24] What does it mean to be alienated or marginalized? What would it be like to not have access to healthcare when you need it most? These are the kinds of questions that are difficult to answer through traditional didactic lectures as they require exploration and conversation. Engagement with the arts and the kind of indirect teaching they offer, on the other hand, can reveal new truths to students and in novel ways, thereby destabilizing students and opening them to new ways of thinking and seeing.[25]

Whether it is a literary work, painting, sculpture, film, or poem, a work of art can reveal a new person or way of life, bringing into relief a different time and place or saying something about our own culture and history—we experience, as Heidegger claims, an opening-up of our world.[26] Artistic expressions offer us truth as unconcealedness (*aletheia*); they uncover a new life-world, engage our imagination, and expose us to a kind of tolerable ambiguity. When we engage with art, we wonder about the person in the story or what is depicted in the painting—we wonder not only at the aesthetics of the work but about what is being expressed. In this wondering, our typical horizons of understanding are expanded, and that which is revealed in the work reconfigures our relation to being. Heidegger describes such a revelation as "the bringing forth of a being such as never was before and will never come to be again."[27] Put simply, art can help us understand what it means to be human in ways that facts, statistics, and objective descriptions never will.

When exposed to new stories outside of biomedicine's master narrative, students can become more sensitive and perceptive to the nuanced moral, interpersonal, and clinical particularities of the situations in which they find themselves. This is because people do not just listen to stories, as Arthur Frank argues, but they "think with them" and get "caught up" in them.[28] Stories can "get under people's skin," as he puts it, and affect what they think, know, and perceive—they teach people what to look for and what to ignore, "what to value and what to hold in contempt."[29] Taking the time to see and hear another allows separate horizons to merge or fuse with each other, resulting in an expansion of each person's particular way of seeing things. It is this "fusion of horizons," which philosopher Hans-Georg Gadamer claims can happen in all human relationships, that leads to a richer knowledge of ways of being in the world.[30] As students engage in an authentic meeting of another and enter into a patient's story, they are granted access to the patient's own interpretive horizon, which may challenge their worldview or at least broaden their own horizon in order to take in the story of the patient.[31] This fusion of horizons can even transcend the exchange between two people and the situation at hand. According to Gadamer, what occurs in an authentic encounter can, in fact, lead to a shared understanding of the human experience.

The Need for Reflection

Engaging with the humanities can also provide learners with the language and skills to reflect on their own feelings and emotions, thereby helping "to heal the nascent healer."[32] It is important for students to take the time to reflect on these stories, which might include engaging in formal reflective writing.[33] The incorporation of reflective writing into medical education is lauded for its capacity to interrupt the automaticity of taken-for-granted thoughts and assumptions, slowing students down so that they might begin to process the vast experiences with the human condition that are made uniquely available to them as doctors in training.[34] Both producing and reading reflective writing require a kind of meditative thinking where truth is uncovered, revealed, and co-created, rather than readily discerned as an objective, observable fact. The movement or freedom within this thinking allows for ambiguity, contradiction, and multiple interpretations. Thus, medical students, in the act of narrating and reflecting on their experiences, might change the stories they tell, gain access to other cultural scripts outside of contemporary medicine, or come to know themselves differently.

The freedom provided by reflective writing is particularly important for medical students who so often become mired down and disoriented by the constrictive cognitive frameworks and patterns of medical culture.[35] Reflecting on how experiences with patients cause them to react or feel allows students to think outside of the prescriptive and limiting language of medicine that all too often renders profound experiences inconsequential and can help them authentically dwell within the affective experience of patient care. Moreover, such writing can offer students an opportunity to express the moral distress they experience when the realities of medicine defy their expectations or when they struggle to offer compassionate care in a medical system that is too often economically inequitable and socially unjust.

Reflective writing can also bring attention to the process of socialization itself, thereby making one attuned to how and in what ways one is being formed by the culture of medicine and medical education. Writing about personal experiences can bring elements of the hidden curriculum into focus and can draw attention to—and perhaps even rally against—implicit and injurious modes of professional identity formation. In reflecting on such experiences, students can embrace their own values and emotions, while also challenging or rejecting what they find problematic within the normative culture of medicine.[36] As Delese Wear and colleagues argue, reflection can be both personally expressive and critically attuned, pointing outward toward issues of oppression and inequality.[37] Reflection can be powerful and transformative, and thus, we agree with these authors that reflection ought to be approached as an ongoing *process* infused throughout medical education as an ethos of medical culture, rather than a singular event or pedagogical tool.

Teaching in Action

These kinds of pedagogical changes, though they require students to slow down and consider the texture of patients' lives, can be easily introduced, even within the established curriculum. In our own teaching, we have found ways to incorporate narrative understanding and personal reflection wherever possible. At the start of my classes, for example, I (N.M.P.) ask my students to write a short, informal reflection about the day's assigned readings, encouraging them to express their own interpretations—what the readings mean to them; how they might challenge or reaffirm their assumptions, biases, or beliefs; or what frustrated, confused, or delighted them. Not only does such reflection help students crystallize their perspectives, but it engenders richer dialogue for the remainder of the class. What is more, the readings assigned in the course are a mix of theoretical, critical, and philosophical pieces that are presented alongside narratives (poetry, film, and stories) created by patients, caregivers, and healthcare professionals. Presenting the material in this way can express to students the embodied, lived experience of medicine in a way that primary philosophical pieces or critical social theory alone may not. I also use shorter patient narratives, such as online essays and blogs, which can compellingly express the complex dynamics of life that shape subjectivities and inform patient decision-making. For instance, in her blog post "Why I Make Terrible Decisions, or, Poverty Thoughts," Linda Tirado points out the barriers to accessing "free" healthcare:

> "Free" only exists for rich people. It's great that there's a bowl of condoms at my school, but most poor people will never set foot on a college campus. We don't belong there. There's a clinic? Great! There's still a copay. We're not going. . . . "Low-cost" and "sliding scale" sounds like "money you have to spend" to me, and they can't actually help you anyway.[38]

She goes on to describe the "unhealthy" decisions she makes that provide her with fleeting moments of pleasure in a life defined by the unrelenting stress of poverty:

> I smoke. It's expensive. It's also the best option. You see, I am always, always exhausted. It's a stimulant. When I am too tired to walk one more step, I can smoke and go for another hour. When I am enraged and beaten down and incapable of accomplishing one more thing, I can smoke and I feel a little better, just for a minute. It is the only relaxation I am allowed. It is not a good decision, but it is the only one that I have access to. It is the only thing I have found that keeps me from collapsing or exploding.

Presenting students with authentic narratives that challenge their presumptions about "non-compliance" and "personal responsibility" offers the opportunity to engage them in conversations about the sociopolitical forces and structural violence that radically condition the lives of some of the patients they will encounter in their life in medicine. These stories—more so than any statistics—are what will begin to shift entrenched perspectives about poverty and the social determinants of health.

The importance of narrative for understanding the lived experiences of health and illness is made all the more clear when, midway through the semester, students are asked to identify someone they know (perhaps themselves) with a serious, chronic, or terminal illness who is willing to share his or her story (see Pedagogy Exercise Section). With the express permission of this person, students then write an illness narrative that illustrates this person's struggles, triumphs, and fears, which the students share with the rest of the class. Such assignments require an element of vulnerability—and bravery—in the classroom, on the part of both students and educators. The hope is that such curricular experiences open students up to new ways of seeing and knowing and that they begin to imagine what it might be like to live a life that may be so different from their own.

At the University of Michigan Medical School, one of us (A.K.K.) designed and directed a required, narrative-based undergraduate medical school program, the Family-Centered Experience (FCE), in which pairs of first- and second-year medical students were matched with families living with chronic or serious medical conditions.[39] Over a two-year period, the student pairs would make scheduled home visits with the families in order to listen to the stories the volunteers would tell of their illness and its care. Home visits were combined with small group discussions, reflective writing, reading of literature, essays, short films, theater, and the creation of art to explore the experience of illness, the human dimensions of healthcare, and the ethical obligations of physicianship.[40] Many of the conversations and small group discussions focused on issues of equity, healthcare access, and healthcare-related financial difficulties. Considering these themes with a narrative approach made them more personal and relevant for the learners. A case in point: in a form of "PhotoVoice"[41] one of the FCE volunteers, a young African American photographer with sickle cell disease, documented her life, including her health crises, through a camera's lens. Using the photographs as a launching point for a discussion about health and illness, patients and doctors, and race and stigmatization, she gave these themes a depth and poignancy that took them out of the abstract and impersonal and prompted the students to consider their own responsibility as physicians in addressing prejudice and injustice.[42]

While we work to maintain appropriate boundaries with students within our classrooms and clinical environments, we also know that asking students to reflect on who they are becoming and who they want to be requires our own personal reflection and vulnerability. These reflections may be disturbing and even traumatic for learners, and institutions must take responsibility for addressing them with sensitivity, thoughtfulness, and support rather than avoid them, as is often the case.[43] Wear and Zarconi remind us that "mentoring for fearlessness" in medical education—encouraging students to be self-reflective, critical, and outspoken regarding the forces that shape them—requires mentors who speak openly to students about their own successes and shortcomings and who are not afraid to use words like *compassion* and *kindness*.[44] Attempting to promote real transformation and growth among our students requires us to address the hierarchy and to abandon archaic ideals that privilege the dominance of the clinician or professor in educational spaces.

If they are perceived as worthwhile, mentoring for fearlessness and encouraging reflective practice, imagination, and wonder can easily become part of medical education, especially if educators and students come to see critical thinking and reflection as complementary, rather than extraneous, to scientific thinking and clinical care. The hope is that an exposure to stories—whether real-life encounters or written accounts—coupled with opportunities to reflect on such experiences will help develop students who are attuned to the lived experience of illness and suffering, who understand the obstacles posed by social determinants of health, who think critically about the systems in which they participate, and who identify themselves as leaders in social justice and advocates for health for all.

Can This Learning Be Assessed?

Activist and feminist writer bell hooks argues that the classroom is a "radical space of possibility" where both students and educators learn about how to live in the world as "whole people" and should be a place where excitement is co-created with students—students whose presence and voices are valued.[45] This view applies equally to the clinic. Getting students engaged and excited about what we teach requires us to be humble and to recognize that, as educators, we learn from our students and that we, too, can change and grow from our experiences in the classroom and clinic. In emphasizing the educational *process* more than quantifiable outcomes, educators can begin to trouble traditional hierarchies between themselves and students, reconnect students to the social import of their current and future work, and reveal the emancipatory potential of education.[46]

Undoubtedly, a "slow medical education" that is committed to ideas of process and growth presents problems in a medical education system that values measurable outcomes and assessments based on observable competencies.

Because the wisdom the humanities offer falls outside the major epistemological framework of medical education, the humanities are particularly well suited for cultivating meditative thinking and creative modes of learning; yet, it is for this same reason that the humanities have struggled to find a central place in medical curricula. Although over the past decade or so the Liaison Committee on Medical Education (LCME) has made additions to its standards for accreditation, mandating that medical schools must provide educational opportunities for learning about end-of-life care, medical ethics, "societal problems," healthcare disparities, and communication skills, there are few specifications about how such educational goals should be met. Also, there is no mention of the humanities per se in the LCME standards.[47]

As a result, whether and how humanities courses are incorporated into medical curricula vary widely; and at some institutions, the medical humanities remain largely on the periphery of the predominant educational focus.[48] This is in part a result of the perennial—and very contentious—problem faced by medical humanities supporters: proving the efficacy of the pedagogy.[49] It has been suggested that the "outcomes" of humanities courses might best be assessed using more qualitative methodologies, and some researchers have done so by facilitating focus groups or analyzing student narratives after the completion of a course or program.[50] Such studies do, indeed, suggest that courses in the humanities are "effective," in that students' self-reports point to a development of self-awareness and personal growth; an understanding of the larger context of medicine; an increase in empathy, compassion, and social skills; an attention to care for oneself; a development of critical thinking skills; and an appreciation for community and connection.[51]

These studies are helpful for illuminating what it is the humanities do for medical students, but one might wonder if such findings are even intelligible in the world of academic medicine where calls for rubrics and observable competencies abound. Without clear and replicable evidence that the humanities "work," it becomes difficult to fund, create, and sustain efforts to change medical practice and education.[52] Ousager and Johannessen, for example, argue that the lack of "empirical evidence" and "measurable learning outcomes" will hinder the humanities from gaining and holding a firm position in medical education.[53] "After all," they say, "the present trend of evidence-based learning . . . requires that the study of the humanities, like any other curricular activity within medical education, should in principle be able to justify its existence with evidence of its effectiveness."[54] Although we recognize the need for the medical/health humanities to demonstrate their value in terms that are meaningful to stakeholders and decision-makers in academic medicine, when we feel pressured to measure the intrinsic value of the humanities in the same terms as the rest of the medical world, we run the risk of falling victim to narrow notions of "success" that only further embed us into closed, calculative understandings of being-in-the-world. The situation is reminiscent of Heidegger's saying about how thinking may be judged: "Thinking is judged by a standard that doesn't measure up to it. Such judgment may be compared to the procedure of trying to evaluate the essence and powers of a fish by seeing how long it can live on dry land."[55] If the medical humanities intend to challenge the epistemological assumptions of traditional medical education, then measuring their efforts against criteria borne of this epistemology misses the mark entirely.

This does not mean, however, that one should not present a persuasive argument for why the humanities are critical to medical education and do so in rhetorically effective ways, something that can be achieved with more qualitative studies and by learning to speak the language of academic medicine. For instance, we might make the case for a pedagogy that encourages the cultivation of the self by identifying the qualities we intend to engender and then mapping these qualities onto LCME standards or onto an institution's existing list of competencies.[56] That said, however, when it comes to "proving" the efficacy of the humanities, we may never be able to offer the kind of results that the system demands of us, as it usually asks us to quantify the unquantifiable. Continuing our efforts to measure outcomes via calculative standards of success puts us at risk for measuring the wrong things—namely, demonstrable behaviors (that may or may not emanate from deeper values) that serve as reductionist surrogates for character. An emphasis on observable outcomes simply might be the wrong tool for assessing the development of a professional way of being-in-the-world; indeed, it may even threaten to reduce the profound human interactions inherent in the act of healing into overly simplified standards and checklists.[57]

Although an emphasis on standards and behaviors fails to fully and authentically reflect the educational goals or "outcomes" of the humanities, this does not mean there is no way to assess a student's growth toward becoming a healer. Indeed, a pedagogy that embraces more tacit ways of knowing and teaches through stories, reflection, and art can more readily access and assess students' formative processes than most other pedagogical approaches. Reflective work such as narratives and essays, for instance, can display the development of certain virtues, such as remaining open, being willing to listen to and become absorbed in a patient's story, managing uncertainty and ambiguity, and pushing against prescriptive and restrictive ways of knowing. Reading a detailed narrative account, for instance, allows a mentor to approach an understanding of a student's way of being-in-the-world-with-others, as opposed to the student's adherence to codes or ability to exhibit observable "professional" behavior.

Reflective work—including writing essays, journal entries, or short stories; keeping a "parallel chart"; and creating artwork or film—that explores the lived experience of medicine can cultivate meditative thinking, encouraging shifts in perspective and personal growth.[58] This kind of "assessment" is *formative* in nature rather than summative: instead of assessments *of* learning at the end of a clinical rotation that allow for little to no in-the-moment guidance and feedback, formative assessments account *for* learning, allowing educators and mentors to "impart information, instill values, and inspire excellence and ongoing learning" throughout educational experience.[59] Creating and facilitating this kind of pedagogy are not easy tasks; both supporting personal growth and assessing it require that educators *engage* with students—that is, offer meaningful and intentional feedback, pose difficult questions, listen intently, and initiate honest dialogue. Feedback should be seen as an opportunity to engage in conversation with students, commending them for their accomplishments, addressing areas for improvement, and helping them question some of their own assumptions, as well as the assumptions of contemporary Western medicine more generally.

Conclusion

Humanities teaching in medical education is becoming more prevalent and we hope more robust and immersive. In sharing our own theoretical and political positions and our own pedagogical approaches, we have tried to show why the humanities are critical in medical education and how this kind of teaching can be enacted. Such pedagogical approaches cannot look like a "parachute humanities," where the educator drops in for abbreviated, discrete lectures taught in the antiquated didactic fashion of medical education; this, undoubtedly, will do little to challenge the dominant epistemology of medicine. Rather, the humanities must be incorporated uniquely and experientially throughout all four years of the curriculum and should encourage open dialogue and reflection about who students are becoming and what kind of doctors they want to be. The practice of medicine is an extraordinary opportunity for students and clinicians to engage in life's moments that make us most fully human; it is an opportunity for them to become courageous healers and thoughtful advocates in a broken healthcare system—and these future healers deserve an education that prepares and encourages them to do just that.

PEDAGOGY EXERCISE SECTION

ILLNESS NARRATIVE ASSIGNMENT

For this writing assignment, you will write an illness narrative that expresses the lived experience of illness, whether your own or the experience of another (e.g., friend, acquaintance, family member) whom you will interview. The person's illness/injury/disability should be one that significantly affects/has affected his or her life—that is, one that has changed or disrupted his or her way of being in the world. You will then construct a narrative (no less than 600 words) describing and analyzing the illness experience, drawing on texts from this class. The primary goal of this assignment is to better understand—and then express to others—the lived experience of illness (or of caring for someone with a serious illness), as well as the social issues affecting health and illness.

Interview

You do not need a formal structure for the interview; it can take the form of an open-ended conversation. However, you should consider in advance the topics/questions you want to explore.

Potential themes you might consider:

- Emotions expressed when talking about the illness (fear, sadness, shame, hope, loneliness, etc.)
- How the individual makes sense of the causes of his or her condition
- Life changes that resulted from the illness and how the illness affects personal relationships
- Ease of, or problems with, access to medical care
- Experience receiving care for the illness, including interactions with healthcare professionals
- Psychological and social stressors that may exacerbate the illness
- Strategies used to cope with the illness
- Sources of emotional and social support
- How social factors such as race, age, gender, and socioeconomic status might affect the individual's experience of illness

Some of these topics can be sensitive, and the person you are interviewing may not want to discuss them. Be mindful of how you engage him or her: do not pressure the person to talk about anything he or she does not feel comfortable with, and ask your questions gently and respectfully. Tell the person before you begin the interview that he or she is in no way obligated to answer anything he or she does not want to, that he or she can stop the interview at any time, and that his or her story will not be used for research or publication and will not leave the walls of your classroom. However, be sure the person knows that his or her story will be shared with your class, and ask her for permission to share it.

Narrative

After the interview, you will construct the person's experience as a narrative, presenting the individual's story, along with your own observations and interpretations, using direct quotes where appropriate. Feel free to be creative—perhaps you write the narrative from the first-person rather than the third-person perspective, perhaps you also include a poem, photos, or art, anything you feel expresses the lived experience of illness.

Confidentiality

Because you will be sharing your narrative with the class, you should avoid using any identifying information in your narrative, unless your interviewee gives explicit permission. You may use a pseudonym to protect the privacy of your interviewee.

Notes

1. Ronald A. Carson, Chester R. Burns, and Thomas R. Cole, *Practicing the Medical Humanities: Engaging Physicians and Patients*, ed. Ronald A. Carson, Chester R. Burns, and Thomas R. Cole (Hagerstown, MD: University Publishing Group, 2003), introduction.

2. Daniel M. Fox, "Who We Are: The Political Origins of the Medical Humanities," *Theoretical Medicine* 6, no. 3 (October 1985): 329.

3. Carson, Burns, and Cole, *Practicing the Medical Humanities*.

4. Craig M. Klugman, "A Survey of Medical Humanities Teaching in North American Allopathic and Osteopathic Medical Schools," Paper presented at the Sixth Annual Health Humanities Conference, Health Humanities Consortium, Houston, TX, March 2017.

5. Belinda Jack, "The Rise of the Medical Humanities," *Times Higher Education*, accessed October 21, 2016, https://www.timeshighereducation.com/features/the-rise-of-the-medical-humanities/2018007.article.

6. Johanna Shapiro et al., "Medical Humanities and Their Discontents: Definitions, Critiques, and Implications," *Academic Medicine* 84, no. 2 (2009): 192–98.

7. Arno K. Kumagai and Monica L. Lypson, "Beyond Cultural Competence: Critical Consciousness, Social Justice, and Multicultural Education," *Academic Medicine* 84, no. 6 (2009): 782–87.

8. Donald A. Schön, *The Reflective Practitioner: How Professionals Think in Action* (New York: Basic Books, 1983), 10–11.

9. Arno K. Kumagai, "From Competencies to Human Interests: Ways of Knowing and Understanding in Medical Education," *Academic Medicine* 89, no. 7 (2014): 978–83; Thirusha Naidu and Arno K. Kumagai, "Troubling Muddy Waters: Problematizing Reflective Practice in Global Medical Education," *Academic Medicine* 91, no. 3 (2016): 317–21.

10. Frederic William Hafferty, "Professionalism and the Socialization of Medical Students," in *Teaching Medical Professionalism*, ed. Richard L. Cruess, Sylvia R. Cruess, and Yvonne Steinert (New York: Cambridge University Press, 2009), 53–70.

11. Ibid., 54, 59.

12. Ibid., 63, emphasis in original.

13. Ibid., 64, emphasis in original.

14. Kathryn Montgomery, *How Doctors Think: Clinical Judgment and the Practice of Medicine* (New York: Oxford University Press, 2005), 167.

15. Paul Komesaroff, "The Many Faces of the Clinic: A Levinasian View," in *Handbook of Phenomenology and Medicine*, ed. S. Kay Toombs (Dordrecht, The Netherlands: Kluwer Academic, 2001), 317.

16. Montgomery, *How Doctors Think*, 173.

17. Lorraine J. Daston and Peter Galison, *Objectivity* (New York: Zone Books, 2010).

18. Montgomery, *How Doctors Think*.

19. Martin Heidegger, "Memorial Address," in *Discourse on Thinking*, trans. John M. Anderson and E. Hans Freund (New York: Harper and Row, 1969), 46.

20. Ronald A. Carson, "Educating the Moral Imagination," in *Practicing the Medical Humanities: Engaging Physicians and Patients*, ed. Ronald A. Carson, Chester R. Burns, and Thomas R. Cole (Hagerstown, MD: University Publishing Group, 2003), 26. Related to the moral imagination is what sociologist C. Wright Mills called the "sociological

imagination"—the ability to consider the larger social, historical, and economic background of the people we encounter and to shift one's perspective from individuals to the larger context in which they find themselves. Both of these imaginative capacities are critical for caring for patients. See C. Wright Mills, *The Sociological Imagination* (New York: Oxford University Press, 1959).

21. H. M. Evans, "Wonder and the Patient," *Journal of Medical Humanities* 36, no. 1 (2014): 47–58.

22. Carson, "Educating the Moral Imagination," 31.

23. Ibid., 26, 28.

24. Thomas R. Cole, Nathan S. Carlin, and Ronald A. Carson, *Medical Humanities: An Introduction* (New York: Cambridge University Press, 2014).

25. See, for example, Craig M. Klugman and Diana Beckmann-Mendez, "One Thousand Words: Evaluating an Interdisciplinary Art Education Program," *Journal of Nursing Education* 54, no. 4 (2015): 220–23.

26. See Martin Heidegger, "The Origins of a Work of Art," in *Poetry, Language, Thought*, trans. Albert Hofstadter (New York: Harper Perennial, 1975), 15–86.

27. Ibid., 60.

28. Arthur W. Frank, *Letting Stories Breathe: A Socio-Narratology* (Chicago: University of Chicago Press, 2010).

29. Ibid., 48.

30. Hans-Georg Gadamer, *Truth and Method*, trans. Donald G. Marshall and Joel Weinsheimer (New York: Bloomsbury Academic, 2004); Arno K. Kumagai, "Acts of Interpretation: A Philosophical Approach to Using Creative Arts in Medical Education," *Academic Medicine* 87, no. 8 (2012): 1138–44.

31. Kumagai, "Acts of Interpretation."

32. Ayelet Kuper, "Literature and Medicine: A Problem of Assessment," *Academic Medicine* 81, no. 10 (October 2006): S130.

33. Delese Wear and Joseph Zarconi, "Challenging the Profession: Mentoring for Fearlessness," in *Mentoring in Academic Medicine*, ed. Holly Humphrey (Philadelphia: American College of Physicians Press, 2010), 51–66.

34. Delese Wear, Joseph Zarconi, Arno Kumagai, and Kathy Cole-Kelly, "Slow Medical Education," *Academic Medicine* 90, no. 3 (2015): 289–93.

35. Johanna Shapiro, Deborah Kasman, and Audrey Shafer, "Words and Wards: A Model of Reflective Writing and Its Uses in Medical Education," *Journal of Medical Humanities* 27, no. 4 (26, 2006): 231–44.

36. Ibid.; Hedy S. Wald et al., "Professional Identity Formation in Medical Education for Humanistic, Resilient Physicians: Pedagogic Strategies for Bridging Theory to Practice," *Academic Medicine* 90, no. 6 (2015): 753–60.

37. Delese Wear et al., "Reflection In/And Writing: Pedagogy and Practice in Medical Education," *Academic Medicine* 87, no. 5 (2012): 603–609.

38. Killer Gibsons, "Why I Make Terrible Decisions, or, Poverty Thoughts," *KillerMartinis* (blog), October 22, 2013, accessed November 13, 2015. http://killermartinis.kinja.com/why-i-make-terrible-decisions-or-poverty-thoughts-1450123558. The author of this blog, Linda Tirado, has recently published a book related to this topic. See Linda Tirado, *Hand to Mouth: Living in Bootstrap America* (New York: G. P. Putnam's Sons, 2014).

39. Arno Kumagai, "The Patient's Voice in Medical Education: The Family Centered Experience Program," *Virtual Mentor* 11, no. 3 (2009): 228.

40. Ibid.; Arno K. Kumagai, "A Conceptual Framework for the Use of Illness Narratives in Medical Education," *Academic Medicine* 83, no. 7 (2008): 653–58.

41. Caroline C. Wang and Cheri A. Pies, "Family, Maternal, and Child Health through Photovoice," *Maternal and Child Health Journal* 8, no. 2 (2004): 95–102.

42. Paula T. Ross et al., "Commentary. Sickle Cell Vision: A Patient's Photographic Illustration of Coping," *Academic Medicine* 85, no. 7 (2010): 1210–11.

43. Arno K. Kumagai, Brittani Jackson, and Saleem Razack, "Cutting Close to the Bone: Student Trauma, Free Speech, and Institutional Responsibility in Medical Education," *Academic Medicine* 92, no. 3 (2017): 318–23.

44. Wear and Zarconi, "Challenging the Profession."

45. bell hooks, *Teaching to Transgress: Education as a Practice of Freedom* (New York: Routledge, 1984).

46. Kenneth Saltman and Alexander Means, "Students as Critical Citizens/Educated Subjects but not as Commodities/Tested Objects," in *The Sage Guide to Curriculum in Education*, edited by Ming Fang He, Brian D. Schultz, and William H. Schubert (Thousand Oaks, CA: Sage, 2015), 284–92.

47. Liaison Committee on Medical Education, "Structures and Functions of a Medical School: Standards for Accreditation of Medical Education Programs Leading to the MD Degree," March 2016, accessed October 12, 2016, http://lcme.org/publications/.

48. Ayelet Kuper, "Literature and Medicine: A Problem of Assessment," *Academic Medicine* 81, no. 10 (2006): S128–37; Cheryl J. Erwin, "Development of a Medical Humanities and Ethics Certificate Program in Texas," *Journal of Medical Humanities* 35, no. 4 (2014): 389–403.

49. Rafael Campo, "'The Medical Humanities,' for Lack of a Better Term," *JAMA* 294, no. 9 (September 7, 2005): 1009–11.

50. See, for example, Antoinette S. Peters et al., "Long-Term Outcomes of the New Pathway Program at Harvard Medical School: A Randomized Controlled Trial," *Academic Medicine* 75, no. 5 (2000): 470–79; Erwin, "Development"; Eliza Miller et al., "Sounding Narrative Medicine: Studying Students' Professional Identity Development at Columbia University College of Physicians and Surgeons," *Academic Medicine* 89, no. 2 (2014): 335–42; Lloyd Rucker and Johanna Shapiro, "Becoming a Physician: Students' Creative Projects in a Third-Year IM Clerkship," *Academic Medicine* 78, no. 4 (2003): 391–97.

51. Erwin, "Development."

52. Campo, "'The Medical Humanities.'"

53. Jakob Ousager and Helle Johannessen, "Humanities in Undergraduate Medical Education: A Literature Review," *Academic Medicine* 85, no. 6 (2010): 988.

54. Ibid., 988.

55. Martin Heidegger, "Letter on Humanism," in *Basic Writings*, ed. David Farrell Krell (New York: Harper Perennial Modern Classics, 2008), 219.

56. David S. Jones et al., "Making the Case for History in Medical Education," *Journal of the History of Medicine and Allied Sciences* 70, no. 4 (2015): 623–52.

57. Kumagai, "From Competencies."

58. In "parallel charts" students are encouraged to write about aspects of patient care that do not fit into the confines of the typical medical chart but that should be considered

and written down somewhere. Doing so can help attune students to the hermeneutic situation of the patients they encounter. See Kuper, "Literature and Medicine," S134. Another practical means of assessment is the "Health Professional Ethics Rubric," which is used to assess students' open-ended responses to moral dilemmas in healthcare. See Nathan Carlin et al., "The Health Professional Ethics Rubric: Practical Assessment in Ethics Education for Health Professional Schools," *Journal of Academic Ethics* 9, no. 4 (2011): 277–90.

59. Lyuba Konopasek, John Norcini, and Edward Krupat, "Focusing on the Formative: Building an Assessment System Aimed at Student Growth and Development," *Academic Medicine* 91, no. 11 (2016): 1492–97.

Works Cited

Campo, Rafael. "'The Medical Humanities,' for Lack of a Better Term." *JAMA* 294, no. 9 (2005): 1009–11.

Carlin, Nathan, Cathy Rozmus, Jeffrey Spike, Irmgard Willcockson, William Seifert, Cynthia Chappell, Pei Hsuan Hsieh, et al. "The Health Professional Ethics Rubric: Practical Assessment in Ethics Education for Health Professional Schools." *Journal of Academic Ethics* 9, no. 4 (2011): 277–90.

Carson, Ronald A. "Educating the Moral Imagination." In *Practicing the Medical Humanities: Engaging Physicians and Patients*, edited by Ronald A. Carson, Chester A. Burns, and Thomas R. Cole, 25–38. Hagerstown, MD: University Publishing Group, 2003.

Carson, Ronald A., Chester R. Burns, and Thomas R. Cole, eds. *Practicing the Medical Humanities: Engaging Physicians and Patients*. Hagerstown, MD: University Publishing Group, 2003.

Cole, Thomas R., Nathan S. Carlin, and Ronald A. Carson. *Medical Humanities: An Introduction*. New York: Cambridge University Press, 2014.

Daston, Lorraine J., and Peter Galison. *Objectivity*. New York: Zone Books, 2010.

Erwin, Cheryl J. "Development of a Medical Humanities and Ethics Certificate Program in Texas." *Journal of Medical Humanities* 35, no. 4 (2014): 389–403.

Evans, H. M. "Wonder and the Patient." *Journal of Medical Humanities* 36, no. 1 (2014): 47–58.

Fox, Daniel M. "Who We Are: The Political Origins of the Medical Humanities." *Theoretical Medicine* 6, no. 3 (1985): 327–41.

Frank, Arthur W. *Letting Stories Breathe: A Socio-Narratology*. Chicago: University of Chicago Press, 2010.

Gadamer, Hans-Georg. *Truth and Method*. Translated by Donald G. Marshall and Joel Weinsheimer. New York: Bloomsbury Academic, 2004.

Hafferty, Frederic W. "Professionalism and the Socialization of Medical Students." In *Teaching Medical Professionalism*, edited by Richard L. Cruess, Sylvia R. Cruess, and Yvonne Steinert, 53–70. New York: Cambridge University Press, 2009.

Heidegger, Martin. "Letter on Humanism." In *Basic Writings*, edited by David Farrell Krell. New York: Harper Perennial Modern Classics, 2008.

Heidegger, Martin. "Memorial Address." In *Discourse on Thinking*. Translated by John M. Anderson and E. Hans Freund, 43–57. New York: Harper & Row, 1969.

Heidegger, Martin. "The Origins of a Work of Art." In *Poetry, Language, Thought*. Translated by Albert Hofstadter, 15–86. New York: Harper Perennial, 1975.

hooks, bell. *Teaching to Transgress: Education as the Practice of Freedom*. New York: Routledge, 1994.

Jack, Belinda. "The Rise of the Medical Humanities." *Times Higher Education*. Accessed October 21, 2016. https://www.timeshighereducation.com/features/the-rise-of-the-medical-humanities/2018007.article.

Jones, David S., Jeremy A. Greene, Jacalyn Duffin, and John Harley Warner. "Making the Case for History in Medical Education." *Journal of the History of Medicine and Allied Sciences* 70, no. 4 (2015): 623–52.

KillerGibsons. "Why I Make Terrible Decisions, or, Poverty Thoughts." *KillerMartinis* (blog). October 22, 2013. Accessed November 13, 2015. http://killermartinis.kinja.com/why-i-make-terrible-decisions-or-poverty-thoughts-1450123558.

Klugman, Craig M. "A Survey of Medical Humanities Teaching in North American Allopathic and Osteopathic Medical Schools." Paper presented at the Sixth Annual Health Humanities Conference, Health Humanities Consortium, Houston, TX, March 2017.

Klugman, Craig M., and Diana Beckmann-Mendez. "One Thousand Words: Evaluating an Interdisciplinary Art Education Program." *Journal of Nursing Education* 54, no. 4 (2015): 220–23.

Komesaroff, Paul. "The Many Faces of the Clinic: A Levinasian View." In *Handbook of Phenomenology and Medicine*, edited by S. Kay Toombs, 312–30. Dordrecht, The Netherlands: Kluwer Academic, 2001.

Konopasek, Lyuba, John Norcini, and Edward Krupat. "Focusing on the Formative: Building an Assessment System Aimed at Student Growth and Development." *Academic Medicine: Journal of the Association of American Medical Colleges* 91, no. 11 (2016): 1492–97.

Kumagai, Arno K. "A Conceptual Framework for the Use of Illness Narratives in Medical Education." *Academic Medicine: Journal of the Association of American Medical Colleges* 83, no. 7 (2008): 653–58.

Kumagai, Arno K. "Acts of Interpretation: A Philosophical Approach to Using Creative Arts in Medical Education." *Academic Medicine: Journal of the Association of American Medical Colleges* 87, no. 8 (2012): 1138–44.

Kumagai, Arno K. "From Competencies to Human Interests: Ways of Knowing and Understanding in Medical Education." *Academic Medicine: Journal of the Association of American Medical Colleges* 89, no. 7 (2014): 978–83.

Kumagai, Arno K. "The Patient's Voice in Medical Education: The Family Centered Experience Program." *Virtual Mentor* 11, no. 3 (2009): 228.

Kumagai, Arno K., Brittani Jackson, and Saleem Razack. "Cutting Close to the Bone: Student Trauma, Free Speech, and Institutional Responsibility in Medical Education." *Academic Medicine: Journal of the Association of American Medical Colleges* 92, no. 3 (2017): 318–23.

Kumagai, Arno K., and Monica L. Lypson. "Beyond Cultural Competence: Critical Consciousness, Social Justice, and Multicultural Education." *Academic Medicine: Journal of the Association of American Medical Colleges* 84, no. 6 (2009): 782–87.

Kuper, Ayelet. "Literature and Medicine: A Problem of Assessment." *Academic Medicine: Journal of the Association of American Medical Colleges* 81, no. 10 (2006): S128–37.

Liaison Committee on Medical Education. "Functions and Structure of a Medical School: Standards for Accreditation of Medical Education Programs Leading to the MD Degree." March 2016. Accessed October 12, 2016. http://lcme.org/publications/.

Miller, Eliza, Dorene Balmer, Nellie Hermann, Gillian Graham, and Rita Charon. "Sounding Narrative Medicine: Studying Students' Professional Identity Development at Columbia University College of Physicians and Surgeons." *Academic Medicine: Journal of the Association of American Medical Colleges* 89, no. 2 (2014): 335–42.

Mills, Wright C. *The Sociological Imagination*. New York: Oxford University Press, 1959.

Montgomery, Kathryn. *How Doctors Think: Clinical Judgment and the Practice of Medicine*. New York: Oxford University Press, 2005.

Naidu, Thirusha, and Arno K. Kumagai. "Troubling Muddy Waters: Problematizing Reflective Practice in Global Medical Education." *Academic Medicine: Journal of the Association of American Medical Colleges* 91, no. 3 (2016): 317–21.

Ousager, Jakob, and Helle Johannessen. "Humanities in Undergraduate Medical Education: A Literature Review." *Academic Medicine: Journal of the Association of American Medical Colleges* 85, no. 6 (2010): 988–98.

Peters, Antoinette S., Rachel Greenberger-Rosovsky, Charlotte Crowder, Susan D. Block, and Gordon T. Moore. "Long-Term Outcomes of the New Pathway Program at Harvard Medical School: A Randomized Controlled Trial." *Academic Medicine: Journal of the Association of American Medical Colleges* 75, no. 5 (2000): 470–79.

Ross, Paula T., Heather L. Davis, Arno K. Kumagai, Andrew D. Campbell, and Monica L. Lypson. "Commentary. Sickle Cell Vision: A Patient's Photographic Illustration of Coping." *Academic Medicine: Journal of the Association of American Medical Colleges* 85, no.7 (2010): 1210–11.

Rucker, Lloyd, and Johanna Shapiro. "Becoming a Physician: Students' Creative Projects in a Third-Year IM Clerkship." *Academic Medicine: Journal of the Association of American Medical Colleges* 78, no. 4 (2003): 391–97.

Saltman, Kenneth, and Alexander Means. "Students as Critical Citizens/Educated Subjects but not as Commodities/Tested Objects." In *The Sage Guide to Curriculum in Education*, edited by Ming Fang He, Brian D. Schultz, and William H. Schubert, 284–92. Thousand Oaks, CA: Sage, 2015.

Schön, Donald A. *The Reflective Practitioner: How Professionals Think in Action*. New York: Basic Books, 1983.

Shapiro, Johanna, Jack Coulehan, Delese Wear, and Martha Montello. "Medical Humanities and Their Discontents: Definitions, Critiques, and Implications." *Academic Medicine: Journal of the Association of American Medical Colleges* 84, no. 2 (2009): 192–98.

Shapiro, Johanna, Deborah Kasman, and Audrey Shafer. "Words and Wards: A Model of Reflective Writing and Its Uses in Medical Education." *Journal of Medical Humanities* 27, no. 4 (2006): 231–44.

Tirado, Linda. *Hand to Mouth: Living in Bootstrap America*. New York: G. P. Putnam's Sons, 2014.

Wald, Hedy S., David Anthony, Tom A. Hutchinson, Stephen Liben, Mark Smilovitch, and Anthony A. Donato. "Professional Identity Formation in Medical Education for Humanistic, Resilient Physicians: Pedagogic Strategies for Bridging Theory to Practice." *Academic Medicine: Journal of the Association of American Medical Colleges* 90, no. 6 (2015): 753–60.

Wang, Caroline C., and Cheri A. Pies. "Family, Maternal, and Child Health through Photovoice." *Maternal and Child Health Journal* 8, no. 2 (2004): 95–102.

Wear, Delese, and Joseph Zarconi. "Challenging the Profession: Mentoring for Fearlessness." In *Mentoring in Academic Medicine*, edited by Holly Humphrey, 51–66. Philadelphia: American College of Physicians Press, 2010.

Wear, Delese, Joseph Zarconi, Rebecca Garden, and Therese Jones. "Reflection in/and Writing: Pedagogy and Practice in Medical Education." *Academic Medicine: Journal of the Association of American Medical Colleges* 87, no. 5 (2012): 603–609.

Wear, Delese, Joseph Zarconi, Arno Kumagai, and Kathy Cole-Kelly. "Slow Medical Education." *Academic Medicine: Journal of the Association of American Medical Colleges* 90, no. 3 (2015): 289–93.

3

The Health Humanities in Nursing Education

Jamie Shirley and Sarah Shannon

Introduction

Nursing is a practice discipline, a body of knowledge and skills that are learned within educational settings for the purpose of being applied to real people, facing sometimes cruel choices, in an often unjust world. Society grants the profession the right to determine the educational standards necessary to prepare the next generation—and the responsibility to oversee that educational process to both protect the public and ensure an adequate supply of competent future professionals. Teaching nursing goes beyond imparting facts or theories or providing training on motor or verbal techniques to include assisting students to develop clinical judgment: to think like a nurse.

In this chapter, we discuss how the health humanities can create a space for nursing students to explore the range of human emotions they will encounter when faced with the intimacy of health and illness. Our goal is to show how this space allows nursing students to explore their own judgments, to learn critical reasoning skills and moral imagination, and to develop a voice that allows them, as nurses, to fully contribute to all aspects of their patients' care and to the development of a just and equitable healthcare system.

Nursing Education

Nursing was originally set up on an apprenticeship model; students worked alongside expert nurses to gain basic and specialized nursing skills, generally in hospital-based programs.[1] The role of the nurse was viewed largely as a technical one, requiring minimal education and with limited career opportunities. Over time, nursing was increasingly viewed as a profession, with similar responsibilities and privileges to other professions, including self-governance, coordination with other professions, and generation of new knowledge for the field.[2] In the United States, these differing perspectives continue to be embodied in the two pathways to educational preparation for the entry-level role in nursing: the registered nurse (RN). Students can qualify to become an RN by earning an associate degree at a community or technical college or by earning a baccalaureate degree at a university.

Increasingly, the profession is becoming unified in supporting nurses to progress to the baccalaureate degree—if not as the direct entry degree, then at least as a subsequently required pathway.[3] The reasons for this shift are multiple—as with other health professions, the body of knowledge in nursing is expanding rapidly, so the need for a longer and more complex educational path is needed. Additionally, there is increasing pressure throughout the system to ensure that all providers are practicing at the top of their license. Research has shown that hospitals with higher proportions of baccalaureate-prepared RNs have better patient outcomes.[4] The mechanism for this difference is not clear; however, the presumption is that the additional time spent in the university setting gaining the classic advantages of a liberal education, including critical thinking skills, is the source of this difference.

The continued existence of these dual pathways for entry to nursing is, in part, a reflection of the profession's commitment to social justice. Nursing always was, and remains, a predominantly female profession. In its early days, it was a path for the "daughters of educated men" to escape the confines of socially constricted lives.[5] Over time, nursing has similarly been a path for diverse families to find economic stability. Nursing has many students who are first in their family to earn a college degree, who identify as having grown up "poor," or who come from socially or economically disadvantaged backgrounds. Like all the healthcare professions, nursing schools have struggled to increase the racial and ethnic diversity of their students; however, programs have shown an upward trend in recent years.[6] As a career, nursing offers the opportunity for a middle-class income. Nursing is an economic engine for families and communities, and within that context making access to education more difficult by limiting it to the university will continue to be met by resistance.[7]

Nonetheless, it is in the university setting of baccalaureate programs where the inclusion of the health humanities is most likely to appear. It is at this level that programs explicitly focus on preparing nurses for professional practice across complex healthcare systems. This chapter will focus primarily on the pedagogical strategies for teaching nurses at this level.

The Language of Nursing

Nursing students generally come into entry-level nursing education with well-developed virtues of caring and compassion—as well as an orientation toward service that is focused on interpersonal relationships.[8] These students understand emotion as a viable moral resource for responding to the world and to clinical situations. This perspective is created and reinforced by the social messages and media images that "good" nurses are gentle and kind ministering angels, while "bad" nurses are evil and mean battleaxes.[9] They idealize themselves and their future practice within these social constructs. This propensity is reinforced by curricular elements within nursing education that introduce grounding theories focused on caring, such as those proposed by Swanson[10] and Watson.[11]

This perspective, however, does not adequately prepare them for the realities of health and illness, of human strength and frailty. Nor does it offer them strategies to analyze and negotiate the power dynamics of hierarchical healthcare organizations for both patients and themselves. The ideal of feeling compassionate and caring may be strained by encounters with angry, fearful, ungrateful, and, occasionally, dangerous patients—particularly in the institutional context of understaffing, fraught interprofessional dynamics, and limited resources. Without language to articulate a more ethically complex worldview, the response of novice nurses may be silence.

The inclusion of the health humanities in nursing education can provide resources to overcome this silence. The social positioning of nursing students, combined with the undergraduate level of nursing programs within the academy, means that these students are in particular need of building skills in critical reading and developing the breadth of their moral imagination.

Critical Reading

The introduction of health humanities into the curriculum offers nursing students an opportunity to learn skills of critical reading—and particularly narrative analysis. While students may be well attuned to what they feel, they can gain insight into why they feel that way—and how the elements of a narrative construct those emotions through close reading and careful analysis.[12]

One text I[13] use to develop these skills is Tillie Olsen's *Tell Me a Riddle*.[14] The novella offers the story of Eva, an elderly Russian Jewish woman who is dying of cancer. The story begins prior to her diagnosis and concludes with her death. Eva is not an easy person to like—for either the reader or the other characters in the story. She is angry about the many shattered hopes in her life and now, in old age, is retreating more and more into silence and a preference for solitude. The reader travels with her as her various family members make one last attempt to connect with her before her death. Along the way, the reader learns how her experiences of immigration, motherhood, and poverty created the character we now meet.

On a pragmatic level, I assign this text to the students so that they have a common story to practice summarizing into a case presentation.[15] Too often students are presented with brief case studies and are asked to provide an ethical analyses based on minimal data. Not only do these cases offer insufficient depth for a complete analysis, but students do not gain the skills of selecting the pertinent data from a complex and messy whole to form a simpler narrative. Real people do not neatly present themselves in a three-paragraph synopsis. In practice, clinicians are sometimes presented with incomplete or insufficient information—and at other times with a deluge of conflicting information about the patient. Sorting through the available information to identify the critical elements—and to notice what is still unknown—is a key feature of clinical decision-making.

Olsen's novella is also a multivocal text. In the story we hear from Eva's husband and children—all of whom have their own hopes and disappointments about the role this woman has played in their lives. These versions of the protagonist are contrasted with her own internal narrative, allowing the reader to see that multiple versions of the story need not be understood as more or less true—but as a source of complexity. Similarly in the clinical setting, families often come to us telling multiple stories about a patient, and students need to be prepared to listen to them all—not so they can evaluate which is the "true" story but to understand them as multiple authentic aspects of the family's story.

In the process of doing this exercise, the gap between the lived experience of a person like Eva and this fifty-page narrative version—and then their two-page summary—is made visible. It becomes abundantly clear to students how much must be left out in the telling of any story; the author is always making choices of what to include and what to leave out. That process of selection inherently shapes the story and thus the judgments that are subsequently made in the analytic process.[16]

Upon completion, students exchange their summaries and discuss how their versions converge and diverge. No two summaries are exactly the same; each student emphasizes different aspects of the story as key to understanding the case. Comparing their summaries provides an opportunity to discuss which elements of the story are established as factual and which are mutable based on perception and perspective. They challenge each other to justify their choices not only of the details they chose to include but also of the language used to describe Eva. Is she difficult? Bitter? Angry? Sad? Tired? Tenacious? How do those linguistic choices construct the reader's understanding of Eva and her situation?

Having experienced this process of construction themselves, students can then go back and evaluate the ways in which the larger text was constructed by the author. Olsen's text is frustrating to many students on a purely textual level. Olsen often eschews standard punctuation and elides the distinction between internal thoughts and spoken dialogue. The difficulty of the text makes Olsen's choices all the more prominent to students. A text that flows in expected ways and is easy to understand feels natural to students and thus is difficult for them to deconstruct. Here, the odd disjunctures are obvious, and students can more readily identify and question them. Understanding this novella is hard work! But so too, I remind students, is the effort to understand the complex patients and families we encounter in the clinical setting. They also resist easy reading and sometimes intentionally frustrate our efforts to understand them as they work to maintain their privacy and dignity in a setting that threatens to rob them of these things.

Another aspect of this assignment is to help students go beyond their initial emotional reaction ("I liked Eva" or "I wouldn't want her as my patient!"). Asking students to find the details that trigger those emotions can help them be more sophisticated readers (and ultimately more sophisticated clinical listeners). Students generally have a strong and immediate emotional response to Eva. The majority are put off by her bitterness and anger; a substantial minority admire her for her grit and strength. Students can evaluate the elements of the story that generated their particular emotional response to the character. What in their own experience led them to focus on the bitterness or the strength? How can this self-knowledge inform their practice?

I discuss that regardless of how one views her, it would be easy to see her as a difficult and ungrateful patient. When I ask the students if they would like to take care of her as a patient, they acknowledge that she would be a patient of few rewards and probably not well liked.[17] Yet in the concluding section of the novella, the reader comes to understand that beneath her gruff exterior Eva is not a pessimist, and she is not a woman who has given up on the world; instead, she is an optimist—against all odds, she still believes in a utopian vision of the future, and it is her disappointment at seeing this vision unfulfilled that creates her bitter affect. This discussion can lead to a productive exploration of strategies they might use to avoid judging patients by their presenting demeanor. Given that nurses value a self-image based in caring and compassion, how can the students develop a reflective practice of identifying the obstacles and triggers that prevent them from expressing these virtues? Olsen's novella provides a rich source for strengthening the students' skills of critical reading.

Another exercise I use to achieve similar goals is to pair two stylistically dissimilar films on the same topic and assist students to explore their divergent responses.[18] One particularly fruitful pairing is Mark Romanek's film *Never Let Me Go*[19] matched with Nick Cassavetes' *My Sister's Keeper*.[20] Both films address the topic of the intentional creation of children genetically matched to be biological donors for others. The film *Never Let Me Go*, based on Kazuo Ishiguro's novel of the same name,[21] posits a dystopian recent past in which cloned children are raised for the express purpose of donating vital organs until they "complete." *My Sister's Keeper*, an adaptation of Jodi Picoult's novel,[22] is based on a "savior sibling" premise of a younger daughter genetically engineered to be matched as a tissue donor for her older sibling.

Beyond these distinct plots, the formal elements of these films present the viewer with wildly differing styles and tones. Surprisingly bright and sunny in presentation, *My Sister's Keeper* is a classic medical melodrama that pulls in the viewer and manipulates his or her emotional responses. Most students are willingly drawn into the story, identify with the characters, and are swept along by the familiar devices of popular film. In striking contrast, the muted *Never Let Me Go* holds the audience at an uncomfortable distance. With a color palette all in grays and greens and blues and characters who rarely display strong emotions, students are uncertain of how to respond to this film. Although students sympathize with the plight of the three main characters, they do not as easily align themselves with these young people.

Exploring different responses to these films provides productive multilayered classroom discussions. I generally begin the discussion with the ethics of the organ procurement decisions being made in the films. When I first taught these two films together, it seemed more natural to begin with their emotional responses. Over time, however, I found that if I began there, the students would try to explain their emotions by referencing arguments about the ethical dilemmas. They failed to see that the strategic decisions of the filmmakers had constructed the conditions for them to experience particular emotions. But when we discuss the ethics first—using ethical theories and strategies of argumentation to debate the questions of organ procurement—they are better able to subsequently unpack their emotional responses to the films as distinct objects for analysis.

Even with this sequencing of the discussion, students initially tend to explain their preferences for one film or the other based on the plot and how the characters behave and make decisions—mostly their preferences match the degree to which the students think the characters act the way they would themselves in the situation! To go beyond this sort of analysis, students need to be provided with the language of the formal elements of film: mise en scène, cinematography, editing, and sound.[23] Most students have never been taught to "read" a film; they have watched films primarily for content and have generally been fairly passive observers. Once they have this language—and have been prodded a bit—they can engage more actively with the viewing experience. This allows them to be insightful about the ways in which the genesis of their emotional responses comes from the construction of the films themselves, rather than from their idiosyncratic responses to the material. A consequence of their past passivity with films is that it is often necessary to remind students that one of the learning goals is to build their critical discernment skills. Most students have been asked to carefully analyze written texts before and so anticipate the request for close reading, but many are frankly puzzled as to what they are supposed to learn from a careful analysis of a single scene in a film.

Both of these teaching strategies—a deep reading of a complex text and contrasting two related films—help students to develop their critical reading skills by building on their already sophisticated moral resources of emotional engagement. The academy too often devalues what nursing students bring with them to their studies. They are too often told to put aside their emotions and to instead pursue logical reasoning. Use of the health humanities reframes this positioning and enables them to see that their emotional skills are positive attributes on which they can build. Noticing their emotional responses to situations can be the basis for a critical reflective practice that explores more deeply the source and meaning of those reactions. These kinds of exercises allow them to build increasingly complex expertise rather than creating a dichotomous choice.

Moral Imagination as a Resource for Judgment

A second goal of health humanities strategies for nursing students is to help them expand their moral imagination as a resource for judgment. Due to their age and social position, nursing students often have limited life experience. One of the functions of the educational process is to help them expand and develop complexity in their moral imagination. Giving students tools to help them slow down and stay in the stage of listening can facilitate their understanding that there are other perspectives, other ways of seeing the world, besides their own.

A quote I often use with students is from Milan Kundera, who writes that "Man . . . has an innate and irrepressible desire to judge before he understands."[24] I explain that while this is a call to listen and to embrace uncertainty and ambiguity, it is not an argument against using judgment. Congruent with their basic orientation toward caring, nursing students are generally quick to take up a position of acceptance of multiple perspectives—but often do so through a naive approach that simply acknowledges that others may see a situation differently without engaging deeply in that alternate viewpoint to truly understand the other. They often refuse to judge among available views or to take a position of their own. They fail to distinguish between the honorable commitment to provide care to all patients without judgment and the necessary social obligation to judge among competing ideas. "I've never been the parent of a severely disabled child. . . . I've never had to make the decision about the appropriate timing of the death of my parent . . . so I can't judge. *We shouldn't even be talking about this.* . . . we weren't there."

While we honor the impulse behind this kind of statement—the commitment to respect for persons and to providing meaningful options to patients and families—students also need to learn to form defensible and well-reasoned opinions of their own. As healthcare providers—and even more as citizens—they have an obligation to participate in the social conversation about health, healthcare, and the creation of health policy. Such participation requires nurses to make meaningful and substantive judgments. The 2010 Institute of Medicine report *The Future of Nursing*[25] calls for nurses to be more involved in structuring the healthcare system—to take a seat at the table. In order for nurses to engage in this work as equals with other providers and administrators, they need to be able to articulate, share, and effectively support their positions. But the precursor to having well-founded opinions is fully understanding the perspectives of others. Nurses need to be able to listen to and ask good questions of viewpoints that are distant from their own.

The expansion of moral imagination is often associated with having students read great literature as a window into the life experiences of others. Unfortunately, in a clinical curriculum, the opportunity to find time for students to read novel-length literature is limited. However, students can be offered multiple perspectives on the topics otherwise integral to the curriculum.

In one such exercise, I assign the students to read multiple websites about advance directives. I intentionally choose sites from organizations that span the political spectrum on this topic, such as Focus on the Family, the National Hospice and Palliative Care Organization, and Compassion and Choices. All of the sites project a tone that appears purely informative, providing assistance to laypeople to understand their choices and complete variously modified versions of advance directive forms.

In general, regardless of their political beliefs and attitudes toward end-of-life decisions, the students are distressed by the site from the right-to-life organization. What they discover through close reading is that their distress does not arise from their disagreement with the opinions expressed—they are willing to accept that different people have different perspectives on end-of-life choices—and indeed many of them are in alignment with the beliefs of the organization. What distresses them is that embedded in this site's arguments is a pervasive distrust of healthcare providers. Once they are able to identify this, we can discuss the prevalence of and reasons for patient distrust of the healthcare system and healthcare providers. Nurses are particularly fond of citing the finding that they are the "most trusted profession"[26] and feel justified in having earned this approbation. Having patients express suspicion feels unwarranted and unfair—and yet many patients have good reasons for their cynicism about this system for which nurses are often the most available face. Not only do patients fear that they may differ from their providers on their approach to specific health decisions, but they also have well-founded concerns about systemic racial and economic discrimination.[27] Deconstructing this distrust can help students to respond with understanding and acknowledgment, rather than defensiveness in the clinical setting.

Similarly, in a unit on end-of-life care, I present students with a collection of short videos of people who are dying expressing their perspectives on death. While this might have once been a difficult task fraught with the perils of patient confidentiality and sensitivity, there are now innumerable examples on the Internet to choose from.[28] I generally present the students with a curated and briefly annotated list of videos with as broad a range of viewpoints as I can find and ask them to choose four or five videos to view and consider. While watching the videos, they are directed to reflect on how the views expressed are different from their own—and different from each other. What questions would they like to ask of the speakers to more fully understand their positions? What are their own experiences and assumptions about what they would want for themselves at the end of life? What do they see as the source of these perceptions? I ask them to consider *why* their beliefs and desires might be different from those expressed by the speakers in the videos.

Once they arrive in class, I break them into small groups to discuss the videos and their reflections. The outcome of these small group discussions is to move beyond sharing their personal reflections to begin to look for patterns. What are the consistent themes that arise, and how are these themes addressed by the speakers? Which speakers articulated beliefs and values that were difficult to hear or to reconcile with their own? Using the evidence from the videos and from the reflections of their colleagues, what can they understand, if anything, about the sources of these differing values? Did hearing these other perspectives cause them to alter their own positions?

Finally, we conclude the exercise with a large group discussion that shifts away from the views of the speakers and toward an application to clinical practice. I ask the students to discuss together how the iterative reflection done with the videos and their small groups might be similar to the work they do with patients and colleagues in the clinical setting. What skills did we explore here that might be useful in patient encounters? How can the openness to alternate perspectives they cultivated in this exercise be carried into practice?

Conclusion

The health humanities offer multiple benefits to nursing students in the classroom, but the two we have focused on here are the development of moral imagination and the integration of critical analytic skills with the students' preexisting emotional resources. The application of these skills challenges students and faculty in contradictory ways. We want nurses to be good speakers *and* good listeners. We want students to find and develop their own voice and to build confidence in presenting themselves as full members of the healthcare team with important and unique insights and knowledge to offer. We want them to understand that as nurses they have not only the right but the obligation to make judgments, argue for positions, and be heard. At the same time, we want them to acquire the skill of listening, of listening carefully and deeply, of slowing down and making sure they have heard the other completely before making a judgment. The health humanities can create opportunities for students to practice both of these skill sets—and most importantly to understand that they are fundamentally the same. It is by reading and listening carefully that we become proficient writers and speakers ourselves.

Integrating the health humanities into the curriculum enables us to teach nursing students that as much as emotions are a legitimate moral resource, they need not be their only resource. Being attuned to their feelings is valuable for recognizing and responding to issues in practice. However, the systematic consideration of any practice issues also involves thoughtful analysis and reflection. Emotional responses to a case are not the same as careful ethical analysis; good choices in ethics do not always feel good. To teach students this important balance, we use a nautical metaphor: our guts (emotions) are good barometers, signaling when an ethical disturbance exists. But we need good compasses (critical discernment) to point us in the right direction for strong ethical practice. Both are required to successfully navigate the murky waters of contemporary healthcare practice.

PEDAGOGY EXERCISE SECTION

Narrative Summary and Analysis: "Tell Me a Riddle" by Tillie Olsen

PREPARATION

Tillie Olsen (1912–2007) is considered one of the great American writers. She is most famous for her collection of four short stories, *Tell Me a Riddle*. We will be reading one of the stories in that collection—also called "Tell Me a Riddle." At about fifty pages, it is actually considered a novella (a short novel). You will need to plan to read it twice. The first time, read it through quickly—just picking up the gist of the story and learning the rhythm of her writing. Olsen's prose is almost more like poetry in some places; she uses punctuation idiosyncratically, and you may have difficulty following the story at first. Just keep going and read through it the first time. On the second reading, you will want to slow down and pay attention to the details of the story. Also read Joan Liaschenko's article "Making a Bridge: The Moral Work with Patients We Do Not Like."

ASSIGNMENT

Prepare a two-page case summary of Eva using the Jonsen, Siegler, and Winslade model at the moment in the story just after she has had surgery. See https://depts.washington.edu/bioethx/tools/4boxes.html for a reminder of the key aspects of the model.

Carefully consider which details of the story you will include. You want your reader to have a vivid and complete picture of Eva, but you only have two pages. What will you include, and what will you leave out? Think carefully about the language you use to describe Eva and her circumstances—make sure that your words accurately describe her as you understand her from the story.

Bring two hard copies of your summary with you to class to share with your classmates.

IN-CLASS INSTRUCTIONS

Small Group Work

Meet in your small groups, and exchange summaries with your colleagues. Each of you should have two different summaries to read. As you read them, notice the ways in which the three summaries (yours and your two colleagues' papers) are the same or different.

Once you have all read your two cases, discuss the similarities and differences among your summaries.

- Did you choose different information to include?
- Did you have different understandings of the facts of the case?
- Did you use different language to describe the case?
- How did each of you handle the ambiguities or contradictions in the original story?
- What questions did you want to ask? (What were the gaps in your knowledge?)

Large Group Work

As a class, discuss some of the following questions:

How did the structure of the original text lead to the differences in the summaries?

How is this different or the same as clinical practice?

When reading the novella, you learn much more about Eva's interior life than you would as her nurse. What kinds of probing questions might you want to ask a patient to learn some of this? Or would you?

How did you feel about Eva? Would you like her to be your patient? Provide some details from the story that led you to feel that way. You will note that there is a range of opinions in the classroom about Eva. Why do you think you feel the way you do about her? What is it about who you are that makes you either disdain or admire her?

How ought we approach patients we do not particularly like or find difficult to care for? What are some strategies you have used to manage your negative feelings toward particular patients? If you liked Eva, what might you say to a colleague who found her difficult?

Notes

1. Susan M. Reverby, *Ordered to Care: The Dilemma of American Nursing, 1850–1945* (Cambridge: Cambridge University Press, 1987).

2. Pamela Abbott and Liz Meerabeau, "Professionals, Professionalization, and the Caring Professions," in *The Sociology of the Caring Professions*, 2nd ed., ed. Pamela Abbott and Liz Meerabeau (London: UCL Press, 1998), 1–19.

3. Approximately 50% of nurses entering the profession in 2014–2015 obtained their first nursing degree at the B.S.N. level. Among those who entered with A.A. degrees, 50% expected to subsequently earn a baccalaureate degree. See Christine T. Kovner et al., "Diversity and Education of the Nursing Workforce 2006–2016," *Nursing Outlook* 66, no. 2 (2018): 160–67.

4. The landmark study in this area is Linda H. Aiken et al., "Educational Levels of Hospital Nurses and Surgical Patient Mortality," *JAMA* 290, no. 12 (2003): 1617–23. Subsequent research in this area is summarized in the American Association of Colleges of Nursing's fact sheet "The Impact of Education on Nursing Practice," last modified August 2017, http://www.aacnnursing.org/News-Information/Fact-Sheets/Impact-of-Education.

5. Reverby, *Ordered to Care*. The phrase "daughters of educated men" is a reference to Virginia Woolf's *Three Guineas*.

6. Kovner et al., "Diversity and Education."

7. Admittedly, not all of this resistance is grounded in social justice motivations. Healthcare institutions, always looking to decrease the costs of the labor force, have exerted substantial pressure to limit the educational requirements of nurses—and thus the compensation for the role.

8. Monica E. Bjorkstrom, Inger S. Johansson, and Elsy E. Athlin, "Is the Humanistic View of the Nurse Role Still Alive—In Spite of an Academic Education?" *Journal of Advanced Nursing* 54, no. 4 (2006): 502–10.

9. Julia Hallam, "Angels, Battleaxes and Goodtime Girls: Cinema's Images of Nurses," in *Signs of Life: Medicine & Cinema*, ed. Graeme Harper and Andrew Moor (London: Wallflower Press, 2005), 105–19.

10. Kristen M. Swanson, "Nursing as Informed Caring for the Well-Being of Others," *Image: The Journal of Nursing Scholarship* 25, no. 4 (1993): 352–57.

11. Jean Watson, "The Theory of Human Caring: Retrospective and Prospective," *Nursing Science Quarterly* 10, no. 1 (1997): 49–52.

12. A particularly useful text for faculty preparing to teach narrative analysis is Tod Chambers, *The Fiction of Bioethics: Cases as Literary Texts* (New York: Routledge, 1999).

13. After considerable debate and revision, the co-authors chose to use the singular pronoun "I" when describing teaching strategies. The use of "the first/second author" third-person phrasing felt awkward, and the inclusive "we" felt disingenuous; these strategies are not used by both of us. We ask the reader's indulgence for eliding our identities in this way.

14. Tillie Olsen, "Tell Me a Riddle," in *Tell Me a Riddle* (New York: Delta, 1994), 63–116.

15. I use the Jonsen, Sigler, and Winslade four-box model.

16. Chambers, *The Fiction of Bioethics*.

17. I always have students read this wonderfully titled paper: Joan Liaschenko, "Making a Bridge: The Moral Work with Patients We Do Not Like," *Journal of Palliative Care* 10, no. 3 (1994): 83–89. Her work helps students to acknowledge that feeling and understand the damage we can do both to patients and to our own character by failing to address it directly.

18. Any list of potential films is inevitably already out of date by the time of publication, but a useful resource for identifying films on particular topics is Henri Colt, Silvia Quadrelli, and Lester Friedman, *The Picture of Health: Medical Ethics and the Movies* (Oxford: Oxford University Press, 2011).

19. Mark Romanek (director), *Never Let Me Go* (Century City, CA: Fox Searchlight, 2010).

20. Nick Cassavetes (director), *My Sister's Keeper* (Los Angeles: New Line Cinema, 2009).

21. Kazuo Ishiguro, *Never Let Me Go* (New York: Vintage, 2005).

22. Jodi Picoult, *My Sister's Keeper* (New York: Washington Square Press, 2004).

23. A brief introduction to the formal elements of film with lots of helpful prompts for discussion is provided in Timothy Corrigan, *A Short Guide to Writing about Film*, 8th ed. (Boston: Pearson, 2012). I provide this analytic material before they watch the films.

24. Milan Kundera, "The Depreciated Legacy of Cervantes," in *The Art of the Novel*, trans. Linda Ascher (New York: Perennial Classics, 2003), 3–22.

25. Institute of Medicine, *The Future of Nursing: Leading Change, Advancing Health* (Washington, DC: National Academies Press, 2010).

26. Megan Brenan, "Nurses Keep Healthy Lead as Most Honest, Ethical Profession," Gallup News, December 26, 2017, http://news.gallup.com/poll/224639/nurses-keep-healthy-lead-honest-ethical-profession.aspx.

27. Institute of Medicine, *Unequal Treatment: Confronting Racial and Ethnic Disparities in Health Care*, ed. Brian D. Smedley, Adrienne Y. Stith, and Alan R. Nelson (Washington, DC: National Academies Press, 2002).

28. Although we are using the example of perspectives on dying here, this exercise might be adapted for any number of clinical conditions or diagnoses. Though we probably should be used to it by now, we continue to be amazed at the things people share with strangers on the Internet.

Works Cited

Abbott, Pamela, and Liz Meerabeau. "Professionals, Professionalization, and the Caring Professions." In *The Sociology of the Caring Professions*, 2nd ed., edited by Pamela Abbott and Liz Meerabeau, 1–19. London: UCL Press, 1998.

Aiken, Linda H., Sean P. Clarke, Robyn B. Cheung, Douglas M. Sloane, and Jeffrey H. Silber. "Educational Levels of Hospital Nurses and Surgical Patient Mortality." *JAMA* 290, no. 12 (2003): 1617–23.

American Association of Colleges of Nursing. "The Impact of Education on Nursing Practice." Last modified August 2017. http://www.aacnnursing.org/News-Information/Fact-Sheets/Impact-of-Education.

Bjorkstrom, Monica E., Inger S. Johansson, and Elsy E Athlin. "Is the Humanistic View of the Nurse Role Still Alive—In Spite of an Academic Education?" *Journal of Advanced Nursing* 54, no. 4 (2006): 502–10.

Brenan, Megan. "Nurses Keep Healthy Lead as Most Honest, Ethical Profession." Gallup News. December 26, 2017. http://news.gallup.com/poll/224639/nurses-keep-healthy-lead-honest-ethical-profession.aspx.

Cassavetes, Nick (director). *My Sister's Keeper*. Los Angeles: New Line Cinema, 2009.

Chambers, Tod. *The Fiction of Bioethics: Cases as Literary Texts*. New York: Routledge, 1999.

Colt, Henri, Silvia Quadrelli, and Lester Friedman. *The Picture of Health: Medical Ethics and the Movies*. Oxford: Oxford University Press, 2011.

Corrigan, Timothy. *A Short Guide to Writing about Film*, 8th ed. Boston: Pearson, 2012.

Hallam, Julia. "Angels, Battleaxes and Goodtime Girls: Cinema's Images of Nurses." In *Signs of Life: Medicine & Cinema*, edited by Graeme Harper and Andrew Moor, 105–19. London: Wallflower Press, 2005.

Institute of Medicine. *The Future of Nursing: Leading Change, Advancing Health*. Washington, DC: National Academies Press, 2010.

Institute of Medicine. *Unequal Treatment: Confronting Racial and Ethnic Disparities in Health Care*, edited by Brian D. Smedley, Adrienne Y. Stith, and Alan R. Nelson. Washington, DC: National Academies Press, 2002.

Ishiguro, Kazuo. *Never Let Me Go*. New York: Vintage, 2005.

Jonsen, Albert, Mark Siegler, and William Winslade. *Clinical Ethics: A Practical Approach to Ethical Decisions in Clinical Medicine*, 7th ed. New York: McGraw Hill, 2010.

Kovner, Christine T., Maja Djukic, Jin Jun, Jason Fletcher, Farida K. Fatehi, and Carol S. Brewer. "Diversity and Education of the Nursing Workforce 2006–2016." *Nursing Outlook* 66, no. 2 (2018): 160–67.

Kundera, Milan. "The Depreciated Legacy of Cervantes." *The Art of the Novel*. Translated by Linda Ascher, 3–22. New York: Perennial Classics, 2003.

Liaschenko, Joan. "Making a Bridge: The Moral Work with Patients We Do Not Like." *Journal of Palliative Care* 10, no. 3 (1994): 83–89.

Olsen, Tillie. "Tell Me a Riddle." In *Tell Me a Riddle*, 63–116. New York: Dell, 1994.

Picoult, Jodi. *My Sister's Keeper.* New York: Washington Square Press, 2004.

Reverby, Susan M. *Ordered to Care: The Dilemma of American Nursing, 1850–1945*. Cambridge: Cambridge University Press, 1987.

Romanek, Mark (director). *Never Let Me Go.* Century City, CA: Fox Searchlight, 2010.

Swanson, Kristen M. "Nursing as Informed Caring for the Well-Being of Others." *Image: The Journal of Nursing Scholarship* 25, no. 4 (1993): 352–57.

Watson, Jean. "The Theory of Human Caring: Retrospective and Prospective." *Nursing Science Quarterly* 10, no. 1 (1997): 49–52.

4

Shine a Light Here, Dig Deeper Over There

INTEGRATING THE HEALTH HUMANITIES IN ONLINE BIOETHICS EDUCATION

Amy M. Haddad

Introduction

Health science professionals and others who work in healthcare-related disciplines are increasingly interested in augmenting their basic education in bioethics. Often, this interest moves beyond independent study or continuing professional education to seek out graduate education. However, for these adult learners, graduate programs in bioethics must be flexible and fit into the restricted work schedules and the other responsibilities that fill their busy lives. There are also economic considerations regarding work and professional commitments that have an impact on whether a potential student will enroll in a graduate program. Picking up and moving to a new community to attend a face-to-face program carries a high price tag. Adult learners have more complex work and family obligations than younger students, which makes moving to a new location to attend graduate school more difficult. The interest in graduate work in bioethics by adult learners has motivated the development of hybrid programs that combine on-campus and online methods as well as fully online bioethics programs.

Although in the minority among bioethics graduate programs in the United States, fully online, asynchronous (student-centered learning on their own schedules) programs allow maximum flexibility for learners. The Master of Science in Health Care Ethics (MSHCE) program at Creighton University, the program that will be used as the reference point for discussion in this chapter, was designed from the outset to be a fully online, asynchronous program, that is, a program that would not require any on-site experiences at the university or real-time course work with peers or faculty. The three-hour courses were designed to be delivered in eight-week sessions. An underlying assumption was that students worked full-time at some other occupation so that they would generally only take one course at a time. The program started with nine required three-hour courses and one three-hour elective. Since the start of the program in 2009, a three-hour required scholarly reading and writing course has been added to the program, for a total of thirty-three hours. Required courses are generally offered three times a year, electives once or twice a year. As predicted by national trends in graduate education, the demographics of learners in the MSHCE program have ranged from a minority of students in their twenties who just completed undergraduate degrees or were taking time to pursue graduate work before entering a health professions program to a majority of mature students well established in their careers. The mean age of students in the MSHCE program is 45. Average time to completion of the degree is a little less than two years. So, the interest of diverse adult learners in flexible online education in bioethics has been one of the drivers of the development of online programs like the MSHCE program. The second driver for online programs in higher education is the development of user-friendly instructional technology.

Over the past two decades, there have been significant advances in computer technology, in general, and instructional technology, in particular.[1] Students and faculty of all ages are more facile and comfortable with computers and other types of technology including work-related and personal-use software and applications for communication, retrieval and sharing of information, word processing, and other tasks. Additionally, best-practice standards have been developed and promulgated for online higher education.[2] Thus, students and faculty are now able to actively participate in online courses with minimal equipment and basic computer skills. Faculty can now refer to standards for online course design and delivery. Faculty development programs have also been established to help faculty design courses and teach in the online environment, which requires different skills and competencies from traditional classroom teaching.[3]

Although face-to-face delivery models of graduate education are still considered the standard to which online graduate courses are compared, there are unique benefits to online education. First, there is the previously mentioned flexibility of asynchronous online learning. Students can be separated by geography and time zones yet still participate at their convenience in a course in an asynchronous program. Students can print assigned readings or use mobile devices that allow them to take their coursework almost anywhere. They can engage with other students and the instructor in the course through structured and informal discussions when it is convenient for them. Students can also choose to work and discuss coursework outside of the course management system through their personal email, texting, chat or video applications, or other social media. Online education offers the opportunity for students from diverse professional backgrounds and geographic locations to attend a graduate program that does not exist in their local community. Thus, there is more equitable access to bioethics programs for those who live in remote or smaller communities that do not have a college or university with such a program.

Online learning, especially in a program that focuses on complex and controversial topics such as those that arise in bioethics, requires a structure that engages learners with the content, peers, and the instructor that is more intimate and inclusive in many ways than a traditional classroom or graduate seminar environment. In other words, to overcome the "distance" in online education, courses and learning experiences have to be specifically constructed to engage individual learners while making them feel they are a part of a community of learners. As we have noted in a previous publication about discussions in online courses, a promising conceptual framework for online graduate programs in bioethics is the community of inquiry (CoI) model.[4] In brief, the CoI framework proposes three elements in online learning: 1) cognitive presence, in which students interact with each other and source materials in critical and analytic ways; 2) social presence that speaks to the interaction of students with each other including formal and informal communication, sharing, and building trust; and 3) teaching presence that manages the learning experience and facilitates understanding.[5] A thorough review of the literature on CoI is beyond the scope of this chapter, but in summary the three presences proposed in CoI "offer a significant framework by which to understand how communities of inquiry in online environments are established and function to foster collaborative processing of course content."[6] As will be noted in the "Designing for the Online Environment" section in this chapter, the MSHCE program is designed to foster collaborative learning by attending to the cognitive, social, and teaching presences.

Although the benefits of online programs can be significant, there are also special challenges. There are more resources today to assist faculty in the transition to teach online, yet faculty still struggle with adapting to the demands of the online teaching environment. Several studies have indicated that online courses require more instructor time, specifically in the areas of planning, course design, delivery, monitoring of student interactions, providing individual and collective feedback, engagement with students in the course and real time such as scheduled phone calls or computer-assisted interaction like videoconferencing, and grading.[7] Developing courses for the online environment is particularly challenging because so much has to be anticipated and built into the course before it is offered to students. Changes on the fly are difficult to make and confusing to learners, so thoughtful planning is essential to a well-designed course. For example, it is easy to ask students to exchange papers with their neighbors in a face-to-face environment but complicated in the online setting. In short, the design and layout of a course are critical elements in planning for an online course. Prior to deciding on an appropriate and consistent format, decisions must be made about content to meet course and program learning goals.

Determining Essential Content in a Graduate Bioethics Program

One planning sequence for curricular design that leads to better student performance, particularly when the content is complex and abstract, is the backward design process developed by Wiggins and McTighe.[8] As the name of the process indicates, the planning process starts with the identified results, then determines evidence of learning, and finally moves to planning learning experiences and activities. In other words, you start where you want learners to end up at the conclusion of the program or course. For example, there are ten program objectives for the MSHCE program that all learners should know, do, or understand at the end of the program of study.[9] Each course in the program includes course objectives that indicate the desired result at the end of the course and link back to the overall program objectives. Learning objectives, whether for a program or course, encompass a great deal of possible content that could be covered, so the next step in program design after deciding on overall outcomes is to determine what content is essential and what would be important to know.

Wiggins and McTighe propose four filters to determine when material or content is worthy of understanding and thus included in a program of study. The material should 1) be enduring or have value beyond the classroom, 2) be at the heart of the discipline, 3) require explanation and unpacking, and 4) offer potential for engagement.[10] These elements are especially important given the time constraints of the eight-week course model in the MSHCE program. There is no room for content that does not explicitly contribute to enduring understandings that are the outcome of the program and the focus of learning goals. Regardless of the length of a course, there will always be a limit to the amount of time that can be spent on any topic, so faculty must make difficult choices about what really needs to be covered in a course and why. Table 4.1 offers some examples of determining priorities in a graduate bioethics program using the four filters.

To grapple with the big ideas in bioethics, various strategies need to be employed to assist learners to discern ethical concepts from other factors in the complex world of healthcare. Because the health humanities can play such an important role in this discernment, a specific program goal in the MSCHE program focuses on the health humanities: "Draw upon the humanities and liberal arts in the process of ethical reflection about the structures of health care."[11] This program goal is a reminder to instructors to incorporate health humanities in a way that is relevant to the overall aims of the courses that they design.

The inclusion of health humanities content in a bioethics program helps students to see a novel way into ethical issues. Students can draw on their imaginations and emotions to go deeper into clinical, ethical issues than is possible with traditional philosophical ideas and concepts in ethics. It is also

TABLE 4.1
Filters for Selected Understandings

Filter	Application to Bioethics
Enduring	In general, big ideas in bioethics, ideas that endure beyond the current headlines and technology in healthcare, include questions about what makes right actions right, distinguishing between ethical and non-ethical evaluations, discerning what constitutes ethically sound decisions, and examining what it means to be a moral person.[a] Specifically, two big concepts in the MSHCE program are vulnerability and social justice.[b]
At the heart of the discipline	Justification of ethical judgments is at the heart of the discipline of bioethics, which requires skills in critical thinking and moral reasoning.[c]
Requires explanation and unpacking	Misconceptions in bioethics are numerous, but some of those that seem to occur with greatest frequency are underestimating the complexity of an idea or situation, disregarding tensions between moral goods, and assuming that good intentions or strong opinions are sufficient justification for moral decisions.
Potentially engaging	Ideas that are interesting to graduate students in a healthcare ethics program relate strongly to the realities of their life and work experiences, especially from healthcare settings. In other words, the learning experiences that are designed for students to develop skills in moral reasoning should be the ones they encounter in their lives.[d]

Adapted from Wiggins and McTighe, *Understanding by Design*. Amy Haddad, "Teaching for Enduring Understandings in Ethics," *Journal of Physical Therapy Education* 19, no. 3 (2005): 73–77.

[a] Robert Veatch, Amy Haddad, and Dan English, *Case Studies in Biomedical Ethics* (New York: Oxford University Press, 2014), 3–19.

[b] Christy Rentmeester et al., "Teaching and Learning Health Justice: Best Practices and Recommendations for Innovation," *International Journal of Teaching and Learning in Higher Education* 28, no. 3 (2016): 440–50.

[c] Denise Dudzinski, Rhonda Rhodes, and Autumn Fiester, "Pedagogical Goals for Academic Bioethics Programs," *Cambridge Quarterly of Healthcare Ethics* 22, no. 3 (2013): 284–96.

[d] Lisa Lee, Hillary Wicai Viers, and Misti Ault Anderson, "The Presidential Bioethics Commission: Pedagogical Materials and Bioethics Education," *Hastings Center Report* 43, no. 5 (2013): 16–19.

important to note that the goals of a bioethics program are enriched by learning goals commonly included in the desired outcomes of medical humanities education. Such learning goals as fostering empathic relationships, promoting professionalism, developing compassion and openness to alternative views, and enhancing personal well-being are all relevant to bioethics as well.[12] The next step in designing an effective online graduate course in bioethics is to attend to the special challenges of the online environment to support students' success.

Designing for the Online Environment

There are entire books on effective design of online courses, so the following are selected key points to consider when beginning the process. In designing online courses in bioethics, especially those that aim to do more than just deliver information, it is important to try and see the course from the student's perspective. Students can get overwhelmed if the content is not presented in an organized, clear manner. Think about how a course would progress in a face-to-face environment if on the first day the instructor introduced himself or herself and then just dumped a stack of all the reading assignments, instructions, lecture notes, etc. on the students' desks and then left the room, with no opportunity for additional explanation or questions. To avoid student and instructor frustration and information overload, students need to be oriented to the online environment in general, including discussion of the technical skills and time required to complete assignments, resources to help the student succeed, and how best to communicate with the course instructor.

In addition, the course content needs to be logically organized according to the course learning goals and to build within a course so that the students can see connections between learning activities from week to week. Content should be "chunked" into manageable modules or components that provide a solid foundation on a topic before moving on to the next point. The format of courses within a program should be consistent as well so that students know where to look for certain common information such as course readings that are on e-reserve, links to writing resources, or support services for technical problems. Consistency in design saves time and provides a sense of familiarity between courses in a program. A quiz or scavenger hunt within the course can be a useful tool to encourage exploration of the various elements in a course that the students will need to successfully complete their work.

Effective and open communication is essential to establish a community of learners. It is safe to say that an instructor cannot overcommunicate with students in an online course. Clear language regarding instructions for assignments, participation in discussions, and grading including rubrics with detailed explanations are essential in on online course. Students also appreciate templates or examples of what a short version of a completed assignment looks like on a comparable topic to the one assigned. In so doing, students get a concrete idea of expectations.[13] Improving clarity in an online course is a never-ending task as every iteration provides an opportunity to revise instructions or content and provide different ways to frame a question or explain the purpose of a reading or assignment. Other types of communication within an online course are equally important such as that between instructor and students, whether that takes the form of a message or an announcement to all students in a course when there appears to be collective confusion about an assignment or reading or individual conversations with students online or on a phone call. Finally, it is important to humanize the course.[14] Humanizing a program and content begins with providing a welcoming environment to learners and offers information about the person who will be teaching the course beyond content expertise and academic credentials. To establish a community of inquiry, students and teachers need to trust each other. To build trust, participants in the course must get to know each other in a more personal way than merely exchanging information, such as appropriate sharing of personal information in a student lounge or other non-assignment space as well as drawing on the expertise and experiences of others in assignments. As has been stated previously, one can also humanize bioethics by integrating the health humanities. A specific course in the MSHCE program will be used to illustrate how the health humanities can be incorporated into a sample writing assignment and discussion on bioethics content in the clinical setting.

Context: A Course in Clinical Bioethics

The types of health humanities content used in the MSCHE program include documentary films, creative non-fiction, art, music, poetry, and short stories. MHE 607 Practical Ethics in Health Care Settings is a required course that "provides the opportunity to apply foundational concepts of ethics to a variety of health care settings. Additionally, the use of deliberative methods to think through and discuss the unique features presented by different health care settings and professional conduct is an integral component of the course."[15] The general purpose of the course is to move students through the functions of institutional healthcare ethics committees: case review and consultation, policy development, and education in a variety of clinical delivery settings such as home care, skilled nursing facility, and critical care. Generally, there are fifteen to twenty students from a variety of disciplinary backgrounds enrolled in the course. Two assignments are used as examples. The first assignment is briefly explained here, regarding how the health humanities are used to highlight subtle points in bioethics that could otherwise be ignored or hidden. The full instructions for this learning activity from week 2 of the course are included at the end of this chapter.

In the week 2 module of the course, the overarching question for the week that frames learning activities is, How do different frameworks of moral reasoning influence how we talk about ethics? The readings for week 2 include dramatically different views of moral reasoning and clinical ethics, such as foundational content on the functions of ethics committees from one of the required textbooks in the course, an article on authority of the clinical ethicist, Margaret Urban Walker's piece on keeping moral spaces open, and a short story by Lorrie Moore.[16] The assignment purposefully integrates objective, abstract, philosophical readings with a short story, thereby linking cognitive and affective approaches to learning. The clinical encounter that is the focus of the assignment is not a standard "case study" format that students are used to in bioethics. Rather, the story highlights a view and a voice that are often absent in case studies. Students are drawn into the story of overwhelmed, almost frantic parents facing a cancer diagnosis for their seemingly healthy baby. Question 1 asks the students to identify instances of miscommunication in the short story.

The students' responses include not only where communication breaks down but also the students' personal engagement with the story and its characters. For example, one student responded as follows:

> This story really hits home for me, as I am a pediatric oncology nurse. The mother's words speak volumes. Mom talks of the staff calmly iterating and reiterating that "this is normal," it is normal to a nurse, but it is the furthest thing from normal for a family going through this.

This student's response reflects that connection between the short story and her clinical experience as a nurse, that is, what is routine for her is not for the parents of critically ill children. Also, the story uses the shorthand language of clinical settings in which the mother is designated as "Mom" rather than by her given name. This language is familiar to clinicians, and it is the rare student who notes what this labeling does to parents.

Another student highlighted her role in similar situations:

> Recognizing when one is on ethical ground is a vital step that seems frighteningly easy for too many healthcare providers to miss. As a nurse, I kept waiting for Baby's nurse to realize how poorly informed the parents were and step in to correct the situation.

Here, the student, also a nurse, waits for the character in the story to "step in" and reflects on her own actions as well.

Finally, a medical student in the course noted not only examples of miscommunication but unpacked a metaphor about decision-making in the story that would be out of place in a traditional case study:

> The Mother alludes throughout the story that she feels overwhelmed with the entire process and that she is filled with questions about the "overwhelming strangeness of everything around her." Although there is some discussion of the decision that she and her Husband face in deciding upon different treatment options for their son, she metaphorically explores the process behind making such difficult decisions through an analogy to shopping at Marshall Fields. Here, the manager of the store appears as the authoritative presence, the one who holds the power and wisdom; the manager is a god-like entity in this metaphor, and it is with him that the Mother strikes up bargaining. She herself claims that she is not a shopper; making decisions does not come easily to her. Instead, the process of shopping or decision making initiates the process of grieving at which she remains firmly in the "bargaining" stage.

In the second example of an assignment that focuses on the humanities, poetry is used in small group discussions. The assignment is in direct contrast with the previous week's work on an ethics consultation workup of a complex, standard case study with specific questions about prognosis, value conflicts, treatment options, etc. Students work in small discussion groups of four or five. To simplify the assignment, each student is assigned one poem[17] to read and respond to, but they often read all of the poems. The directions for the discussion assignment are as follows. First, read the piece "What Poetry Does" by Marilyn Chandler McEntyre.[18] Then read your assigned poem. Then write a response to the following questions for your initial post: choose one of the "things" that poetry does from McEntyre's list and apply it to the poem you read. Now think about what a "case study does." In other words, how does this differ from reading a poem? Then you have the opportunity to discuss what others in the small group had to say about their poems and the insights, surprises, or ways of seeing the poem provoked.

The reactions to the poems and the realizations of the students about what "poetry does" as opposed to case studies create a dynamic exchange that often includes a common fear of poetry. Using a poem instead of a traditional ethics case causes the students to look at clinical ethics with new eyes, or what Kumagai and Wear refer to as "making strange" or trouble assumptions.[19] The poems do the trick of troubling assumptions as the students have had difficulty with this assignment over many offerings and iterations of the course until the piece by Marilyn McEntyre was recently included in the instructions. McEntyre's ten examples of what poetry does give students options and ways to look at a poem and see what the poem does or does not do. Furthermore, students are encouraged to collaborate for deeper understanding of content in small group discussions. In sum, student reactions to the various poems they read indicate that poetry works differently from case studies in raising ethical issues, power dynamics, emotional connections, etc. Students were honest about their dislike of poetry but generally found at least one "thing" that the poems did that made sense to them. As one student noted,

> I agree with you, as I have been enjoying reading the posts also. I have never really enjoyed reading poetry, nor have I taken the time to analyze the deeper meaning of a poem. I am a fairly black and white person, and poetry is clearly not that. The "things" that McEntyre addresses in the article *What Poetry Does*, have helped me to look at poetry differently and gain a better understanding of its intention. I have found it interesting how differently people interpret the assigned poems, but I like the deeper insight I have gained by reading the posts!

Another student dug a bit deeper into parts of a peer's poem regarding what "stopped me short":

> It seems like in poetry and in case studies understanding where the "characters" are coming from is central to the whole thing. I appreciated your poem too, and the idea of being stopped short. I think two things in the poem stopped me short. They both came right at the end of the poem.

> First, I think it's interesting when he looks at his brother in a way that says "Did you get what you came for?" I think it brings up an aspect of ethics that is frequently present when a parent or guardian/representative of some kind has a role in the decision-making process. Anytime a loved one is involved, for better or worse, the question can be asked: "Is this for me or for them?" an important ethical ideal, loosely represented in the poem. The other part that caught my attention was the idea of leaving paper crumbs so that someone could come and find him. I found that very moving and I think not just in the psychiatric setting but in the presence of any burdensome condition, the idea of waiting to be found to be rescued.

However, not every student understands the underlying reasons to include poetry in a course on clinical ethics. Several students in each course attempt to "fix" the poem to turn it into a case study, a genre that they are used to in clinical practice and in ethics. They literally strip the poem of emotions, voice, imagery, etc. Also, the following comment is almost always found in the final course evaluations, "I don't understand why we read poetry in week 6." Thus, this discussion needs further refinement so that students understand the purpose of including poetry and the connection to bioethics and clinical realities. The underlying lesson here for the course design is to trouble assumptions but not so much that students are lost and frustrated or at the very least to warn them that they will likely feel lost and frustrated but that is part of the process of reading poetry and unraveling bioethical issues.

Conclusion

The health humanities generally have an underlying moral function that helps bioethics students question their own underlying assumptions, values, and behaviors as well as offering a "nuanced and integrated perspective on the fundamental aspects of illness, healing and suffering."[20] For example, the health humanities can help students understand what is happening in a situation by examining the plot of a story or play. Students can learn about who is talking or thinking in a poem or story by attending to voice. Bioethics content is inherently complex, so by working through the ambiguity that the humanities introduce students will have the skills to analyze ambiguities in bioethics material. This chapter has included practical suggestions as well as theoretical background information for educators on how the health humanities could be used in teaching bioethics in the online environment. Methods to design or redesign courses, from determining essential content to formatting material for online delivery, were presented. The opportunities and challenges in online education were enumerated along with examples of integrating health humanities content into bioethics courses that draw on the strengths that underlie both disciplines.

PEDAGOGY EXERCISE SECTION

Learning Exercise

Focus question for the week: How do different frameworks of moral reasoning influence the way we talk about ethics?

Writing assignment instructions: Read the short story "People Like That Are the Only People Here: Canonical Babbling in Peed Onk" by Lorrie Moore[21] and reflect on the story in light of the article by Walker[22] on creating moral space. Then individually respond to each of the following three questions using all of the assigned readings in a well-constructed paragraph or two.

Question 1: Cite an example in the story that indicates miscommunication or differing understanding regarding language. Why is this ethically important? Explain.

Question 2: Are there any references in the story to decision-making capacity? Explain.

Questions 3: Walker speaks about the responsibility of an ethics consultant to create "moral space" in literal and figurative terms. Cite places in the short story where the creation of moral space would help the individuals in the short story and explain why.

Notes

1. Kyong-Jee Kim and Curtis J. Bonk, "The Future of Online Teaching and Learning in Higher Education: The Survey Says . . ." *Educause Quarterly* no. 4 (2006): 22–30.

2. Quality Matters, Specific Review Standards from the QM Higher Education Rubric, Sixth Edition Accessed August 20, 2016. https://www.qualitymatters.org/sites/default/files/PDFs/Standardsfromthe QMHigherEducationRubric.pdf.

3. Morris Sammons, "Exploring the New Conception of Teaching and Learning in Distance Education," in *Handbook of Distance Education*, ed. M. G. Moore and W. G. Anderson (Mahwah, NJ: Lawrence Erlbaum Associates, 2003), 387–400.

4. John Stone et al., "Discussion in Graduate Online Bioethics Education: Best Practices and Ongoing Challenges," *International Journal of Ethics Education* 2, no. 1 (2017): 17–36.

5. D. Randy Garrison, Terry Anderson, and Walter Archer, "Critical Inquiry in a Text-Based Environment: Computer Conferencing in Higher Education," *Internet and Higher Education* 2, nos. 2–3 (2000): 87–105.

6. Michael S. Putman, Karen Ford, and Susan Tancock, "Redefining Online Discussions: Using Participant Stances to Promote Collaboration and Cognitive Engagement," *International Journal of Teaching and Learning in Higher Education* 24, no. 2 (2012): 151–67.

7. Gail Lindsay, Janet Jeffrey, and Mina Singh, "Paradox of a Graduate Human Science Curriculum Experienced Online: A Faculty Perspective," *Journal of Continuing Education in Nursing* 40, no. 4 (2009): 181–86.

8. Grant Wiggins and Jay McTighe, *Understanding by Design* (Alexandria, VA: Association for Supervision and Curriculum Development, 1998).

9. Creighton University, "Master of Science in Health Care Ethics, Program Learning Goals," accessed August 31, 2016 https://gradschool.creighton.edu/program/health-care-ethics-ms.

10. Wiggins and McTighe, 23.

11. Creighton University, "Master of Science."

12. Arno Kumagai and Delese Wear, "'Making Strange': A Role for the Humanities in Medical Education," *Academic Medicine* 86, no. 7 (2014): 973–77. David Doukas, Laurence McCullough, and Stephen Wear, "Medical Education in Medical Ethics and Humanities as the Foundation for Developing Medical Professionalism," *Academic Medicine* 87, no. 3 (2012): 1–8.

13. Poonan Kumar and Marilyn Skrocki, "Ensuring Student Success in Online Courses," *Online Classroom* 15, no. 6 (2015): 3–4, 8.

14. Ibid., 4.

15. Master of Science in Health Care Ethics, "MHE 607 Practical Ethics in Health Care Settings Syllabus."

16. D. Micah Hester and Toby Schonfeld, "Introduction to Healthcare Ethics Committees," in *Guidance for Healthcare Ethics Committees*, 2nd ed., ed. D. Micah Hester and Toby Schonfeld (New York: Cambridge University Press, 2012), 1–8. David J. Casarett, Frona Daskal, and John Lantos, "The Authority of the Clinical Ethicist," *Hastings Center Report* 28, no. 6 (1998): 6–11. Margaret Urban Walker, "Keeping Moral Spaces Open: New Images of Ethics Consulting," *Hastings Center Report* 23, no. 2 (1993): 33–40. Lorrie

Moore, "People Like That Are the Only People Here: Canonical Babbling in Peed Onk," in *Birds of America* (New York: Picador Press, 1998), 212–48.

17. The following poems are presently used in MHE 607 for the week 6 assignment: Anne Caston, "The Good We Do," *Prairie Schooner* 76, no. 2 (2002): 27–28; S. Hazen-Hammond, "Let Me Breathe," *The Healing Muse: A Journal of Literary & Visual Arts* 8, no. 1 (2008): 14; Jeanne LeVausseur, "Old Man in Bed Clothes," *JAMA*, 276, no. 24 (1996): 1928; Jeanne LeVausseur, "Danny Boy," in *Between the Heartbeats*, ed. Cortney Davis and Judy Schaefer (Iowa City: University of Iowa Press, 1995), 106; Peter Schmitt, "Thanksgiving: Visiting My Brother on the Ward," *Bellevue Literary Review* 6, no. 2 (2006): 90–91.

18. Marilyn Chandler McEntyre, "What Poetry Does," n.d., accessed August 31, 2016, http://alphaomegaalpha.org/pdfs/WhatPoetryDoes.pdf.

19. Kumagai and Wear, "'Making Strange.'"

20. Johanna Shapiro et al., "Medical Humanities and Their Discontents: Definitions, Critiques, and Implications." *Academic Medicine* 84, no. 2 (2009): 192–98.

21. Moore, "People Like That."

22. Walker, "Keeping Moral Spaces Open."

Works Cited

Casarett, David J., Frona Daskal, and John Lantos. "The Authority of the Clinical Ethicist." *Hastings Center Report* 28, no. 6 (1998): 6–11.

Creighton University. "Master of Science in Health Care Ethics, Program Learning Goals." Accessed August 31, 2016. https://gradschool.creighton.edu/program/health-care-ethics-ms.

Doukas, David, Laurence McCullough, and Stephen Wear. "Medical Education in Medical Ethics and Humanities as the Foundation for Developing Medical Professionalism." *Academic Medicine* 87, no. 3 (2012): 1–8.

Dudzinski, Denise, Rhonda Rhodes, and Autumn Fiester. "Pedagogical Goals for Academic Bioethics Programs." *Cambridge Quarterly of Healthcare Ethics* 22, no. 3 (2013): 284–96.

Garrison, D. Randy, Terry Anderson, and Walter Archer. "Critical Inquiry in a Text-Based Environment: Computer Conferencing in Higher Education." *Internet and Higher Education* 2, nos. 2–3 (2000): 87–105.

Haddad, Amy. "Teaching for Enduring Understandings in Ethics." *Journal of Physical Therapy Education* 19, no. 3 (2005): 73–77.

Hester, D. Micah, and Toby Schonfeld. "Introduction to Healthcare Ethics Committees." In *Guidance for Healthcare Ethics Committees*, 2nd ed., edited by D. Micah Hester and Toby Schonfeld, 1–8. New York: Cambridge University Press, 2012.

Kim, Kyong-Jee, and Curtis J. Bonk. "The Future of Online Teaching and Learning in Higher Education: The Survey Says . . . " *Educause Quarterly* 29, no. 4 (2006): 22–30.

Kumagai, Arno, and Delese Wear. "'Making Strange': A Role for the Humanities in Medical Education." *Academic Medicine* 86, no. 7 (2014): 973–77.

Kumar, Poonan, and Marilyn Skrocki. "Ensuring Student Success in Online Courses." *Online Classroom* 15, no. 6 (2015): 3–4, 8.

Lee, Lisa, Hillary Wicai Viers, and Misti Ault Anderson. "The Presidential Bioethics Commission: Pedagogical Materials and Bioethics Education." *Hastings Center Report* 43, no. 5 (2013): 16–19.

Lindsay, Gail, Janet Jeffrey, and Mina Singh. "Paradox of a Graduate Human Science Curriculum Experienced Online: A Faculty Perspective." *Journal of Continuing Education in Nursing* 40, no. 4 (2009): 181–86.

McEntyre, Marilyn Chandler. "What Poetry Does." n.d. Accessed August 31, 2016. http://alphaomegaalpha.org/pdfs/WhatPoetryDoes.pdf.

Moore, Lorrie. "People Like That Are the Only People Here: Canonical Babbling in Peed Onk." In *Birds of America*, 212–48. New York: Picador Press, 1998.

Putman, Michael S., Karen Ford, and Susan Tancock. "Redefining Online Discussions: Using Participant Stances to Promote Collaboration and Cognitive Engagement." *International Journal of Teaching and Learning in Higher Education*, 24, no. 2 (2012): 151–67.

Quality Matters. Specific Review Standards from the QM Higher Education Rubric, Sixth Edition Accessed August 20, 2016. https://www.qualitymatters.org/sites/default/files/PDFs/StandardsfromtheQMHigherEducationRubric.pdf.

Rentmeester, Christy, Helen Chapple, Beth Furlong, Amy Haddad, and John Stone. "Teaching and Learning Health Justice: Best Practices and Recommendations for Innovation." *International Journal of Teaching and Learning in Higher Education* 28, no. 3 (2016): 440–50.

Sammons, Morris. "Exploring the New Conception of Teaching and Learning in Distance Education." In *Handbook of Distance Education*, edited by M. G. Moore and W. G. Anderson, 387–400. Mahwah, NJ: Lawrence Erlbaum Associates, 2003.

Shapiro, Johanna, Jack Coulehan, Delese Wear, and Martha Montello. "Medical Humanities and Their Discontents: Definitions, Critiques, and Implications." *Academic Medicine* 84, no. 2 (2009): 192–98.

Stone, John, Helen Chapple, Amy Haddad, Sarah Lux, and Christy Rentmeester. "Discussion in Graduate Online Bioethics Education: Best Practices and Ongoing Challenges." *International Journal of Ethics Education* 2, no. 1 (2017): 17–36.

Veatch, Robert, Amy Haddad, and Dan English. *Case Studies in Biomedical Ethics*. New York: Oxford University Press, 2014.

Walker, Margaret Urban. "Keeping Moral Spaces Open: New Images of Ethics Consulting." *Hastings Center Report* 23, no. 2 (1993): 33–40.

Wiggins, Grant, and Jay McTighe. *Understanding by Design*. Alexandria, VA: Association for Supervision and Curriculum Development, 1998.

5

Moral Imagination and More

TEACHING HEALTH HUMANITIES IN THEOLOGICAL EDUCATION

Melinda A. McGarrah Sharp

Introduction

"I didn't have time to read this book," said one student, who had in the past reported a personal goal of reading no more than 20% of assigned reading and skimming the rest, "but I couldn't put it down and actually read the whole thing." In many classes I teach, I include at least one novel, work of historical fiction, memoir, or autobiographical narrative to activate moral imagination broadly and to narrow in on particular issues of moral distress and moral responsibility.[1] If medical schools make little time for health humanities by assigning few hours of class time and little to no academic credit to ethics education, theological schools devote plenty of class time hours and course credit for ethics and reflection on responsible practice.[2] However, health humanities can still be difficult to address within the required curriculum of a seminary.

In order to awaken the theme of moral imagination when teaching health humanities within theological education, I regularly assign two novels, José Saramago's *Blindness* in an introductory required theological ethics class and Edwidge Danticat's *Brother, I'm Dying* in an elective practical theology course on death and dying.[3] These two texts serve efficient and effective pedagogies of health humanities within theological education. In this essay, I begin by identifying moral imagination as key to my commitments to bridging theology and health humanities. Then, I describe my pedagogical context and outline how I teach the texts by Saramago and Danticat in this context. Within theological education, I locate health humanities in the intersections between theological ethics and practical theology. The remaining sections of the essay show, in the face of student and curricular time pressures, how Saramago and Danticat work well as authors who help activate and probe moral imagination as significant to teaching health humanities in theological education.

Moral Imagination: Bridging Theology and Health Humanities

My first academic conference lecture outside of a university was to a group of licensed clinical psychologists who were not uniformly thrilled to attend what I thought was a fantastic panel on health humanities. The panel was organized to "count" for one hour of required continuing education in ethics and included case studies in rapid fire with provocative dilemmas and discussion of best-practice responses. As a seminary professor, I now teach required and elective ethics and practical theology courses every semester. I have more time to dwell in the moral conundrums and complexities of case studies and to suspend the need for response, giving students time to wrestle and wonder. The purpose is to equip my students to respond quickly and with moral imagination when they put this slower-paced study in service of their various vocations in the world.

Theological schools draw a variety of kinds of students, many of whom will move into professions where they will serve a prominent role in healthcare decisions within their communities. Some current students—with little to no formal bioethics training—already serve on hospital boards, some students are regularly invited into the sacred room of a dying community member, and some students already speak up at public events in times of crisis. All of these contexts will demand future contribution of my students who are not already so engaged.

One might think that I do not have the same pressures to find a way to engage health humanities deeply with my students as colleagues teaching health humanities in other departments or professional schools. However, after including diverse religious traditions, attending to denominational standards, and embodying my commitment to emerging voices and issues in addition to traditional figures and themes, I only have a few hours of any semester-long class to devote to health humanities per se. Yet, I am still morally obligated to make sure that I include health humanities in my teaching because of the prominence of spiritual health, bodies, communities, and intercultural dynamics in a vocational calling to support faithfulness, responsibility, wholeness, and well-being.[4] Narrative—attending to the ways human beings tell each other nonfictional and fictional stories about their lives—becomes an integrative resource for supporting an intersectional approach to health and well-being.[5]

I have found narrative genres to help quickly open depth when teaching health humanities in theological ethics. I often assign these so-called non-theological texts to provide students and myself a way into the difficult work of activating and engaging moral imagination. *Blindness* and *Brother, I'm Dying* in particular work well as opening books in a unit of study because of the vivid moral landscape that each portrays. Saramago and Danticat both masterfully illustrate a much larger range of interconnected moral dilemmas than could be addressed in a given semester. Assigned at the beginning of a course of study, these texts open space for addressing health humanities in theological education while also providing an on-ramp into the semester's learning process.

Many Ways In

As I consider how I became invested in teaching health humanities in theological education, I learned the importance of structuring "a way in" at the beginning of each class.[6] My health humanities training began when I was in middle school and served as a "candy-stripe" volunteer[7] in my local children's hospital. Regularly attending the hospital gift shop cashier, I bore witness to varieties of human yearning in clinical settings. Later, I gained formal training as a premedicine and religious studies major. As a hospital volunteer during this time I was regularly and miraculously invited into the sacred work of listening to life stories in hospital hallways and rooms of suffering and healing. Biomedical ethics, philosophy, and medical anthropology bridged the two disciplines of medicine and theology for me then and continue to do so today.

Of note, I trained at three different schools espousing three different philosophies and theologies of medicine. I first studied principle-based ethics with Dr. James Childress at the University of Virginia, where I learned to love health humanities. This school of ethics provides a way in to moral dilemmas through clarifying and using a matrix of robust principles, especially autonomy, nonmaleficence, beneficence, and justice.[8] I then studied liberationist and feminist ethics with Dr. Margaret Farley at Yale University, where I learned to foreground questions of power within health humanities. This way in to moral dilemmas makes room for noticing the silent, silenced, underrepresented, minoritized, or missing voices in complex situations.[9] In doctoral work, I studied phenomenological approaches with students of Dr. Richard Zaner at Vanderbilt University, where I learned to probe moral responsibilities within health humanities. This third way in to moral dilemmas balances astonishment at the possibilities of understanding what is going on in creative tension with a commitment to clarity and precision regarding myself, other(s), and larger contextual political and social forces.[10]

Shaped by three schools of thought, I find that a generous approach to each methodology helps me identify and teach the importance of method in relation to students' concepts and experience of moral imagination. All three schools of thought, while offering diverse ways in and through the moral conundrums of health humanities, require moral imagination. While I want my students today to know and consider implications of their embedded and deliberative habits of engaging health humanities from within their role as theologian,[11] the desire to awaken the concept and experience of moral imagination drives my pedagogy of health humanities in theological education.

Health Humanities at the Intersection of Theological Ethics and Practical Theology

Theological education and health humanities education both address human vulnerabilities and anxieties. The enduring presence of loss, systemic and interpersonal violence, global interconnectedness, and social-political anxieties can be heightened and/or made invisible in and beyond the distinct faith, chaplaincy, and non-profit communities where theological students often will work. A primary pedagogical goal is not only to expand students' exercise of moral imagination in general but to awaken moral imagination to serve *empathic imagination*, or the ability to remain simultaneously present to oneself, another human being, complex contextual factors, and a divine presence or ultimate reality.[12] The quality of presence and resultant shared narrative fragments can contribute to harm or well-being.[13] Often, folks ask whether it is possible or responsible to offer care in relationship with another person whose life experience, race, marital status, experience of loss, gender identity, childbearing or infertility experience, and so on and so forth, differ. While sustaining this important question in the classroom, I believe that empathic imagination allows the possibility of presence in the first place, whether such differences are more or less pronounced.

As a theological educator, rather than an entire class focused specifically on health humanities, I address health humanities within both theological ethics and practical theology courses. First, I understand theological ethics to be oriented toward thoughtful and intentional reflection on what it means to be an embodied human being who acts rightly and justly in community as a participant in all of creation. The partnership of ethical reflection and embodied action is expressed in practices of moral discernment. Moral discernment is not to be confused with being moralistic or judgmental about what I and other people should and should not do but rather to be morally engaged with my participation in the good life, in general, and in a helping and healing vocation, in particular.

Teaching and learning to activate moral imagination in oneself in service of the empathic imagination that facilitates responsible interactions with others requires disciplined and courageous practices of self-awareness. Courses of study then need to incorporate invitations to probe meanings, intentions, and consequences of human actions in communities. Theologians, like bioethicists, contemplate what it means to be a moral person in theory and practice. Theologians look to sacred texts, structures of communal life such as law and class, and the world around them to identify gaps between the way the world is and the way the world ought to be.

Building on traditional figures from fourth-century Augustine of Hippo to fourteenth-century Thomas Aquinas, contemporary modern philosophers and theologians have framed moral discernment in terms of right relationship (Buber), discipleship (Bonhoeffer), justice (Rawls), consequences (James,

Rorty), value (Gilkey), virtue (Gustafson, MacIntyre), God's divine command (Mouw), realism (Barth, Reinhold Niebuhr), agape love (Kierkegaard), responsibility (H. Richard Niebuhr), ecclesial communities (Hauerwas), obligation (Kant), and commitment (M. Farley)—and the list goes on.[14] The drive to fashion faithful Christian ethics has been robust and continues to benefit from new methods and new perspectives.

Careful moral discernment is one place where practical theology intersects with theological ethics. Practical theology involves making and examining theological claims about practices of life, both religious practices and other meaningful and mundane practices that contribute to a life, such as meals, care of the dying, parenting, human migration, or gardening. As a theological educator, I see health humanities residing in intersections between theological ethics and practical theology. For example, examining the practices of teaching and learning key figures who have shaped theological ethical study practice, such as the list sketched above, shows how various histories of ethics have knowingly and unknowingly pushed many people to "the margins" of mainstream life by ignoring their presence in the human family or participating in other dehumanizing strategies—a concern shared in the interdisciplinary work of health humanities.[15]

Today, theological ethicists and practical theologians, such as Miguel de la Torre, Stacey Floyd-Thomas, Evelyn Parker, Phillis Sheppard, and Christie Neuger, theorize the margin itself as a significant resource and corrective in identifying right and just ways of life. Feminist and liberationist approaches ask which voices are missing and what populations are excluded from any process or rule of moral discernment (Russell, Farley). Womanist ethicists make space for the unique experiences and contributions of African American women's experiences (Parker, Townes, West, hooks). As more voices are granted access to publication and positions of teaching and learning, wide diversities of life stories continue to impact expressions of moral imagination within academic theology.

The classroom with all its present diversities and missing diversities becomes a laboratory for practicing moral reflection in public, both in and beyond the public of any one class. The idea of inviting students to address a public, theorized in practical theology by David Tracy, has become its own specialized field of public theology.[16] The idea is that any care provider is tasked to address multiple publics simultaneously: in the case of theology, students train to address faith communities, academic communities, and the public square. While students often leave theological education for a variety of kinds of work, from traditional church ministries to new forms of faith expressions to nonprofit justice work, the classroom equips students for speaking in public policy conversations, local activism, and responsible participation in various social movements as a global citizen. Emerging scholarship and pedagogical reflection pay particular attention to the politics of power that impinges on literacies of reading, interpreting, and reshaping narratives of life and death both historically and today.[17]

Narrative approaches to theological ethics and practical theology foster careful attention to the ways in which storied accounts of lived experience are ordered so as to make sense of choices and actions across a lifetime in a particular community with implications for the global neighborhood in which human beings share in creation. Pedagogically, this involves inviting students into a practice of careful listening through reading narratives and reading each other's words in order to understand the nature of moral reflection. Specifically, I draw on narrative to solicit and expand moral imagination because of how narrative beckons attention to the moral dilemmas and moral distress that emerge when choices and actions come into conflict with what one thinks is a right and just way to live in the world. The following sections outline two pedagogical examples.

PEDAGOGICAL EXAMPLE 1: READING SARAMAGO'S *BLINDNESS* TO AWAKEN MORAL IMAGINATION

Summary of *Blindness*

Portuguese writer José Saramago's 1995 book *Blindness* moves from an ordinary day in ordinarily frustrating stop-and-go traffic to the inception of a mysterious epidemic of blindness. The first case of blindness manifests in a driver right in the midst of driving a familiar car in familiar traffic. A logistical question is activated by this sudden blindness: how does a just-stricken-blind driver drive or even stop driving? Almost at the same time, a moral question is also activated: who can and should the just-stricken-blind driver trust and under what conditions? The just-stricken-blind man fears, "obviously he would not invite a complete stranger to come in who, after all, might well be plotting at that very moment how to overcome, tie up and gag the poor defenseless blind man, and then lay hands on anything of value. There's no need, please don't bother, he said, I'm fine, and as he slowly began closing the door, he repeated, there's no need."[18]

Seemingly the epidemic of sudden blindness spreads from this one man to the stranger he entertained entrusting with his newfound need—the very trust which was both questioned and then perhaps violated perhaps confirming the man's fears. After the terrifying image of blindness erupting in the midst of stop-and-go traffic, Saramago takes the reader to the optometrist's office. What happens, the reader quickly wonders, if the optometrist becomes blind? What then is the role of the eye doctor struck blind? Does the eye doctor's own experience of blindness offer special insight to understanding the disease process or disrupt medicine entirely? Without knowing the names of any characters—another significant moral dilemma—the epidemic quickly moves into wider and wider circles of human life: air traffic control, the United Nations, policing, health policymaking.

While huge and terrifying implications play out in the background, the reader is thrust into the complexities of quarantining the just-stricken-blind from the temporarily sighted. Where do blind persons who have previously learned to navigate social structures fit into this new fear-based dichotomy of the haves and have-nots? How do human practices like meals, communication, movement, sickness and health, access to resources, birth, and burial work? What happens to human institutions like transportation, government, family, hospitals, military, education, media, and socially acceptable rules of engagement? What happens to accountabilities for violating laws, codes of conduct, or moral commitments? What is the role of race, class, nationality, gender, age, ability, and other intersectional identity markers?

In his provocative thought experiment, Saramago disrupts driving as the first physical and metaphorical context of how a mass blindness epidemic could affect the systems and institutions that structure life—traffic laws, car safety protocols, the rough sense of knowing where one is going. From the first words of the book, Saramago foreshadows this disruption on the page with run-on sentences and unconventional punctuation. Sharpening moral dilemmas around human dignity, Saramago's characters remain both deeply engaging and nameless. How might empathy manifest in this strange new world? The reader is left with more questions than answers, making *Blindness* a wonderful candidate for providing students a way into learning about and activating the concept and experience of moral imagination.

How I Teach *Blindness*

I teach *Blindness* in order to awaken moral imagination in the required theological ethics introductory course at the level of master's and doctoral education. When the book list is posted months before the semester, I indicate that this will be the first text used. I then assign the whole book on the first day of class to be read before the second class meeting of the semester. I ask students to take note of two things as they read: first, any moral dilemmas. Before we get into how histories, practices, and approaches to ethics shape moral imagination in particular situations, I also invite students to notice any unwritten and/or pronounced goals, rules, and virtues that play out in the novel.

The in-class exercise the second week of class can be done in either one hour or two hours. Of note, I also follow each of the same steps in online classes through a combination of whole class and small group discussion boards and preparing annotated images that summarize each step through a brief screencast. Here I will describe the steps as they unfold in an on-campus course. In order to break the ice in the first five minutes—to provide a way in to the particular class for all voices—I ask class participants to turn to their neighbor and identify a striking line or image from the book. Then, I issue a challenge: previous classes have noticed more than one hundred moral dilemmas in the novel *Blindness*. Almost immediately in every class so far, someone will say that while there are lots of moral dilemmas in *Blindness*, there is no way there are one hundred. So, we begin with one example.

I solicit moral dilemmas from the class, writing the list on the board. It does not take long to name one hundred examples. The last time I taught this class, the class came up with one hundred and eighty-five examples of moral dilemmas from the text in about twenty minutes. Here are a few examples: authority, human rights, boundaries, belonging, charity, childcare, social class, coercion, criminality, care of the dying, dehumanization, clean/profane, distribution of resources, discipline, human nature, forgiveness, dignity, following orders, the good life, pleasure, hatred, inclusion, hygiene, hospitality, leadership, identity, law, mental health, militarization, who is my neighbor, paternalism, obedience, sexualized violence, rituals, security, voice, just war, weapons, suffering, suicide, and trust. And this is the twenty-minute version. Each moral dilemma is pertinent not only in the intersection of health humanities and theological study but indeed also in each student's unique vocational context. As the class continues, a landscape of moral dilemmas on the board provides a backdrop for both the particular class period and the whole semester.

In the next fifteen to twenty minutes, I break the class into three groups: rules, goals, and virtues. Again, while some students loved and/or were deeply troubled by the book and are therefore eager to engage in this exercise, even the more skeptical students quickly shift from thinking that there is not much to say to a more detailed list than they imagined possible. This accomplishes at least two things: first, it reiterates the importance of conversation and consultation in the work of activating moral imagination. Second, students can pinpoint goals, rules, and virtues more quickly than often is possible in more traditional philosophy or theology textbooks that review teleological, deontological, and virtue ethics. For example, discernible goals in *Blindness* include survival, human dignity, justice, safety, order, health and healing, pleasure, and communal cohesion; discernible rules include utilitarianism, containment, proper burial of the dead, policies and procedures, and noticing that power shifts in response to change; and discernible virtues include loyalty, bravery, persistence, generosity, honesty, and sacrifice. Without being prompted, each group can point to pages and passages to support its claims.

In the last portion of class, as each group reports on goals, rules, and virtues that they notice, I summarize by writing keywords around the edges of the board. As a group, we discuss connections students notice between their own work and vocational plans and any of the identified moral dilemmas, goals, rules, or virtues. Nearly all students remain engaged. I typically have to cut off conversation for the sake of time. One hallmark of a great class is feeling that it ended too soon. Every class where I have used this exercise at the beginning of the semester has included references to the *Blindness* text and class discussion later in the semester, even in the final paper or exam twelve weeks later.

PEDAGOGICAL EXAMPLE 2: READING DANTICAT'S *BROTHER, I'M DYING* TO FOCUS MORAL IMAGINATION

Summary of *Brother, I'm Dying*

In *Blindness*, every predictable and strategic element of infrastructure begins to fail, creating unforeseen opportunities for pain, suffering, and healing. In contrast, *Brother, I'm Dying* unmasks suffering perpetuated by systems working exactly as they are designed. While *Blindness* unpacks a terrifying thought experiment—Saramago reports literally having the book unfold from a thought that occurred to him one day over lunch[19]—*Brother, I'm Dying* courageously and clearly reports real-life terror. Celebrated Haitian American author Edwidge Danticat opens this autobiographical account with the all too human set of contrasts between Danticat learning that she is pregnant the same day that she travels to escort her ill father to a hospital pulmonologist in Brooklyn, New York, and learns that he is dying. An additional complicating factor between this convergence of possible impending birth with possible impending death that is less common for many folks is Danticat's foreshadowing of the less than miraculous events that would befall her dear Uncle Joseph after a health miracle when his throat nearly closed. "This [book] is an attempt at cohesiveness," writes Danticat, "and at re-creating a few wondrous and terrible months when their lives and mine intersected in startling ways, forcing me to look forward and back at the same time. I am writing this only because they can't."[20]

With possibilities of life and death in the foreground, Danticat reviews Haiti's difficult and unique history while also telling her family's story of living in Haiti with Uncle Joseph from age four to twelve while her parents migrated to New York before, like many immigrants, only able to reunite with their children many years later. Uncle Joseph not only was a courageous public speaker aware and involved in civic life in Haiti but also preached and led a church in Bel Air, committed to this work even after an emergency radical laryngectomy. "Still," reports Danticat, even though he learned to speak with the assistance of a voice box, "there were times when it was painfully clear how much he missed the full participation his voice allowed him."[21] The next hundred pages of text probe the complexities of health and sickness, healing and suffering, for an extended family living partly in New York, partly in Bel Air, Haiti, and partly traveling between the two places.

Complex intersections of migration and immigration with health, illness, healing, and suffering come alive and are made more concrete in Danticat's family history. However, a turn to terror unfolds slowly with the increasing violence in Bel Air, culminating when eighty-one-year-old Uncle Joseph is caught in the middle of a confusing local, national, and United Nations–backed armed dispute in post-Aristide Bel Air. In the midst of a situation too volatile to clarify his role as clergy who tries to maintain a politically neutral stance regarding mounting deaths and destructions, Uncle Joseph urgently flees Haiti for New York under cover of night's darkness. Instead of his usual responses about his intentions of temporarily entering a legal port of entry to US customs and immigration officials at Miami International Airport for a visit, which his visa allowed, this time Uncle Joseph requests temporary asylum.

In response to the recorded question "Why exactly are you requesting . . . political asylum in the United States today?" Uncle Joseph is recorded as responding, "Because they burned down my church in Haiti and I fear for my life."[22] Without his voice, voice box, or medications, Uncle Joseph quickly becomes "Alien 27041999" within Krome Detention Center, one of the many detention centers in the United States where undocumented persons are held as if imprisoned. Uncle Joseph's medical condition deteriorated quickly and access to communication, medical care, or even the medicines he had at the time of fleeing were made inaccessible in the detention infrastructure. By the end of *Brother, I'm Dying*, Danticat re-creates another heartbreaking set of convergences, just months from the first chapter of the book but seemingly ages later: the death and burial of Uncle Joseph, the birth of her daughter Mira, and the last days of her father's life.

How I Teach *Brother, I'm Dying*

I teach *Brother, I'm Dying* in the practical theology classroom in order to provide a narrative way in to some of the complex intersections and interconnections of immigration, suffering, health, and well-being. The specific course in which I have taught this book is a pastoral care elective that focuses on discerning an ethics of practice around accompanying persons and families through death, dying, and grief. While *Blindness* helps to depict a broad landscape of moral dilemmas and the goals, rules, and virtues that shape and are shaped by moral imagination, *Brother, I'm Dying* focuses moral imagination on a complex yet specific intersection of immigration, yearning for life, and death and dying. Rather than the first book of the course, I begin with a unit of study on general grief theory, and then I teach *Brother, I'm Dying* as the first text in a unit on the theme of "complicated grief," which analyzes several issues that further complicate already complex situations of grief work.

The following in-class exercise can be done in a little over an hour or extended to a three-hour course block. Each of the following steps also translates well online using a mixed media approach and engaging the class through discussion board features of the learning management platform. While I have used the exercise in an intensive weekend model of the course with success, I have found that it works best in the middle of a semester-long study of death, dying, and grief work. For obvious reasons, death, dying, and grief work not only are relevant to the professional lives of students and myself but also intersect in predictable *and unpredictable* ways with our various personal life histories, present circumstances, and near-future opportunities and challenges. I teach this book through five steps: quotes and questions, policy review, book study, public prayer practice, and a summative exercise.

Before meeting, I ask students to identify a few moving, challenging, or disturbing quotes and either email to me ahead of class or bring to class. I also ask students to raise two substantial questions that include reference to the text in connection with the student's own previous experiences or newly awakened concerns or insights. At the beginning of the class, I ask each student to share one quote. This serves two pedagogical commitments: to honor the student's experiences of reading in preparation for the class and to invite all voices into the space as equally worthy. If two students choose the same quote, that is fine. Because I am asking for reading a brief excerpt from the text and not yet students' interpretations, even students who have been able to spend less time with the book before class can participate fully in this portion of the exercise.

The second twenty to thirty minutes is devoted to a brief immigration policy review. Because I also regularly teach an elective intensive immigration immersion seminar on the US–Mexican border, a course offered at many seminaries, I draw on current narrative, film, and policy information to review some legal, economical, and political elements of immigration before moving into a more specifically theological reflection later in the class session. Helpful resources for this portion of the exercise include the current State Department report on immigration,[23] the current resource list posted by educational institutions located at physical borders,[24] and/or charts and policy briefs from local policy institutes. In addition to highlighting some of the many push-and-pull factors that I do not attempt to be able to cover in just a brief review, two important factors that I make sure to convey are the length of time for migrants to move through the formal legal immigration process (up to twenty years or more given access to money, language proficiency, and personal connections) and the huge role of for-profit detention centers in the economy of immigration in relation to the United States. Including images or brief film excerpts enriches this portion of the course because of the power of connecting "the immigration debate" to actual lives involved in the flux and flow of immigration as a way of life and death.

I then solicit questions that students identified from the text *Brother, I'm Dying.* In addition to a variety of connections and concerns of current class members, the class quickly raises the issues of risk and vulnerability in relation to immigration. What kinds of risks and vulnerabilities—from translation services to consent to risk of deportation and indefinite familial separation—must likely be negotiated when immigrants or undocumented persons are in dire need of medical care? Who can and should be trusted and not trusted? What kinds of choice do various actors have in relation to trust? What kind of communication is possible in detention centers when access to resources is urgent? What counts as urgent suffering that demands access to a medical intervention, and who decides? Who shapes and is shaped by narratives of distinct families affected? Where might and where should narratives and policies intersect?

The last twenty to forty minutes of the class session include two activities, which can be wrapped up into the first when time is more limited. Unlike many deaths in detention centers, Danticat's Uncle Joseph's death at the Krome Detention Center garnered national attention when it happened in 2004. Therefore, I invite students as individuals, pairs, or small groups to compose a portion of a public prayer that they might contribute to a local vigil held to mark this particular kind of complicated grief. This exercise can be rather short, where prayers only include a few words or phrases, or it can be extended to begin composing a communal public prayer, drawing on words and phrases suggested by different class members and groups. The class can end liturgically with the verbal sharing of these prayers out loud. Or, before or after a liturgical moment, I sometimes ask class members to offer one take-home learning summary on complicated grief surrounding immigration after pausing for a moment for silent reflection on their quotes and questions connecting immigration to complicated grief in their own work and life, policy discussion, experience of reading and discussing text, and contemplations about making public offering.

Pragmatic Concerns and Three "More" Things

The novel *Blindness* and the autobiography *Brother, I'm Dying* both meet a standard for books I hope students will purchase for their bookshelves—they are challenging enough to bear reading and rereading over time. I am not alone in this assessment as Saramago's *Blindness* won the Nobel Prize for literature and Danticat's *Brother, I'm Dying* won the National Book Critics Circle Award for autobiography. In addition to the pedagogical outlines mentioned here, both texts can support teaching health humanities in briefer and in more sustained engagements.

For semesters without enough room to assign a full-length text, *Blindness* is also available as a 2008 feature-length film with the same title[25] and Danticat's *Brother, I'm Dying* appears in briefest outline in a *Nation* article entitled "Not Your Homeland."[26] An Internet search leads quickly to many versions of structured discussion guides for each book. Further, both authors have granted engaging interviews about these texts. I recommend reading Saramago's interview in the *Paris Review*,[27] where he outlines the origin and writing process that created *Blindness*, and Danticat's 1996 interview in *Callaloo*, where she traces the themes of absence and recovery from absence as moral and familial concerns.[28] It is possible to use shorter excerpts to begin to awaken moral imagination without the before-class preparation or with less face-to-face time than the present outlines require.

When time allows, it is also possible to do more with these texts. I began this chapter reflecting on my own formation as a scholar-teacher through three different, even competing, methodologies for discerning how to employ and deepen my exercise of moral imagination. In all three methods and amid many different theorists, I have encountered work by the philosopher of religion and leading contributor to the field of modern psychology William James. Like many trying to clarify the science of psychology while noticing cultural forces that impinge on human experiences of suffering and healing, from Sigmund Freud to Frantz Fanon, William James intertwined science and what he identified as "more" than what can be reduced to science.

What might James mean by *more*? Among the most moving of James's writing is where he stops to notice suffering within his philosophical reflections on health and the science of healthcare. While "matter is indeed infinitely and incredibly refined" and can therefore be studied as an object of serious science, James writes, in *Pragmatism*, matter also incarnates something more than mere science. He continues, "To any one who has ever looked on the face of a dead child or parent the mere fact that matter *could* have taken for a time that precious form, ought to make matter sacred ever after [. . . . matter] lends itself to life's purposes. That beloved incarnation was among matter's possibilities."[29] I imagine James's ability to notice that the uniquely moral and existential character of *this* moment is influenced by the tragic death of his six-month old son, Herman, in 1885. Doing *more* can simply denote the power of presence in moments of anguish and uncertainty, beauty, and love.

What more is required for moral imagination to serve empathic imagination and responsibility in the face of moral dilemmas? How shall educators teach students to be prepared for it? In the seminary classroom, I am interested in the *more* that will awaken and help shape pastoral practices toward empathic imagination. I teach health humanities in theological education so that moral imagination can be awakened and focused in service of paying attention to the more. Both Saramago and Danticat provide a way in to the topic of presence in the face of deep and unsettling uncertainties. I know that students will not leave these novels knowing what to say and do, but I hope that students will feel more courageous in knowing how important it is to stay present to stories that are crying out to be told, heard, and shared.

The *more* often resides at the hinge between clarifying what is known and knowing what to do next. Three "more" things that could be explored in the process of teaching health humanities with the texts *Blindness* and *Brother, I'm Dying* include probing the character of the mystery, hope, and misunderstanding that accompany the awakening and directing of moral imagination. What happens to the eye doctor who becomes blind or the preacher who loses their voice is a matter of technical response and treatment, professional identity, and much more. First, the more can be probed in relation to the kind of *mystery* that involves confronting the limits of knowing what to do, whether the uncertainty resides in moral imagination, technical proficiency, or both. Second, the more can be probed in relation to the *hope* that recognizes that the next best thing to do is created in the doing itself.[30] Third, the more can be probed in relation to *misunderstandings* that beckon staying in the room, staying in human communities through the process of better understanding each other for the sake of well-being. Learning to pay attention to *more* is significant for vocations of ministry and medicine that aim toward addressing and transforming pain, celebrating and supporting life, and knowing what to do in the vast hinges in between.

Conclusion

My basic pedagogical goal of asking students to read José Saramago's 1995 novel *Blindness* is to awaken moral imagination with specific examples of moral dilemmas, goals, rules, and virtues alive and in the room at the beginning of a semester of in-depth study. The broad landscape of moral dilemmas that emerges through engaging this text brings many concerns of health humanities alive within theological education. Edwidge Danticat's 2007 autobiography *Brother, I'm Dying* brings pedagogical attention to more focused intersections of immigration, suffering, and well-being, unmasking some political dimensions of death and dying where social forces, public and national policies, and individual human bodies and families intersect.

Both texts offer a way in to moral imagination, whether pressed for time or when time allows opportunities to go deeper. Both texts raise a number of complex issues with vivid, heartbreaking imagery. Both books are hard to put down because of enlisting readers' imaginations from the first page, when the first driver is struck blind in *Blindness* and when pregnancy accompanies midwifery of death in *Brother, I'm Dying*. Both texts illustrate that moral imagination can both increase empathy and mislead moral actors into collusion, architecture, and/or enforcement of policies and practices that more likely harm rather than heal.

How do I attend to suffering and inspire healing in the complex twenty-first century? Medical humanities and theological education share this question as a matter of life and death. Twentieth-century pragmatic philosopher William James described "the more" that accompanies human loss and suffering as irreducible to physiology. In theology classrooms today, when students engage narratives such as Saramago's *Blindness* or Danticat's *Brother, I'm Dying*, the experience of close reading raises significant questions of attending the spiritual needs and intercultural wrestlings that accompany life-and-death decisions and policy discussions across the life span. These pedagogical examples demonstrate that health and justice are connected in theological education where teaching and learning make room for moral imagination and more.

ACKNOWLEDGMENTS

I acknowledge that policies regarding migration and immigration around the world, and particularly in the United States, are rapidly changing, continuing to place great risk on families and to threaten familial separation. It could be instructive to engage current policies, particularly as they unfold in health care contexts, respecting what is at stake for many children, families, and communities.

PEDAGOGY EXERCISE SECTION

Awakening Moral Imagination

CLASS HANDOUT

Explanation of Exercise: The purpose of this exercise is to awaken moral imagination through (1) rapid brainstorming of moral dilemmas, guiding goals, rules, and virtues and then (2) using these resources to examine one specific moral dilemma. (3) Questions for further conversation may be engaged if time permits or as prompts for written reflections after the exercise. The three-part exercise can be accomplished in an hour or can be expanded to fill more than an hour of class time. The novel *Blindness* by José Saramago[31] and the autobiography *Brother, I'm Dying* by Edwidge Danticat[32] can be used to deepen the following exercise, but they are not required reading for an engaging process of awakening moral imagination. Materials needed include projection with sound, materials for making lists in the front of the classroom, and photocopies of the article "Not Your Homeland."

STRUCTURE OF THE HOUR

Part One: Awakening Moral Imagination through Rapid Brainstorming (Twenty Minutes)

1. (three minutes) Show the *Blindness* film preview.[33]
2. (five to ten minutes) As a whole group, brainstorm and record moral dilemmas that could arise.
3. (five to ten minutes) Split into three groups, brainstorm with assigned scribe from each group to record insights in the front of the room responding to the following three questions:
   a. What goals drive your engagement in moral dilemmas? (example: human dignity)
   b. What rules guide your engagement in moral dilemmas? (example: access to healthcare)
   c. What virtues or personal or communal characteristics discipline your engagement in moral dilemmas? (example: generosity)

Part Two: Probing One Moral Dilemma Using Resources Created in Rapid Brainstorming (Thirty Minutes)

1. (five minutes) Read/review "Not Your Homeland" article by Edwidge Danticat.[34]
2. (fifteen minutes) In small groups, using the dilemmas, goals, rules, and virtues listed in front of the room, practice asking and responding to the following scenario:
   Imagine you are consulting a trusted colleague or mentor on how best to care for Uncle Joseph. Take turns playing the person making the consult

call, the person receiving the call, the person communicating your recommendation to Edwidge Danticat, and the person communicating your recommendation to the officials at Krome Detention Center.

3. (five to ten minutes) Share insights and concerns in the whole group.

Part Three: Questions for Further Discussion (Ten Minutes)

- How do you put the goals, rules, and virtues you value into practice in specific moral dilemmas?
- What practices of moral discernment do you need to hone and use most in your work?
- What would change if moral imagination was awakened in a new way for you?
- How would you know that moral imagination was awakened in a new way in someone else?
- What other questions arise for you in this exercise?

Notes

The author is grateful for the support of M. Y. Perkins, J. DaMetz, T. Sharp, Y. J. Song, and the volume editors O. Banner, T. Cole, and N. Carlin.

1. While novels are not a new pedagogical tool in practical and pastoral theology classrooms and even research (as multiple works by Donald Capps, Nathan Carlin, Carrie Doehring, Chanequa Walker-Barnes, and many more attest), I have drawn on this pedagogical insight and found novels particularly helpful in highlighting intersections of practical theology and ethics.

2. I use the phrase *health humanities* in this chapter because of the biomedical ethics context in which I was trained as a clinical ethics consultant (with appreciation and course credit for health humanities) and because of the theological ethics element of my current teaching profession.

3. José Saramago, *Blindness*, trans. Giovanni Pontiero (London: Harvill, 1997); Edwidge Danticat, *Brother, I'm Dying* (New York: Vintage, 2008).

4. While human flourishing has long been a goal of practical theologies, emphasis on well-being denotes the structural, social, and political elements of sickness and health that accompany individual embodied persons. See Emilie M. Townes, "Ethics as an Art of Doing the Work Our Souls Must Have," in *Womanist Theological Ethics*, ed. Katie Geneva Cannon, Emilie M. Townes, and Angela D. Sims (Louisville, KY: Westminster John Knox, 2011), 35–50.

5. Some examples of narrative theologies include Karen Scheib's *Pastoral Care: Telling the Stories of Our Lives* (Nashville, TN: Abingdon, 2016), Gregory Ellison's *Fearless Dialogues: A New Movement for Justice* (Louisville, KY: Westminster John Knox, 2017), Andrew Lester's *Hope in Pastoral Care and Counseling* (Louisville, KY: Westminster John Knox, 1995), Christie Neuger's *Counseling Women: A Narrative, Pastoral Approach* (Minneapolis, MN: Fortress Press, 2001), Edward Wimberly's *Recalling Our Own Stories* (San Francisco: Jossey-Bass, 1997), Herbert Anderson and Edward Foley's *Mighty Stories, Dangerous Rituals* (San Francisco: Jossey-Bass, 1998), and my own *Misunderstanding Stories: Toward a Postcolonial Pastoral Theology* (Eugene, OR: Pickwick, 2013).

6. Note that it is equally important to structure a way out of a class, but that exceeds the scope of this chapter.

7. This name refers to the red and white–striped uniforms the volunteers historically wore, resembling a candy-cane pattern.

8. See, for example, Tom Beauchamp and James Childress, *Principles of Biomedical Ethics*, 7th ed. (New York and Oxford: Oxford University Press, 2013).

9. See, for example, Margaret Farley, *Just Love: A Framework for Christian Sexual Ethics* (New York: Continuum, 2006).

10. See, for example, Richard M. Zaner, *Conversations on the Edge: Narratives of Ethics and Illness* (Washington, DC: Georgetown University Press, 2004), or the documentary film directed by Shane Bartlett, *A Life in Clinical Philosophy: A Conversation with Richard M. Zaner*, Oral History of Healthcare Ethics, vol. 1 (Los Angeles: Bring Chase Productions, 2016), www.ohhe.org.

11. Theological education attempts to identify embedded theologies at work through the life stories of all persons and work to acknowledge and create more deliberative theologies out of which intentional practices of religious leadership can be framed. See,

for example, Carrie Doehring, *The Practice of Pastoral Care: A Postmodern Approach* (Louisville, KY: Westminster John Knox, 2015), and Howard W. Stone and James O. Duke, *How to Think Theologically* (Minneapolis, MN: Fortress, 2013).

12. Empathy, particularly in contrast to the more paternalistic concept of sympathy, remains a significant concept in practical and pastoral theologies, even though it has come under scrutiny recently in a variety of fields. See my chapter "Misunderstanding Empathy" in *Misunderstanding Stories*.

13. See, for example, Chanequa Walker-Barnes, *Too Heavy a Yoke* (Eugene, OR: Cascade, 2014), in practical theology or Therese Jones, Delese Wear, and Lester D. Friedman, eds., *Health Humanities Reader* (New Brunswick, NJ: Rutgers University Press, 2014).

14. While this list is my own categorization that could be unpacked as a stand-alone research article, many introductory texts in Christian ethics could expound on it. One interesting approach is to invite students to learn classic voices through Miguel A. De La Torre and Stacey M. Floyd-Thomas, eds., *Beyond the Pale: Reading Ethics from the Margins* (Louisville, KY: Westminster John Knox, 2011), which provides a brief and generous introduction to twenty-four classic voices and then outlines foreseen and unforeseen implications on minoritized communities pushed to the margins.

15. In my immersion learning courses on the US–Mexican border and international immersion courses, I often draw on narratives such as Miriam Davidson's *Lives on the Line: Dispatches from the U.S.–Mexico Border* (Tucson: University of Arizona Press, 2000) or Margaret Regan's *Detained and Deported: Stories of Immigrant Families under Fire* (Boston: Beacon, 2016), which help awaken students to vulnerabilities of undocumented persons, while Nancy Mairs's *Carnal Acts* (Boston: Beacon, 1996) and Arthur Frank's *The Wounded Storyteller* (Chicago: University of Chicago Press, 1997) help students identify and reflect on their own expected and unexpected vulnerabilities that impinge on their ethics of practice.

16. See, for example, David Tracy's *The Analogical Imagination* (New York: Crossroad, 1981). An excellent review of practical theology can be found in Bonnie J. Miller-McLemore, ed., *The Wiley Blackwell Companion to Practical Theology* (Oxford: John Wiley and Sons, 2014). For a review of practical theology pedagogy, see Dorothy C. Bass and Craig Dykstra, eds., *For Life Abundant* (Grand Rapids, MI: Eerdmans, 2008).

17. See, for example, the first edited volume on practical theology that takes up the effects of postcolonialism on vitality of life and faith practices, Pui-lan Kwok and Stephen Burns, eds., *Postcolonial Practice of Ministry* (Lanham, MD: Rowman and Littlefield, 2016).

18. Saramago, *Blindness*, 5.

19. Donzelina Barraso, "José Saramago, The Art of Fiction No. 155," *Paris Review* 149 (1998), accessed January 6, 2015, http://www.theparisreview.org/interviews/1032/the-art-of-fiction-no-155-jose-saramago.

20. Danticat, *Brother, I'm Dying*, 26.

21. Ibid., 68.

22. Ibid., 218.

23. The US Department of State publishes a monthly visa bulletin outlining many factors related to immigration including date of visa application being processed in the current month (https://travel.state.gov/content/visas/en/law-and-policy/bulletin/).

24. See, for example, Borderlinks, http://www.borderlinks.org/.

25. Fernando Meirelles (director), *Blindness* (Los Angeles: Miramax, 2008).

26. Edwidge Danticat, "Not Your Homeland," *The Nation*, September 8, 2005, accessed October 30, 2012, https://www.thenation.com/article/not-your-homeland/.

27. Barraso, "José Saramago," 1998.

28. Renee H. Shea, "The Dangerous Job of Edwidge Danticat: An Interview," *Callaloo* 19, no. 2 (Spring 1996): 382–89.

29. William James, *Pragmatism* (Cambridge, MA: Harvard University Press, 1975, 1978), 46–47.

30. Here, the image that "we make the road by walking" is instructive and serves moral imagination. For one explication, see Brenda Bell, John Gaventa, and John Peters, eds., *We Make the Road by Walking: Conversations on Education and Social Change* (Philadelphia: Temple University Press, 1990).

31. Saramago, *Blindness*.

32. Danticat, *Brother, I'm Dying*.

33. Meirelles, *Blindness*.

34. Danticat, "Not Your Homeland."

Works Cited

Anderson, Herbert, and Edward Foley. *Mighty Stories, Dangerous Rituals.* San Francisco: Jossey-Bass, 1998.

Barraso, Donzelina. "José Saramago, The Art of Fiction No. 155." *Paris Review* 149 (1998). Accessed January 6, 2015. http://www.theparisreview.org/interviews/1032/the-art-of-fiction-no-155-jose-saramago.

Bartlett, Shane (director). *A Life in Clinical Philosophy: A Conversation with Richard M. Zaner*. Oral History of Healthcare Ethics, vol. 1. Los Angeles: Bring Chase Productions, 2016. www.ohhe.org.

Bass, Dorothy C., and Craig Dykstra, eds. *For Life Abundant*. Grand Rapids, MI: Eerdmans, 2008.

Beauchamp, Tom, and James Childress. *Principles of Biomedical Ethics*. 7th ed. New York and Oxford: Oxford University Press, 2013.

Bell, Brenda, John Gaventa, and John Peters, eds. *We Make the Roadby Walking: Conversations on Education and Social Change.* Philadelphia: Temple University Press, 1990.

Borderlinks. http://www.borderlinks.org/.

Danticat, Edwidge. *Brother, I'm Dying*. New York: Vintage, 2008.

Danticat, Edwidge. "Not Your Homeland." *The Nation*, September 8, 2005. https://www.thenation.com/article/not-your-homeland/.

Davidson, Miriam. *Lives on the Line: Dispatches from the U.S.–Mexico Border*. Tucson: University of Arizona Press, 2000.

De La Torre, Miguel A., and Stacey M. Floyd-Thomas, eds. *Beyond the Pale: Reading Ethics from the Margins*. Louisville, KY: Westminster John Knox, 2011.

Doehring, Carrie. *The Practice of Pastoral Care: A Postmodern Approach*. Louisville, KY: Westminster John Knox, 2015.

Ellison, Gregory. *Fearless Dialogues: A New Movement for Justice*. Louisville, KY: Westminster John Knox, 2017.

Farley, Margaret. *Just Love: A Framework for Christian Sexual Ethics.* New York: Continuum, 2006.

Frank, Arthur. *The Wounded Storyteller*. Chicago: University of Chicago Press, 1997.

James, William. *Pragmatism*. Cambridge, MA: Harvard University Press, 1975, 1978.

Jones, Therese, Delese Wear, and Lester D. Friedman, eds. *Health Humanities Reader.* New Brunswick, NJ: Rutgers University Press, 2014.

Kwok, Pui-lan, and Stephen Burns, eds. *Postcolonial Practice of Ministry*. Lanham, MD: Rowman and Littlefield, 2016.

Lester, Andrew. *Hope in Pastoral Care and Counseling*. Louisville, KY: Westminster John Knox, 1995.

Mairs, Nancy. *Carnal Acts*. Boston: Beacon, 1996.

Meirelles, Fernando (director). *Blindness*. Los Angeles: Miramax, 2008.

Miller-McLemore, Bonnie J., ed. *The Wiley Blackwell Companion to Practical Theology*. Oxford: John Wiley and Sons, 2014.

Neuger, Christie. *Counseling Women: A Narrative, Pastoral Approach*. Minneapolis, MN: Fortress Press, 2001.

Regan, Margaret. *Detained and Deported: Stories of Immigrant Families under Fire*. Boston: Beacon, 2016.

Saramago, José. *Blindness*. Translated by Giovanni Pontiero. London: Harvill, 1997.

Scheib, Karen D. *Pastoral Care: Telling the Stories of Our Lives*. Nashville, TN: Abingdon, 2016.

Sharp, Melinda McGarrah. *Misunderstanding Stories: Toward a Postcolonial Pastoral Theology*. Eugene, OR: Pickwick, 2013.

Shea, Renee H. "The Dangerous Job of Edwidge Danticat: An Interview." *Callaloo* 19, no. 2 (Spring 1996): 382–89.

Stone, Howard W., and James O. Duke. *How to Think Theologically*. Minneapolis, MN: Fortress, 2013.

Townes, Emilie M. "Ethics as an Art of Doing the Work Our Souls Must Have." In *Womanist Theological Ethics*, edited by Katie Geneva Cannon, Emilie M. Townes, and Angela D. Sims, 35–50. Louisville, KY: Westminster John Knox, 2011.

Tracy, David. *The Analogical Imagination*. New York: Crossroad, 1981.

US Department of State. "Visa Bulletin." n.d. https://travel.state.gov/content/visas/en/law-and-policy/bulletin/.

Walker-Barnes, Chanequa. *Too Heavy a Yoke*. Eugene, OR: Cascade, 2014.

Wimberly, Edward. *Recalling Our Own Stories*. San Francisco: Jossey-Bass, 1997.

Zaner, Richard M. *Conversations on the Edge: Narratives of Ethics and Illness*. Washington, DC: Georgetown University Press, 2004.

PART II

Politics of Pedagogy

6

Medical Education and the Challenge of Race

John Hoberman

Medical education has never engaged with the racial dimension of medicine by integrating racial topics into the required curricula at medical schools in the United States. This race-aversive approach to medical training has contributed to racial health disparities in two ways: first, by fostering ignorance about the history of medical racism and, second, by ignoring the medico-racial folklore that has subverted the process of formulating accurate diagnoses and effective treatments within many medical subdisciplines over many years. Racial health and treatment disparities, meaning inferior care for black patients, have been described across an entire range of medical specialties. The response of organized medicine to the hundreds of peer-reviewed reports that confirm these deficits has fallen far short of what medical ethics and social justice require. This essay offers what is intended as a practical manual of racially motivated diagnostic and therapeutic errors that can be avoided by informed physicians.

Mainstream medicine's public engagement with racially differential diagnosis and treatment dates from the 1980s. John Ayanian has noted that health-care disparities research has developed in three phases: (1) describing the range and magnitude of disparities, (2) identifying specific factors that may promote disparities, and (3) designing interventions that might reduce or eliminate them.[1] *Unequal Treatment: Confronting Racial and Ethnic Disparities in Health Care* (2003), published by the Institute of Medicine, is frequently cited as a pathbreaking document that put health disparities on the medical agenda. Less frequently cited are the shortcomings of this volume, including the systematic use of euphemistic jargon to deflect responsibility away from the individuals and medical institutions that are accountable for decades of substandard care.

Five years before the publication of *Unequal Treatment*, a prominent physician had been more candid about American medicine's treatment of black patients. Dr. Arnold Epstein, then chair of the Department of Health Policy at the Harvard School of Public Health, commented on the silence around medical racism. By this time the medical literature had clearly demonstrated that black patients were getting inferior medical care across many areas. "What is striking," Dr. Epstein said, "is that the findings are not subtle and that we as a country have done nothing about it."[2] Two decades (and hundreds of additional medical reports) later, race-aversive medical training and non-accountability for racially motivated medical harm are still the rule. "It appears that very few medical education programs currently collect the data necessary to understand and ameliorate racial disparities," the *AMA Journal of Ethics* commented in 2015.[3] In summary, medical students should be aware that the medical institutions that are training them continue to avoid the topic of medical racism at the expense of black patients.

Let us first address the knowledge deficit about racial factors in medicine. Modern doctors know little, if anything, about the racial attitudes and behaviors of their twentieth-century predecessors. Without this knowledge doctors will be literally unable to imagine their own capacity for racially motivated thinking and responses to patients of color. A medical profession that remains unaware of the racist legacy of American medicine cannot hope to improve race relations within the medical culture. Navigating cross-racial relationships inside or outside of the medical world requires a capacity for introspection as well as an awareness of the profession's slow development during the twentieth century toward a racially integrated medicine that remains woefully incomplete to this day.

Race relations in medicine require physicians to think about the emotional dynamics of their relationships with patients. This is a demanding exercise for which most doctors have not been prepared. Cross-racial relationships between doctors and patients add an extra dimension of emotional complexity. Self-scrutiny of this kind requires a self-analytical procedure that enables the practitioner to examine his or her feelings about traditionally defined racial differences and how to deal with these feelings in the context of a therapeutic relationship. This requires in turn some historical knowledge as well as an awareness of these problematic feelings and an acknowledgment of their significance for the practice of humane medicine. In the same manner as their fellow citizens, doctors have absorbed and are influenced by the racial folklore generated during the eras of plantation slavery, post-Reconstruction Jim Crow racism, the civil rights revolution, and the current backlash against "politically correct" standards of racial etiquette.

A review of the medical literature indicates that the great majority of doctors are not seriously concerned about the racial dimension of medicine. In cardiology alone, multiple reports since 2005 have documented cardiologists' lack of awareness of or attention to health disparities.[4]

How can medical students prepare for interracial encounters with patients? Medical students will often be unsure of how to relate to and care for patients they have learned to think about as racially different from themselves. How can medical students prepare for these relationships? A useful first step is to see these encounters in their historical context.

As the prominent African American cardiologist Clyde Yancy observed in 2009, "The general awkwardness surrounding racial issues in our society bleeds into medicine."[5] Medical students and doctors must acknowledge the discomfort that persists as a consequence of our racial traumas and learn something about their historical and sociological origins. "We have an aversion to emotional turmoil as medical students that persists in the physician," a medical author wrote in 1988.[6] Understanding the origins of these turbulent emotions, whether or not they express racial discomfort, is the most practical way to deal with their potentially distorting effects on doctor–patient relationships.

Black physicians, too, have sometimes commented on white doctor–black patient scenarios that have been deeply distorted by the lingering effects of racial segregation.[7] They have often pointed to the emotional awkwardness and discomfort that can affect both participants in these relationships. The black psychiatrist Walter A. Adams wrote in 1950 that "a white therapist may feel insecure with his Negro patient [because of] the patient's physical appearance, the therapist's unfamiliarity with Negro culture and problems, and even doubt concerning his patient's ability to pay. In his effort to conceal his insecurity and his guilt feelings, the therapist unwittingly may be oversympathetic and indulgent; he may be patronizing or hostile."[8] David Satcher, a future surgeon general of the United States (1998–2002), wrote in 1973 that "Black patients are almost always called by their first names and they are frequently exploited for teaching sessions."[9] Few in number and politically powerless, black doctors have had little influence on race relations in medicine over the past century. Medical students should be aware of this long-standing imbalance of power and think about its impacts on the medical experiences of black patients. At the same time, medical students must learn to recognize the heterogeneity of the "black patient" population along with the stressful circumstances they have in common.

It goes without saying that black patients differ among themselves as much as any other group of people. What they share is a certain kind of collective experience, a predicament that originates in the racial mores of American society and the polluted reservoir of racial folklore about their anatomical, physiological, and psychological traits that has saturated the American racial imagination.

Optimally effective treatment of many black patients requires an understanding of how their imposed racial predicament and its emotional impacts can affect their feelings and behaviors as patients. For example, the decisions black patients make about whether to undergo specific treatments are commonly referred to as "patient preferences." This term asserts the ideal of patient autonomy that has become a standard part of modern medicine. The problem is that for many years medical authors have used this term in a color-blind manner, based on the assumption that there is no difference between how white and black patients make medical decisions. But the distinctive sociohistorical conditions experienced by African Americans over many generations have made it highly unlikely that black and white patients always perceive the risks and benefits of medical procedures in the same ways since many black patients must deal with the "fear, suspicion, and distrust" that have long undermined confidence in a medical establishment that has always been and is still controlled by white medical personnel. This is important because many physicians have assumed that the treatment "preferences" of black patients help to account for racial disparities in the rates of medical procedures performed on black and white patients, including life-saving techniques such as heart surgeries and organ transplantation. For example, in the case of renal transplantation, one study showed that "two-thirds of the physicians view patient preferences and the availability of living donors as the most important reasons why racial disparities arose in care, and only one in eight physicians reported physician bias as an important factor."[10] In other words, "patient preferences" have been routinely treated as simply one more variable that is comparable to health status, insurance coverage, and other socioeconomic factors that affect how patients weigh their treatment options.

Medical students and doctors should recognize that a patient's preference for one medical solution over another is a subjective rather than an objective variable and that these choices should be interpreted within their historical context.[11] Medical students and physicians must also learn to appreciate the "racial" significance of their own clinical behaviors, of which they may be unaware. The significance of these scenarios is rooted in how the stigmatizing of black people has affected their reactions to being examined by medical personnel. Some patients, for example, want reassurance that doctors and nurses are open to making physical contact with them. It is understandable that some patients would want their caregivers to demonstrate a willingness to touch black skin. (A survey of white racial attitudes toward blacks carried out in 1963 found "that the greater the suggestion of physical contact, the greater the white antipathy—and even revulsion."[12]) This sensitivity about being touched may even apply to the use of the hygienic latex gloves used during physical examinations. "I learned not to glove for black and brown patients a long time ago," a nurse once told me. This extends to doctors' body language and speech habits during clinical examinations, which are also subject to patients' interpretations of how doctors feel about them.

Physician-dominated dialogue or "verbal dominance" appears to be a major obstacle to better relationships between doctors and patients. This verbal imbalance of power may have an even greater effect on the racial scenarios that occur in clinical settings.[13] Medical students' awareness of this "greater clinician domination of the medical dialogue"[14] can prepare them to plan and monitor their own verbal interactions with patients for the purpose of learning as much as possible about how their patients think and feel about their medical treatment.

The result of a physician's "verbal dominance" is likely to be an intimidated and perhaps resentful patient. In fact, passive attitudes on the part of patients are more likely in "racially discordant" doctor–patient relationships in which the patient is black. We know this because the past century's "racially discordant" medical relationships have, until relatively recently, promoted passivity and powerlessness among black patients. Even today, in the eyes of some doctors, the incompetent "Negro patient" of a hundred years ago has his modern counterparts. The greater distrust of doctors by black patients that is widely acknowledged will also promote emotional disengagement from the therapeutic relationship as well as noncompliance with doctors' recommendations. Medical students should know where to look for passive attitudes in patients that can impede therapeutic progress or prevent therapy altogether. As we have seen, the social marginalization of black people can make them unwilling to seek out medical treatment.

The fundamental medical consequence of centuries of sociohistorical trauma is the psychobiological phenomenon known as *stress*. Racist practices from plantation slavery to Jim Crow segregation and the psychosocial racial stressors that continue today have created a pathogenic social universe that has exposed black people to an undetermined number of stressors that can cause premature illness and death. In a 1970 article titled "The Daily Irritations," *Time* magazine pointed to the "seemingly minor irritations that crop up innumerable times during the ordinary business of getting through the day" that are among the unavoidable results of racial inequality.[15] Half a century later we have learned to regard these experiences—now called "micro-aggressions"—as serious threats to the physical and emotional health of African Americans. The relationship between the experience of racism and post-traumatic stress disorder has been called "race-based traumatic stress injury," a diagnosis that proposes "race-based stress reactions can be triggered by events that are experienced vicariously, or externally, through a third party—like social media or national news events." African Americans can be emotionally "worn down by the barrage of reports about black deaths and police brutality."[16] There is scientific evidence that the emotional impacts of neighborhood crime can produce depressive symptoms epigenetically via DNA methylation of a region of a specific gene.[17] Other scientific evidence suggests that "simply perceiving or anticipating discrimination contributes to chronic stress that can cause an increase in blood-pressure problems, coronary-artery disease, cognitive impairment, and infant mortality. Black Americans do not have to directly experience police brutality to experience the negative health ramifications of its possibility."[18]

The "weathering" hypothesis proposed by the medical sociologist Arline T. Geronimus posits that blacks in the United States experience "early health deterioration as a consequence of the impact of repeated experience with social or economic adversity and political marginalization." The weathering process represents the physiological burden imposed by stress that can be measured by two categories of biomarkers. The first consists of "primary mediators, the substances the body releases in response to stress," including norepinephrine, epinephrine, cortisol, and dehydroepiandrosterone sulfate. The second category comprises "the effects that result from the actions of the primary mediators," which include cortisol levels and blood pressure.[19]

The concept of a racially selective "weathering" process accommodates other findings about disproportionate stress loads borne by African Americans. Research on race and cumulative disadvantage incurred over the course of a lifetime includes the impact of "the trauma of premature deaths of blacks in the United States" since "losing a child, spouse, or parent is the most stressful life event people experience and one that affects them for years." Premature death exposures occur much more frequently in black families compared to white families and are likely to produce adverse health effects.[20] Emotional stressors experienced by many black students at American colleges and universities can adversely impact these young people's mental health.[21] Adolescents' loss of trust in important social institutions such as schools, governments, medical institutions, and the police can become a long-term emotional liability.[22] These major (and often unrecognized) disadvantages can create cascading psychosomatic effects that impair both mental and physical health.

Medical students need to recognize the existence and potential medical effects of this pathogenic social universe. The sheer complexity of its dimensions and effects has produced a terminology that confirms how few of its psychobiological mechanisms are understood. For example, a 1997 paper on the presumed relationship between stress and hypertension resorts to vague formulations such as, "It is thought that multiple pathophysiological mechanisms are involved in a complex interaction among factors that are both extrinsic and intrinsic to physiological functioning." Or "[e]xpression of emotion and physiological reactivity to psychosocial stressors may be moderated socioculturally." In this case, the almost total absence of conceptual precision signifies the urgency rather than the futility of this research. "Modifying oppressive environmental stressors and adverse living conditions in African-American communities will take time and may be difficult."[23] This observation is, if anything, an understatement; and medical students should understand that virtually all black patients inhabit this pathogenic social universe to one degree or another. Now that these crucial environmental dimensions have been recognized, medical students must learn to think in an expansive and imaginative way about the social and psychological factors that shape the experiences of the patients they will meet.

The first section of this essay has focused on the personal dimension of medical race relations—how doctors and patients endowed with racial identities interact within the racial force field that surrounds us all. These relationships are shaped by how doctors and patients think and feel about themselves and each other. Their racio-medical identities are formed by what they expect of each other, what they may fear or resent in each other, how they speak (or do not speak) to each other, what they think they know and what they cannot know, and how they make or avoid making fateful medical decisions. All of this amounts to the racial dimension of medicine that consists of our social and emotional selves.

The second part of this chapter examines the racial dimension of medicine that plays out in thinking about human biology and human biological variation that is of potential medical significance.

Human Biological Variation

Doctors make decisions about racially differential diagnoses and treatments based on biomedical evidence that either has been validated, remains speculative, or has been discredited in the medical literature. The medical judgments based on this evidence will often make the difference between those patients who will regain their health and those who will never recover from their medical problems. These judgments are relevant to the problem of racial health disparities because of the racially differential diagnoses and treatments that have done enormous harm to countless black patients and cost many of them their lives. Racially differential diagnoses and treatments can be medically appropriate or inappropriate, depending on the quality of the evidence that has informed them. At the same time, racially differential medical judgments have always been inherently problematic because so many of them have been rooted in an ideological compulsion to dichotomize between black and white human beings. This racial ideology has been an integral part of the Western cultural tradition since the eighteenth century.

The racial biology that persists within modern medicine originates in a Western racial doctrine formulated by European thinkers during the second half of the eighteenth century. During the Enlightenment a scientific theory of race gradually prevailed over the biblical doctrine of human unity and established a hierarchical ranking of the "races" that remains influential to this day. The scientific racism of the nineteenth century produced a racial hierarchy that at times went so far as to define white and black human beings as belonging to different species. The profound influence of this racially dichotomous interpretation of the human organism is evident in twentieth-century medicine and beyond.

Modern medicine is as permeated by the racial folklore we all absorb as any other social sector. As two medical authors commented in 2014,

> The similarity in the prevalence of implicit bias between physicians and the general population is congruent with other studies that have found that physicians hold stereotypes and biases, often unconsciously, based on race, gender and other characteristics. This is not surprising, because like the general population, physicians are human, and are subject to the same socializing influences, such as constant negative portrayals of members of racial/ethnic minorities by popular and social media.[24]

Over many decades, as we shall see, medical thinking has absorbed many societal ideas about racial difference. Medical specialists in various fields have long converted this folkloric material into medico-racial folklore that has distorted many diagnoses and treatments of black patients. Over the past century racially motivated interpretations of human anatomy, physiology, and psychology have infiltrated a range of medical specialties. This essay is intended to serve as a "practical manual" that enables medical practitioners to recognize and correct for these distortions.

Medico-racial folklore produces the racially differential diagnoses and treatments that can do harm to patients whose symptoms and disorders may have been misinterpreted by medical personnel who are not prepared to correct for the distortions that can result from inaccurate ideas about racially differentiated minds and bodies.

The compulsion to employ a racially bifurcating typology that defines blacks and whites as different or even opposite human types has permeated Western thinking and its medical culture. Medical thinking has formulated these binary racial distinctions in several ways. On the level of different categories of human experience, it has produced racially differential interpretations of black infants and children, the black elderly, black athleticism, black musical aptitude, and the black capacity to lose consciousness.[25] On the level of human organ systems, it has imposed racial differentiation on the cardiovascular apparatus, female reproductive organs, the nervous system, lung volumes, blood chemistry, skin thickness, bone density, dental caries, eye diseases, pain sensitivity, and the mental phenomena analyzed and treated by psychiatry.[26] On the level of medical disorders, racially differential theories of disease susceptibilities and immunities were common during the first half of the twentieth century and gradually declined as medical science advanced.[27]

The gradual elimination from the medical literature of fallacious ideas about racial vulnerability or resistance to disease represents a type of scientific progress that confirms the waning influence of pseudoscientific ideas in medicine. It would be mistaken, however, to conclude that medical thinking about racial variation has simply left nineteenth-century racial biology behind.

A much-noted 2016 paper points out that "many white medical students and residents hold beliefs about biological differences between blacks and whites, many of which are false and fantastical in nature."[28]

Racially differential interpretations of human organs and disorders have often ascribed an imagined "hardiness" to the black organism. These erroneous medical judgments have deprived an untold number of patients of proper diagnosis and treatment. Medical students should be aware of the history of false ascriptions of various forms of "hardiness" to black people.[29] These falsely ascribed traits include a purported immunity or special resiliency to disease, injury, or pain. These claims about black biological resiliency provided white doctors with an alibi for neglecting the medical needs and emergencies of an impoverished black population. While the possibility of their continuing influence on the thinking of some physicians is real, this influence tends to be difficult to verify because medical journals will no longer publish speculation based on racial folklore.

Medico-racial folklore about the "hardiness" of the black organism has shaped medical thinking about various human organ and organ systems. The idea that blacks enjoy a partial immunity to heart attacks has had a long career and is contradicted by the fact that they are more vulnerable to heart disease than whites are. "The myth of blacks' 'immunity' to CHD [coronary heart disease], which continues to appear in recent literature, is at best a half-truth and at worst an obstruction to understanding of CHD," a black cardiologist wrote in 1982.[30] The acknowledged influence of hearsay evidence in medicine suggests that this belief in black cardiac immunity has persisted to one degree or another in the minds of some doctors, despite ample evidence to the contrary. The same phenomenon can be observed in the field of psychiatry. Racially differential thinking has flourished within psychiatry, due to the fact that this medical specialty interprets the patient in a uniquely holistic way. No other medical discipline diagnoses a patient's entire sentient and experiencing self. The idea that black people enjoy a relative immunity to clinical depression had a long career during the twentieth century and is likely to persist today in some quarters.[31]

Medical school training in the United States does not address the racial dimension of medicine beyond the widespread "cultural competency" courses most observers have found unsatisfactory. Indeed, after years of doing research in the area of race and medicine, I have never encountered a discussion of what might qualify a "cultural competency" teacher to offer this sort of instruction. Good instruction on race and medicine topics requires a thorough knowledge of medical history and the social dynamics of race in the United States. It is above all a practical curriculum that aims at preventing avoidable diagnostic and therapeutic errors.

In 1996 the prominent physician H. Jack Geiger published a medical liberal's anguished cri de coeur on the alarming racial disparities in medical treatments that could no longer be ignored. How could this be happening? Yet even this conscientious physician could not bring himself to believe that "racially discriminatory rationing by physicians and health care institutions" was occurring in American medicine. What he did say was that "awareness of the dilemmas associated with race and health care should be a part of every physician's training."[32] A generation later the absence of this sort training in American medical schools is one more sign of how thoroughly liberal social policy has failed our black fellow citizens over the past half-century.

Teaching the Racial Dimension of Medicine

During the spring 2017 semester I taught an elective course on race and medicine at the new University of Texas-Dell Medical School in Austin. The class consisted of three first-year medical students, including one of the two African American students in the inaugural class of fifty M1s. The format was a seminar-style combination of lecture and discussion. For each of the ten class topics, including the introduction to the course, I presented a PowerPoint of between ten and twenty slides to reinforce my presentations bearing on the history of medical racism in the United States, along with current issues and problems that often represent modern forms of older, and usually discredited, ideas about racial differences. Two associate deans/physicians periodically attended the class to listen and contribute to our conversations about the assigned topics. It was reassuring to have M.D.s in the room to explain medical matters I could not.

This elective was based on an undergraduate course titled "Race and Medicine in American Life" I have given nine times since 2001 for three different programs within the University of Texas's College of Liberal Arts. Many of these students have gone off to medical school.

My presentation of the racial dimension of medicine is grounded in the history of Western racial doctrine that was formulated in Europe during the second half of the eighteenth century. This doctrine continues to shape our understanding of race in profound ways. The traditional racial hierarchy that places whites at the top and blacks at the bottom remains largely intact and is hugely influential, as is the idea that white and black people represent opposite racial types. As the racial hierarchy doctrine evolved over time, it created a reservoir of racial folklore that has proven to be very tenacious. Medical personnel absorb this racial folklore in the same manner as their non-medical fellow citizens. The result of this process is the medico-racial folklore that has infiltrated its way into every medical subspecialty. This medico-racial folklore produces in turn the racially differential diagnoses and treatments than can cause medical harm.

The topic with which we began the course is "racial health disparities." This is a foundational concept for race and medicine studies because it is both a medical reality and a misleading euphemism. Research on "racial health disparities" has been a cottage industry since the 1980s. The problematic aspect of this term is that it presents these disparities as an enormously complex phenomenon in which human motivations and behaviors play no understandable role. Physicians are neither accountable nor responsible for their unintentional contributions to racial health disparities. This course points out the unwillingness of medical educators to acknowledge and inform medical students about physician misbehaviors that include racially motivated diagnoses and treatments.

The second topic—the racial dynamics of the doctor–patient relationship—and the third topic—racially motivated physician behaviors—take up where unsatisfactory treatments of "racial health disparities" that omit physician accountability leave off. These course segments make two major points about race relations in medicine. First, dysfunctional cross-racial doctor–patient relationships have already been presented and analyzed in the medical literature; most doctors have either missed or ignored these publications. Second, African American physicians have been publishing analyses of interracial doctor–patient relationships for most of a hundred years. The evidence suggests that white doctors have ignored this potentially valuable advice, along with the African American–edited *Journal of the National Medical Association*, which has appeared since 1917, has an impact factor of 1.067, and is seldom cited in other medical journals. Forfeiting such opportunities to learn from African American colleagues is a persisting form of racial segregation in American medicine.

The fourth section of the course examines three stereotypes of "black" disease that have figured prominently in American media. All of these medical topics have had sensationalistic public careers that have been exploited for political purposes by white interest groups bent on stigmatizing or saving black people by associating them with disease. Sickle cell anemia has inspired schemes to subject all African Americans to testing despite the irrationality of these plans. The severe impact of HIV/AIDS on the black population of New York provoked a standoff between the African American community and white public health authorities unaware of the distrust they had created in the past. Hysteria over the black "crack babies" of the late 1980s and early 1990s was a medicalized way for whites to express their fears of black men. These babies had been exposed to crack cocaine in their mothers' wombs. Many whites, including media-savvy conservatives like William Bennett and Charles Krauthammer, claimed these black male babies would turn into conscienceless "super-predators" who would terrify "decent" society. In fact, the period that followed the "crack babies" scare saw a sharp drop in youth crime.

The fifth course topic is "The Racial History of Heart Disease." Medical students should be aware that all of the major medical subdisciplines have been infiltrated by medico-racial folklore that can remain influential even in the twenty-first century. Heart disease is an especially rich topic in this regard. Ideas about racially differential heart problems once flourished, including a reputed black immunity to heart attacks and anginal pain. Racial differentiation included a differential racial psychology in the form of an assumption that heart disease afflicted "civilized" whites rather than "primitive" blacks. Black medical authors struggled to convince their medical audience that blacks were capable of being achievement-oriented Type A personalities who were vulnerable to heart disease. Historical instruction of this kind enables today's medical students to understand that modern doctors, too, are capable of absorbing medico-racial folklore that can lead to misdiagnoses of black patients.

The sixth topic is "Racially Differential Pain Management." Medical publications on the undermedicating of black patients with analgesics have been appearing since the early 1990s. In 2016 the *Proceedings of the National Academy of Sciences USA* published a report on this practice that finally received widespread media coverage. It should be noted that inferior pain treatment in hospitals includes black children as well as adults. Confronting this sort of medical misbehavior ought to provoke medical students to ask how it can be that a quarter-century of medical publications appear to have changed nothing. How is it possible for organized medicine to be so disorganized or, perhaps, unmotivated to abolish malpractice of this kind?

The racial politics of renal transplantation, our seventh topic, presents an especially complex and interesting medical predicament with a racial dimension, in that it combines an uncontroversial biological factor—human leukocyte antigen matching—with both socioeconomic issues and judgments underlying patient selection made by physicians whose decisions can be influenced by their assumptions about black patient behavior. Perhaps more than any other race–medical conundrums, these scenarios offer medical students an opportunity to see how the medical profession can work at and, after years of effort, achieve optimal outcomes for many black patients.

The eighth section of the course addresses the notorious Tuskegee syphilis experiment (1932–1972), during which US Public Health Service doctors abused the medical rights of several hundred black Alabama sharecroppers. Commonly referred to as simply "Tuskegee," this medical scandal has become the universally recognized symbol of American medical racism. Medical students should understand both the ethical failures and the medical consequences of the Tuskegee revelations. First, the sensational exposure of this officially sponsored medical misbehavior has effectively concealed from both lay and medical audiences the many forms of medical racism that occur daily within our medical culture. Second, the Tuskegee scandal alarmed many prospective black patients and thereby further increased the level of doctor avoidance among African Americans. The volume of medical harm caused by "Tuskegee" is, therefore, literally incalculable.

The final section of the course examines how racial stereotypes have functioned within American psychiatry over the past century. The fundamental tenet of Western racism—that black people are less complex than whites—remains influential in psychiatric diagnosis and treatment to this day. Here, as in the racial history of heart disease, is where medical students can learn to appreciate the sheer persistence of medico-racial folklore in a modern medical culture. The ideas that black people are resistant to depression and that they do not require long-term psychotherapy are diagnostic misconceptions that have not disappeared from the profession. In fact, psychiatry is most vulnerable to racial-folkloric illusions precisely because psychiatrists strive for holistic diagnoses of human lives in a way that other medical specialists generally do not. The most familiar racist ideas about blacks focus on psychological phenomena such as personality and intelligence. That is why they are more likely than other physicians to slide down the slippery slope of stereotyping into traditional stigmatizing judgments about their black patients.

Notes

1. John Ayanian, "Determinants of Racial and Ethnic Disparities in Surgical Care," *World Journal of Surgery* 32, no. 4 (2008): 509–15.

2. Quoted in Ford Fessenden, "Blacks Passed By," *Newsday*, November 29, 1998, A55.

3. Brian B. Drwecki, "Education to Identify and Combat Racial Bias in Pain Treatment," *AMA Journal of Ethics* 17, no. 3 (2015): 221–28.

4. A 2008 commentary notes, "Many physicians currently in practice have limited awareness of the legacy of segregation and discrimination in health care—dating from the era of slavery—that affects the perspective of African-American patients seeking care" (Ayanian, "Determinants"). According to a 2005 report, "Cardiologists' level of awareness of racial/ethnic disparities in care remains low. Fewer than one third of cardiologists perceived that racial/ethnic disparities exist in the US health-care system, and even fewer believed that these disparities exist in their own practice settings. The general lack of awareness is a bit surprising given the extent of government agencies' and professional associations' efforts to make physicians aware of this issue" (Nicole Lurie et al., "Racial and Ethnic Disparities in Care: The Perspectives of Cardiologists," *Circulation* 111, no. 10 [2005]: 1267). Surveys of cardiologists and cardiac surgeons had demonstrated by 2008 that "most doctors do not perceive disparities in their own care or that of their clinical colleagues or hospital, despite many studies documenting these disparities over the past two decades" (Ayanian, "Determinants"). A 2014 report concludes, "Given that nearly 200 publications between 1983 and 2003 documented racial and ethnic disparities in the treatment of myocardial infarction, the lack of awareness among fully trained heart specialists and trainees documented in these reports is staggering" (Quinn Capers IV and Zarina Sharalaya, "Racial Disparities in Cardiovascular Care: A Review of Culprits and Potential Solutions," *Journal of Racial and Ethnic Health Disparities* 1, no. 3 [2014]: 171). The 2005 paper also reports a fatalistic attitude among cardiologists toward ever repairing these

inequities since "fewer than 30% of cardiologists felt that increasing provider awareness about disparities or improving the cultural competence of either the provider or the institution would likely be useful in addressing disparities" (Lurie et al., "Racial," 1267).

5. Emily Singer, "Beyond Race-Based Medicine," *MIT Technology Review*, January 16, 2009.

6. Bruce B. Dan and Roxanne K. Young, eds., *A Piece of My Mind: A Collection of Essays from* The Journal of the American Medical Association (Los Angeles: Feeling Fine Programs; Toronto: Random House of Canada, 1988), 62.

7. See, for example, Walter A. Adams, "The Negro Patient in Psychiatric Treatment," *American Journal of Orthopsychiatry* 20 (1950): 309–10; Chester M. Pierce, "Is Bigotry the Basis of the Medical Problems of the Ghetto?" in *Medicine in the Ghetto*, ed. John C. Norman (New York: Appleton-Century-Crofts, 1969): 301–14; David Satcher, "Does Race Interfere with the Doctor–Patient Relationship?" *JAMA* 223, no. 13 (1973): 1498–99.

8. Adams, "The Negro Patient," 308.

9. Satcher, "Does Race Interfere?" 1499.

10. Ayanian, "Determinants."

11. In the case of total knee replacement, for example, blacks with advanced knee arthritis are less inclined to undergo total knee replacement. However, as one medical author noted in 2016, "We should be cautious not to accept these preferences at face value, as they may represent generations of internalized repression and truncated horizons of opportunity" (Jeffrey N. Katz, "Persistence of Racial and Ethnic Differences in Utilization and Adverse Outcomes of Total Joint Replacement," *Journal of Bone and Joint Surgery* 98 [2016]: 1241). As other medical authors put it in 2005, "[T]reatment preferences are formed by experiences with the health care system and the information provided to the patient about the treatment under consideration" (Jennifer J. Griggs and Jerome Engel, "Epilepsy Surgery and the Racial Divide," *Neurology* 64, no. 1 [2005]: 8). The "patient preferences" explanation of black decision-making also exempts doctors from responsibility for their conduct vis-à-vis their patients' medical decisions. One study showed that "physicians markedly overestimated the role of patient preference," thereby minimizing the influence of their own behaviors (ibid.). In this sense, "patient preferences" is one of the euphemisms that have become a familiar category of medical jargon (see John Hoberman, "Medical Racism and the Rhetoric of Exculpation: How Do Physicians Think about Race?" *New Literary History* 38, no. 3 [2007]: 505–25). The alienation of white doctors from black patients is a problem of "patient–physician race concordance." Black patients may experience "less patient-centered" visits than white patients and hear a "less positive affective tone" when doctors address them (John Hoberman, *Black & Blue: The Origins and Consequences of Medical Racism* [Berkeley: University of California Press, 2012], 51). The function of this euphemistic jargon is to insulate white physicians from certain kinds of discomfiting information about their black patients as well as their own limited understanding of what black people are thinking about their white doctors.

12. "How Whites Feel about Negroes: A Painful American Dilemma," *Newsweek*, October 21, 1963, 44–50.

13. A 2004 report thus finds that "[p]hysicians were 23% more verbally dominant and engaged in 33% less patient-centered communication with African American patients than with White patients" (Rachel L. Johnson et al., "Patient Race/Ethnicity and Quality of Patient–Physician Communication during Medical Visits," *American Journal of Public*

Health 94, no. 12 [2004]: 2084). In a similar vein, from a 2011 report, "Providers were more verbally dominant in conversations with black as compared to white patients. This was largely due to black patients' talking less than white patients" (Mary Catherine Beach et al., "Patient–Provider Communication Differs for Black Compared to White HIV-Infected Patients," *AIDS Behavior* 15, no. 4 [2011]: 805).

14. Medical News Today, "Unconscious Racial Bias among Doctors Linked to Poor Communication with Patients, Dissatisfaction with Care," March 16, 2012, https://www.medicalnewstoday.com/releases/242975.php.

15. "The Daily Irritations," *Time*, April 6, 1970, 77–78.

16. Jenna Wortham, "Racism's Psychological Toll," *New York Times*, June 24, 2015.

17. Man-Kit Lei et al., "Neighborhood Crime and Depressive Symptoms among African American Women: Genetic Moderation and Epigenetic Mediation of Effects," *Social Science & Medicine* 146 (2015): 120. "Social scientists have long recognized the important role that neighborhood crime can play in stress-related disease, but very little is known about potential biosocial mechanisms that may link the experience of living in high-crime neighborhoods with depression. The current study introduces an integrated model that combines neighborhood, genetic, and epigenetic factors. Hypotheses were tested with a sample of 99 African American women from the Family and Community Health Study (FACHS). Allele variants of the serotonin transporter gene (5-HTT) interact with neighborhood crime to predict depressive symptoms in a manner consonant with the differential susceptibility perspective. Furthermore, this association is mediated by DNA methylation of the promoter region of the serotonin transporter gene. The findings provide support for an integrated model in which changes in DNA methylation, resulting from neighborhood crime, can result in an increase or decrease in gene activity which, in turn, influences depressive symptoms."

18. Clint Smith, "Racism, Stress, and Black Death," *New Yorker*, July 16, 2016. See also Emma K. Adam et al., "Developmental Histories of Perceived Racial Discrimination and Diurnal Cortisol Profiles in Adulthood: A 20-Year Prospective Study," *Psychoneuroendocrinology* 62 (2015): 279–91.

19. Arline T. Geronimus et al., "'Weathering' and Age Patterns of Allostatic Load Scores among Blacks and Whites in the United States," *American Journal of Public Health* 96, no. 5 (2006): 826–33. See also Sandeep Jauhar, "When Blood Pressure Is Political," *New York Times*, August 6, 2016.

20. Debra Umberson et al., "Death of Family Members as an Overlooked Source of Racial Disadvantage in the United States," *Proceedings of the National Academy of Sciences USA* 114, no. 5 (2017): 915–20.

21. Adrienne Green, "The Cost of Balancing Academia and Racism," *Atlantic*, January 21, 2016.

22. David S. Yeager et al., "Loss of Institutional Trust among Racial and Ethnic Minority Adolescents: A Consequence of Procedural Injustice and a Cause of Life-Span Outcomes," *Child Development* 88, no. 2 (2017): 658–76.

23. Vernon Barnes et al., "Stress, Stress Reduction, and Hypertension in African Americans: An Updated Review," *Journal of the National Medical Association* 89, no. 7 (1997): 465, 466, 468.

24. Joseph Ravenell and Gbenga Ogedegbe, "Unconscious Bias and Real-World Hypertension Outcomes: Advancing Disparities Research," *Journal of General Internal Medicine* 29, no. 7 (2014): 974.

25. See Hoberman, *Black & Blue*, 71–91.

26. Ibid., 92–120.

27. In 1915, for example, the *Southern Medical Journal* reported the frequent "opinion" that "the negro is developing a racial immunity to the [syphilis] infection and that he suffers little from its effects" (Kenneth M. Lynch, Kater McInnes, and G. Fleming McInnes, "Concerning Syphilis in the American Negro," *Southern Medical Journal* 8 [June 1, 1915]: 453). A black "racial immunity" to scarlet fever proposed in 1932 (Harry Bakwin, "The Negro Infant," *Human Biology* 4, no. 1 [1932]: 24) was debunked by the prominent black physician Paul Cornely in 1939 (Paul Cornely, "Morbidity and Mortality from Scarlet Fever in the Negro," *American Journal of Public Health* 29 [September 1939]: 999–1005). In 1953 the *British Medical Journal* announced that "[n]o example of racial immunity to an infectious disease is known in man" ("Disease, Race, and Civilization," *British Medical Journal* 1, no. 4823 [June 13, 1953]: 1320). Medical personnel should be aware that these and other versions of racial biology have had long careers in medicine, and that the assessment of racially differential ideas about human health and disease is an ongoing process.

28. Kelly M. Hoffman, "Racial Bias in Pain Assessment and Treatment Recommendations, and False Beliefs about Biological Differences between Blacks and Whites," *Proceedings of the National Academy of Sciences USA* 113 (2016): 4296–301.

29. See Hoberman, *Black & Blue,* 120–30.

30. Richard F. Gillum, "Coronary Heart Disease in Black Populations. I. Mortality and Morbidity," *American Heart Journal* 104, no. 4 (October 1982): 849.

31. See, for example, Hoberman, *Black & Blue,* 125–30.

32. H. Jack Geiger, "Race and Health Care—An American Dilemma?" *New England Journal of Medicine* 335 (1996): 816.

Works Cited

Adam, Emma K., Jennifer A. Heissel, Katharine H. Zeiders, Jennifer A. Richeson, Emily C. Ross, Katherine B. Ehrlich, Dorainne J. Levy, et al. "Developmental Histories of Perceived Racial Discrimination and Diurnal Cortisol Profiles in Adulthood: A 20-Year Prospective Study." *Psychoneuroendocrinology* 62 (2015): 279–91.

Adams, Walter A. "The Negro Patient in Psychiatric Treatment." *American Journal of Orthopsychiatry* 20 (1950): 305–10.

Ayanian, John Z. "Determinants of Racial and Ethnic Disparities in Surgical Care." *World Journal of Surgery* 32, no. 4 (2008): 509–15.

Bakwin, Harry. "The Negro Infant." *Human Biology* 4, no. 1 (1932): 1–33.

Barnes, Vernon, Robert Schneider, Charles Alexander, and Frank Staggers. "Stress, Stress Reduction, and Hypertension in African Americans: An Updated Review." *Journal of the National Medical Association* 89, no. 7 (1997): 464–76.

Beach, Mary Catherine, Somnath Saha, P. Todd Korthuis, Victoria Sharp, Jonathon Cohn, Ira B. Wilson, Susan Eggly, et al. "Patient–Provider Communication Differs for Black Compared to White HIV-Infected Patients." *AIDS Behavior* 15, no. 4 (2011): 805–11.

Capers, Quinn IV, and Zarina Sharalaya. "Racial Disparities in Cardiovascular Care: A Review of Culprits and Potential Solutions." *Journal of Racial and Ethnic Health Disparities* 1, no. 3 (2014): 171–80.

Cornely, Paul. "Morbidity and Mortality from Scarlet Fever in the Negro." *American Journal of Public Health* 29 (September 1939): 999–1005.

Dan, Bruce B., and Roxanne K. Young, eds. *A Piece of My Mind: A Collection of Essays from* The Journal of the American Medical Association. Los Angeles: Feeling Fine Programs; Toronto: Random House of Canada, 1988.

"Disease, Race, and Civilization." *British Medical Journal* 1, no. 4823 (June 13, 1953): 1320.

Drwecki, Brian B. "Education to Identify and Combat Racial Bias in Pain Treatment." *AMA Journal of Ethics* 17, no. 3 (2015): 221–28.

Fessenden, Ford. "Blacks Passed By." *Newsday*, November 29, 1998, A55.

Geiger, H. Jack. "Race and Health Care—An American Dilemma?" *New England Journal of Medicine* 335 (1996): 815–16.

Geronimus, Arline T., Margaret Hicken, Danya Keene, and John Bound. "'Weathering' and Age Patterns of Allostatic Load Scores among Blacks and Whites in the United States." *American Journal of Public Health* 96, no. 5 (2006): 826–33.

Gillum, Richard F. "Coronary Heart Disease in Black Populations. I. Mortality and Morbidity." *American Heart Journal* 104, no. 4 (October 1982): 839–51.

Green, Adrienne. "The Cost of Balancing Academia and Racism." *Atlantic*, January 21, 2016. https://www.theatlantic.com/education/archive/2016/01/balancing-academia-racism/424887/.

Griggs, Jennifer J., and Jerome Engel. "Epilepsy Surgery and the Racial Divide." *Neurology* 64, no. 1 (2005): 8–9.

Hoberman, John. *Black & Blue: The Origins and Consequences of Medical Racism.* Berkeley: University of California Press, 2012.

Hoberman, John. "Medical Racism and the Rhetoric of Exculpation: How Do Physicians Think about Race?" *New Literary History* 38, no. 3 (2007): 505–25.

Hoffman, Kelly M. "Racial Bias in Pain Assessment and Treatment Recommendations, and False Beliefs about Biological Differences between Blacks and Whites." *Proceedings of the National Academy of Sciences USA* 113 (2016): 4296–301.

"How Whites Feel about Negroes: A Painful American Dilemma." *Newsweek*, October 21, 1963, 44–50.

Institute of Medicine. *Unequal Treatment: Confronting Racial and Ethnic Disparities in Health Care*, edited by Brian D. Smedley, Adrienne Y. Stith, and Alan R. Nelson. Washington, DC: National Academies Press, 2002.

Jauhar, Sandeep. "When Blood Pressure Is Political." *New York Times*, August 6, 2016.

Johnson, Rachel L., Debra Roter, Neil R. Powe, and Lisa A. Cooper. "Patient Race/Ethnicity and Quality of Patient–Physician Communication during Medical Visits." *American Journal of Public Health* 94, no. 12 (2004): 2084–90.

Katz, Jeffrey N. "Persistence of Racial and Ethnic Differences in Utilization and Adverse Outcomes of Total Joint Replacement." *Journal of Bone and Joint Surgery* 98 (2016): 1241–42.

Lei, Man-Kit, Steven R. H. Beach, Ronald L. Simons, and Robert A. Philibert. "Neighborhood Crime and Depressive Symptoms among African American Women: Genetic Moderation and Epigenetic Mediation of Effects." *Social Science & Medicine* 146 (2015): 120–28.

Lurie, Nicole, Allen M. Fremont, Arvind K. Jain, and Thomas Bruce Ferguson, Jr. "Racial and Ethnic Disparities in Care: The Perspectives of Cardiologists." *Circulation* 111, no. 10 (2005): 1264–69.

Lynch, Kenneth M., Kater McInnes, and G. Fleming McInnes. "Concerning Syphilis in the American Negro." *Southern Medical Journal* 8 (June 1, 1915): 453.

Medical News Today, "Unconscious Racial Bias among Doctors Linked to Poor Communication with Patients, Dissatisfaction with Care." March 16, 2012. https://www.medicalnewstoday.com/releases/242975.php.

Pierce, Chester M. "Is Bigotry the Basis of the Medical Problems of the Ghetto?" In *Medicine in the Ghetto*, edited by John C. Norman, 301–14. New York: Appleton-Century-Crofts, 1969.

Ravenell, Joseph, and Gbenga Ogedegbe. "Unconscious Bias and Real-World Hypertension Outcomes: Advancing Disparities Research." *Journal of General Internal Medicine* 29, no. 7 (2014): 973–75.

Satcher, David. "Does Race Interfere with the Doctor–Patient Relationship?" *JAMA* 223, no. 13 (1973): 1498–99.

Singer, Emily. "Beyond Race-Based Medicine." *MIT Technology Review*, January 16, 2009.

Smith, Clint. "Racism, Stress, and Black Death." *New Yorker*, July 16, 2016.

"The Daily Irritations." *Time*, April 6, 1970, 77–78.

Umberson, Debra, Julie Skalamera Olson, Robert Crosnoe, Hui Liu, Tetyana Pudrovska, and Rachel Donnelly. "Death of Family Members as an Overlooked Source of Racial Disadvantage in the United States." *Proceedings of the National Academy of Sciences USA* 114, no. 5 (2017): 915–20.

Wortham, Jenna. "Racism's Psychological Toll." *New York Times*, June 24, 2015.

Yeager, David S., Valerie Purdie-Vaughns, Sophia Yang Hooper, and Geoffrey L. Cohen. "Loss of Institutional Trust among Racial and Ethnic Minority Adolescents: A Consequence of Procedural Injustice and a Cause of Life-Span Outcomes." *Child Development* 88, no. 2 (2017): 658–76.

7

The Power of Black Patients' Testimonies When Teaching Medical Racism

Keisha Ray

Introduction

I have[1] had many odd, seemingly racially motivated experiences with racially uneducated and racially insensitive doctors and nurses, from being told by one of my white physicians that I sound white when I speak to another physician calling me "sista girl" for what seemed like a hundred times during our brief fifteen-minute interaction or another physician who in disbelief kept asking me, "Are you sure you've never been pregnant? It's very rare for a black woman your age to not have had any pregnancies. Maybe you think I mean births, when I mean pregnancies?" Although these stories made for good laughs between my friends and me, there is one experience that I have had with the medical profession that was less comical because my doctor's attitudes about race could have had serious effects on my health.

When I was a senior in college I discovered I had hypertension. I went to see a doctor at a family medicine facility and was prescribed a common hypertension drug. While meeting with the doctor in her office, she was very reassuring and told me not to worry, that this drug has been known to work very well for black people.

But this drug did not work for me at all. Consistently my blood pressure readings were 140/120 (what is considered "normal" varies, but typically 120/80 is the standard). So after taking the drug for a month as instructed, I went back to see my doctor. In that office I encountered an utterly dumbfounded physician. She just could not believe that the drug did not work for me. She kept saying, "I just don't understand. This drug is supposed to work for black people." She even said, "Plus it's cheap, so it's good for poor black people," without ever asking me about my financial status. My doctor then said that she was going to come up with a new game plan, and I was optimistic that something was going to be done about my hypertension. Little did I know that the doctor's "new" game plan was actually the same game plan. Her recommendation: "Let's keep trying because this drug is supposed to work for black people." So I left the doctor's office with a blood pressure of 140/120 (and sometimes higher) and with another month's supply of the same drug and the same dosage because, after all, *this drug is supposed to work for black people*.

Eventually, I went to a new doctor who was willing to try different drugs to help me, and eventually I got my blood pressure controlled. But this experience left a lasting impression on me—because this was only the beginning of a series of encounters with doctors who dispensed overly generalized care and saw me only as a black patient and nothing else.

The above testimony recounts some of my experiences with physicians. I frequently share my experiences with students so that they can learn about the nature of interactions that many black patients have with their doctors and nurses. Olivia Banner argues that narratives, much like my own, can be a beneficial part of antiracist medical humanities education.[2] My own classroom experiences support Banner's arguments as I have found that patients' narratives and testimonies can be a powerful and an educationally meaningful tool when discussing medical racism with either future or current medical practitioners. So rather than just recount medicine's horrifically racist past with black patients, I choose to discuss testimonies from black patients and use them to put a contemporary face on medical racism. But I do so with caution. Medical racism calls on us to be less discriminatory toward black patients, but it also acknowledges that, given black people's experiences with discrimination and prejudices and the adverse effects these have on health, black patients require special consideration from their caregivers. Therefore, when teaching medical racism I try to make sure that I do not send a message of homogenization to my students and give them the impression that all black people require the same kind of special treatment. To do this in my lessons I include testimonies with varying themes, and I also ask my students to participate in a short exercise on intersectionality.

Medical Racism

As described by scholar John Hoberman, *medical racism* is an all-encompassing term that includes racial discrimination that many patients of color experience while receiving care from physicians and nurses and the racial prejudices that physicians employ to treat their patients of color, like that recounted in my testimony.[3] Medical racism also includes the history of racism in medicine that many healthcare workers ignore, downplay, or sometimes deny; the racialization of organs; the health disparities between white patients and patients of color that put patients of color on the losing end; and the racism that many physicians of color experience from their white patients. In general, medical racism is the acknowledgment that black patients are treated differently from white patients and that their skin color, and the prejudices that are associated with their skin color, is the reason for this difference in treatment.

Medical racism also encourages us to recognize the distinct needs that black patients have that are related to their skin color. For instance, the medical community is just now beginning to recognize the detrimental health effects of racial discrimination that some black people experience.[4] The medical community is also recognizing that experience with or even only witnessing racism or violent, racially charged events such as watching videos of police officers using deadly force against unarmed black people can be a cause of post-traumatic stress disorder (PTSD).[5] Given that these are just a few adverse health events that are specific to black people, as educators we also have to teach our students that because of the connection between race, social and cultural factors, and health, black people have special needs that must be taken into consideration when treating them.

Medical racism can be used to bring medicine's historically racist past and present to the forefront of education for students. Medical racism is an acknowledgment that only by understanding and making caregivers aware of medicine's relationship with patients of color, particularly black people, can we change its future relationship with patients of color and ultimately give better care to a population that has typically been disenfranchised by medicine.[6] I have found that relaying the facts of medical racism is not enough to help students understand and reflect on how medical racism can impact patient care but that using patients' testimonies puts a human, contemporary face to medical racism that is more relatable and therefore memorable.

Using Patients' Testimonies

I have found that students are more drawn to black patients' testimonies than to recaps of the historically racist relationship that medicine has had with certain racialized groups such as African Americans, Native Americans, and Hispanics/Latinos. Students are typically appalled and shocked when we discuss the black men who were a part of the Tuskegee syphilis study, or the young Native American girls who were made sterile by American doctors without their or their parents' knowledge or the "bath riots" that resulted from US medical officials authorizing the use of toxic chemicals and extreme heat to sterilize the bodies and clothing of Mexican men and women entering the United States at the US border. But students' shock almost always subsides as soon as our unit on race and medicine is over. It is hard for them to understand the lasting implications that these cases, and countless other similar cases, have on the medical profession, including current patients of color. It is hard for them to "see what the big deal is" because they look at these cases as events that would never happen now. This is generally because students do not understand the structural and systemic nature of racism in institutions like the US healthcare system; they cannot imagine unethical treatment of people of color in the twenty-first century. Therefore, they have a difficult time understanding the purpose of studying medical racism.

When teaching medical racism I prefer to focus on personal testimonies of medical racism that resemble my own in the introduction of this chapter. Patient testimonies can easily be found on the Internet with a quick search. Also, many books about disparities between black and white patients, books concerning other inequities, and books that cover more general topics related to race and medicine also include testimonies from black patients. I have found that patient testimonies encourage meaningful discussion and sophisticated student essays. Following are the typical goals I have for the race unit in my courses:

- Understand the concept of medical racism
- Reflect on the role medical racism plays in caring for black patients
- Reflect on how medical racism affects medical professionals as individuals, as members of a profession, and as caregivers to black patients
- Discuss the various manifestations of medical racism
- Discuss how medical racism affects black patients
- Discuss the reasons medical professionals would be resistant to acknowledging medical racism
- Discuss the value of patient testimonies
- Practice writing our own medical testimonies

The first step to accomplishing these goals is to have students read testimonies from black patients as a group, in class. Rather than assigning testimonies as reading to do outside of class, I have found that reading the testimonies together as a group helps students learn from each other and helps them better process the subtle themes in the testimonies. I have also found that students learn from each other in ways that I could not have imagined. For instance, I have discovered that students learn from the way their classmates read the testimonies, including the words they choose to emphasize or de-emphasize, the changing inflections in their voice, and even their facial reactions. From listening and watching their classmates read the testimonies the students see what other students find important or troubling about the testimony and can compare it to their own reactions.

I typically choose multiple testimonies that can be categorized into specific categories: doctors' experiences with medical racism, patient care, and patients' perceived experiences with racism. For the first category, one testimonial that I use is that of physician and author Damon Tweedy, M.D., as found in his book *Black Man in a White Coat*.[7] In this book Tweedy recounts his experiences with discrimination and prejudices from his instructors, peers, and patients. I typically use Tweedy's book as an example of how to write a testimony and then ask students to write their own medical testimony. Even if they have not had any experiences with medical racism, I have found that every student has a story to tell; and I encourage them to tell whatever story depicts their experience with medicine.

As a part of teaching medical racism, I think it is necessary to teach the importance of patients' perceived racism. Many times students will argue that what patients recount in their testimonies is in fact not racism. Although an adequate response to these kinds of arguments can be complex because it includes an explanation of structural and institutional racism, microaggressions, implicit bias, and an explanation of people of color's lifelong experience with these concepts and social ideals, it also includes the power of perceived racism, particularly the power perceived racism can have on patient compliance.

As an example of the kind of testimonies about patients' experiences with perceived racism from their physicians and/or nurses that I use in my courses, here is the testimony of Mr. King, an elderly black man:

> One day this nurse comes in with this pill between her fingers and says, "Here, take this." Now they usually have little cups like this and they open the medicine without touching it and drop it in the cup. Now why did this woman think it was all right for her to walk in with a pill between her fingers and hand it to me? I don't think she was deliberately being discriminatory, I think she was just racist. She felt that she didn't have to adhere to the customs and mores of healthy practices because my skin was a different color. I'm convinced of this. I don't think she would have done that if I were a White man.[8]

We also discuss patient testimonies like that of Ms. Ellis, a middle-aged black woman who believed that her doctors treated her differently from their white patients:

> I see a lot of White patients come through there and it seems like they listen to them a lot more; they understand them a lot more as opposed to me telling them how I feel and it's like it's blowed [*sic*] over, I'm just more or less going by how they're [white patients] getting treated by the medical assistant. . . . They will help them come in . . . the courtesy and all that. I don't hear them come up to them and tell them . . . I have asked her about this, I have asked her about that . . . you know. I don't hear them saying that [to me].[9]

My goal with using testimonies like that of Mr. King and Ms. Ellis is to have students discuss what these patients are trying to convey about their experience with their practitioners and what should be our take-away message from these testimonies. Additionally, we discuss why it matters less if we think these patients experienced racism and more that these patients believed their treatment was influenced by racism. Namely, I stress that the perception of racism can affect patients' willingness to comply with physicians' treatment recommendations, which ultimately affects their overall health. Lastly, although these are not testimonials of such horrendous acts as unethical experimentation on people of color, they are testimonials of the impact of medical racism on people of color.

Concerns about Empathy and Overgeneralization

Medical racism can be confusing for students because it essentially has two seemingly conflicting threads. On the one hand, it tells us that relying on patients' race too much is considered medical racism and detrimental to patient care. But, on the other hand, it tells us that completely ignoring the race of our black patients can lead us to ignore the unique social factors, like discrimination, that can contribute to their poor health. I typically parse this out for students by characterizing medical racism as a concept that warns against using people's race against them or to their detriment. When race is used as a way to hurl prejudices onto their character, and thus as an excuse to give them subpar treatment, that is medical racism. It is, however, not medically racist to acknowledge that the discrimination and racially motivated violent events that some black people experience can cause them to experience PTSD.

I teach medical racism because I agree with scholars like Hoberman who argue that students, physicians, and nurses need more education about race to be better caregivers to their black patients. Ultimately, the goal is to give better patient care to a group of people who have historically been given inferior care because of the color of their skin. But my concern is that the goals of teaching medical racism will get lost in translation. What we will intend to say is that because of the history of racism in medicine and in the greater public black people have a special relationship with medicine, and we have to recognize that and give them treatment in such a way that recognizes this relationship. But what students will hear is a message of homogenization—that every black person requires the same kind of special treatment simply because they all share the same common feature, dark skin. If the two threads of medical racism are not explained well, black people's individuality and individual needs can get lost. And as a result, when a black person like me walks into a doctor's office, her race will be treated first and her body and mind, second.

Another concern that I have about teaching medical racism is the relationship between race education and a favorite topic of medical humanities instructors—empathy. There is a vast literature concerning the meaning of empathy, with philosophers, sociologists, psychologists, clinicians, and other scholars giving varying definitions. The explanation that Amy Coplan and Peter

Goldie give represents at least one way in which these varying definitions of the meaning of empathy converge: "[a] tool for developing our understanding of others and enabling us to determine what the best thing to do is in real world situations."[10] For these reasons, empathy, or the ability to imagine what it would be like to live in someone else's shoes, is often encouraged as a skill that practitioners can use to be better caregivers.[11] Empathy gives practitioners insights into their patients' ways of being and gives them the tools to respond to their suffering. Indeed, there are empirical studies that link practitioners' levels of empathy to patients' reception of bad news and how well patients recover from medical procedures.[12] Empathy has also been said to be important because it is equated to good listening skills, and if patients feel that their practitioners are listening to them, they may be more likely to reveal information pertinent to their care that they may otherwise have been too afraid to share.[13]

Although we want our physicians and nurses to be empathetic, often, as a part of our empathetic imagination, we will try to find some likeness between the subject and ourselves. We will say things like "If this were me, how would I react?" or "If this were me, what might I consider to be a desirable outcome?" Rebecca Garden calls this "a preoccupation with the self that obscures the other."[14] Garden argues that the preoccupation with the self that is inherent in the act of empathizing can "exclude the patient's suffering and the meaning the patient makes of suffering." This represents an epistemological problem that Garden argues can happen when practitioners *know* characteristics of a culture but do not acknowledge that this does not mean that they *know* a specific member of that culture's individual experience of illness. This epistemological problem is of particular concern when considering that the overwhelming majority of physicians treating black patients are white. Empathetic imagination runs the risk of making whiteness and the white experience the standard by which all black patients and experiences are judged by bringing white physicians' interpretation of black patients' culture and subsequent experience of illness rather than the individual patient's experience of illness to the forefront of their clinical interactions.

Empathy has the ability to exclude black patients' experience of illness from their interactions with their practitioners because when imagining what it is like to be another person we necessarily contemplate the ways that we are different. And while it is important to note what makes us unique individuals, medicine also requires us to not exaggerate our differences, particularly those between black and white patients. Yes, we have to acknowledge how black patients' needs may sometimes differ from those of white patients, but black patients are still people just like their white counterparts. Both black and white patients have desires to be healthy and live the kind of lives that they deem worthy of living. So when adding medical racism to a curriculum that already stresses the importance of empathy, we have to teach both in such a way that does not exaggerate the differences between black and white patients but also recognizes the differences between black and white patients and the individual differences among black patients.

This exaggeration of differences between racial groups and overgeneralization of members within a racial group often happens when people are unwilling to recognize their complicity in racist institutions and unwilling to confront their own racist behaviors; such unwillingness is common, and we should not expect that students will be any different. To help students understand that sometimes practitioners can exaggerate differences between patients yet overgeneralize patients within the same racial group, I also teach intersectionality, particularly how intersectionality can make them better physicians.

Teaching Intersectionality

For the portion of the unit of medical racism in which I teach the concept "intersectionality," I ask students to take out a sheet of paper and use its entire space to draw themselves. (They will usually draw a large stick figure.)[15] Then I ask them to write down the different social and cultural labels that they occupy across the body, such as "woman," "Hispanic," "black," "Catholic," "swimmer," "student," or "father." I also tell them to choose labels that they would be comfortable with other people using to identify them. Typically students find it very easy to cover the entire portrait of themselves. I then ask students to pick only one label that they believe best fits them. This is typically the hard part. Sometimes there is even resistance. Students usually cannot pick just one label, nor do they want to. So I then give them permission to pick two labels. Although there is still resistance, students will usually, albeit uneasily, pick two labels.

When I ask students to discuss why it was difficult to pick just one label, they usually will say because they do not see themselves as just black or just a woman but rather they see themselves as both, and sometimes they will even say that they are committed to social issues that both groups face. I then use their remarks and the exercise to show students that we are all situated within many social and cultural categories, that no person is just one *thing*, nor do we want to be identified by just one part of ourselves. Additionally, we discuss how the labels that we use to describe ourselves are sometimes connected. For instance, a student may share that she identifies as Hispanic and Catholic and tell a personal story detailing how one influences the other in her life. This is how I introduce the concept of intersectionality.

The term, coined by Kimberlé Crenshaw, originated as a way to conceptualize that every person inhabits multiple identity categories, and these interact with discriminatory practices in different ways. For instance, according to intersectionality, the ways in which black women may experience sexism in the workplace are not the same as the ways in which white women may experience sexism in the workplace because their blackness and their womanhood are each the object of discriminatory practices.[16] At the core of intersectionality, however, is the idea that we are not singular people; no one is situated in just one social category. And all of the categories that we are situated in make us uniquely ourselves. If we teach intersectionality as a part of medical education, this sends the message that when patients enter a doctor's office they should be thought of as a whole person made up of multiple social, cultural, and biological parts. Within the context of intersectionality, no patient is just a black patient, but a black woman and academic or a black man, father, and businessman. Teaching intersectionality is a way to help students understand that all parts of a person ought to be taken into consideration when diagnosing and treating disease and that focusing on just any one part of a person, like race, is being a poor practitioner.

Conclusion

Most bioethics textbooks have a problem in the way the authors choose to depict the relationship between race and medicine. Namely, they depict racism as a past phenomenon that has been eradicated from medicine, which unfortunately is not true. Bioethics textbooks are also lacking in their full depiction of medical racism. Teaching medical racism is one of the best ways to teach students about all of the corners of medicine that race can reach. But we have to do it in a way that does not make racism in medicine look like a fossil from our past but an issue that many physicians, nurses, and patients encounter when trying to secure their health. This is why using testimonies that depict patients' experience with racism is a great way to teach students about the experience of so many patients.

Students can relate to testimonies because everyone has a story to tell and everyone wants their story to be heard and understood. By using testimonies from black patients we show students that black patients are just like other patients: they are asking their physicians and nurses to help them be well. Yet testimonies also show that black patients' unique experiences sometimes require a different kind of care from other patients. Testimonies give medical racism human feelings and a human face. Overall, testimonies make medical racism personal, which can be a learning tool that no regurgitation of a few history cases could provide.

PEDAGOGY EXERCISE SECTION

Intersectionality Exercise

GOAL

The goal of this exercise is to get us thinking about how complex humans can be. To do this we will discuss what makes us who we are. For this exercise I want you to give serious thought to all of the parts of your personality, good and bad; your hobbies and interests; your role in your family and circle of friends; your social and spiritual beliefs; your life goals; and the person you are now versus the person you hope to become.

STEPS

1. On a blank sheet of paper I want you to draw yourself. You can draw just your face, or you can draw your entire body. Just try to use as much of the paper as possible for your drawing. Stick figures are acceptable as long as they are large.
2. Next, I want you to write words that you think describe yourself across your picture. Be sure to use words that you would be comfortable with someone else using to describe you. For instance, for myself I may write "black," "woman," "professor," "daughter," "runner," etc. Feel free to use markers or crayons to write each word in a different color. Be sure to write the words large enough for people to see.
3. Now in small groups (three or four students) I want you to hold up your picture for your group to see. Tell them which one term best describes you. If you find this difficult, I give you permission to choose two but no more than two.
4. After each person has had a turn sharing in your small group, I want you all to take turns answering the discussion questions below.
5. Lastly, I want you to share your picture with the entire class and discuss any difficulties you had picking just one word to describe yourself.

DISCUSSION

- Was it difficult picking just one descriptive word?
- Are any of your descriptive words connected to one another?
- Would your friends or family pick the descriptive word that you chose?
- While listening to your peers share their terms were you confused by their chosen term? Did you think that any student should have picked another descriptive word written on the picture to best describe himself or herself?
- Do you think it would be difficult to pick one descriptive word for each of your friends and family members?

Notes

1. Parts of this chapter were originally published at bioethics.net.

2. Olivia Banner, "Structural Racism and Practices of Reading in the Medical Humanities," *Literature and Medicine* 34, no. 1 (2016): 25–52.

3. John Hoberman, *Black and Blue: The Origins and Consequences of Medical Racism* (Berkeley: University of California Press, 2012).

4. Ibid.

5. Monnica T. Williams, "Can Racism Cause PTSD? Implications for DSM-5," *Psychology Today*, May 20, 2013, https://www.psychologytoday.com/blog/culturally-speaking/201305/can-racism-cause-ptsd-implications-dsm-5.

6. See Hoberman, *Black and Blue*.

7. Damon Tweedy, *Black Man in a White Coat: A Doctor's Reflections on Race and Medicine* (New York: Picador, 2015).

8. Paula T. Ross, Monica L. Lypson, and Arno K. Kumagai, "Using Illness Narratives to Explore African American Perspectives of Racial Discrimination in Health Care," *Journal of Black Studies* 43, no. 5 (2012): 527.

9. Ibid., 526.

10. Amy Coplan and Peter Goldie, "Introduction," in *Empathy: Philosophical and Psychological Perspectives*, ed. Amy Coplan and Peter Goldie (New York and Oxford: Oxford University Press, 2011).

11. Rebecca Garden, in "The Problem of Empathy: Medicine and the Humanities," *New Literary History* 38 (2007): 551–67, reviews the literature documenting the conflict between medical educators' theories on the importance of empathy to patient care and clinical practitioners' biomedical approach, which oftentimes focuses on pathology rather than empathy.

12. Jodi Halpern, "Clinical Empathy in Medical Care," in *Empathy: From Bench to Bedside*, ed. Jean Decety, Social Neuroscience (Cambridge: MIT Press, 2012), 229–44; John Ptacek and John J. Ptacek, "Patients' Perceptions of Receiving Bad News about Cancer," *Journal of Clinical Oncology* 19 (2001): 4160–64.

13. Halpern, "Clinical Empathy."

14. Garden, "The Problem of Empathy."

15. See the Pedagogy Exercise Section at the end of this chapter detailing the steps of this exercise.

16. Kimberlé Crenshaw, "Mapping the Margins: Intersectionality, Identity Politics, and Violence against Women of Color," *Stanford Law Review* 43, no. 6 (1991): 1241–99.

Works Cited

Banner, Olivia. "Structural Racism and Practices of Reading in the Medical Humanities." *Literature and Medicine* 34, no. 1 (2016): 25–52.

Coplan, Amy, and Peter Goldie. "Introduction." In *Empathy: Philosophical and Psychological Perspectives*, edited by Amy Coplan and Peter Goldie. New York and Oxford: Oxford University Press, 2011.

Crenshaw, Kimberlé. "Mapping the Margins: Intersectionality, Identity Politics, and Violence against Women of Color." *Stanford Law Review* 43, no. 6 (1991): 1241–99.

Garden, Rebecca. "The Problem of Empathy: Medicine and the Humanities." *New Literary History* 38 (2007): 551–67.

Halpern, Jodi. "Clinical Empathy in Medical Care." In *Empathy: From Bench to Bedside*, edited by Jean Decety, 229–44. Social Neuroscience. Cambridge: MIT Press, 2012.

Hoberman, John. *Black and Blue: The Origins and Consequences of Medical Racism*. Berkeley: University of California Press, 2012.

Ptacek, John, and John J. Ptacek. "Patients Perceptions of Receiving Bad News about Cancer." *Journal of Clinical Oncology* 19 (2001): 4160–64.

Ross, Paula T., Monica L. Lypson, and Arno K. Kumagai. "Using Illness Narratives to Explore African American Perspectives of Racial Discrimination in Health Care." *Journal of Black Studies* 43, no. 5 (2012): 520–44.

Tweedy, Damon. *Black Man in a White Coat: A Doctor's Reflections on Race and Medicine*. New York: Picador, 2015.

Williams, Monnica T. "Can Racism Cause PTSD? Implications for DSM-5." *Psychology Today*, May 20, 2013. https://www.psychologytoday.com/blog/culturally-speaking/201305/can-racism-cause-ptsd-implications-dsm-5.

8

Treating Gender and Illness Together in the Classroom

Lisa Diedrich

I am not a very disciplined teacher and scholar. With an M.A. and Ph.D. in women's, gender, and sexuality studies and with areas of specialization in medical/health humanities, or what I prefer to call critical medical studies, and disability studies, my training, research, and teaching are inter- or transdisciplinary all the way down. Sometimes students are surprised that my classes are women's, gender, and sexuality studies classes. A glance at some of my course titles, such as "Testimonies: Making History and Memory," "Plague Narratives," "Madness and Civilization, 1960–1980," "Documenting Mental Illness," and "Cultures of Disability," causes some students to wonder why the words *women, gender*, and *sexuality* are not in the titles. In designing my classes, I have tried to move away from a model of pedagogy that frames the project of women's, gender, and sexuality studies as discipline-bound, in the sense that we have, simply, to add women, gender, and/or sexuality to the mix in order to change the way a discipline is practiced and the knowledges that emerge from it. While I think this was, and still often is, a necessary correction to the exclusion of women, gender, and sexuality as subjects and objects of research, I also think that the project of the field of women's, gender, and sexuality studies has to be—and indeed already is—much more than this.

Drawing on my multiple interdisciplinary backgrounds, then, in this essay I discuss ways of treating illness and disability in the classroom as I might women, gender, and sexuality or, put differently, treating gender and illness together as categories of analysis that come into being through a multiplicity of archives, discourses, practices, and institutions. By treating illness as analogous to gender, I do not mean to suggest that they are necessarily the same kind of thing in every situation. Instead, by bringing them together, my intention is to multiply how we understand illness and gender, ontologically and epistemologically, through particular pedagogical practices. Thus, rather than stabilize and consecrate an object as belonging to a particular field, I am more interested in attending to the histories, methods, and pedagogies that bring objects and whole fields into being and that sustain, challenge, or transform them. I organize my analysis in this essay around several general transdisciplinary themes—categories, concepts, methods, and spaces—that inform my approach to teaching and scholarship on illness and gender. I also offer specific practical, even personal, pedagogical tactics and strategies—a variety of things I do in my women's, gender, and sexuality studies classroom to treat illness like gender as a multiple and complex object. In doing so, I argue for women's, gender, and sexuality studies as creating an *other space (and time)* for critical health studies, *and vice versa*.

Categories (of Historical Analysis)

In 1986, feminist historian Joan W. Scott published the essay "Gender: A Useful Category of Historical Analysis" in the *American Historical Review*, inaugurating a practice of feminist history interested in "critically understanding how history operates as a site of production of gender knowledge."[1] In this and other work, Scott emphasizes the importance of writing histories of difference, including gender, race, class, sexuality, and, I would add, illness and disability differences. Following Michel Foucault's genealogical approach, Scott argues that "events" are not simply things that happen and are then understood by our existent thought processes applied after the fact to the event; rather, events transform the substance of our thought, and thought itself is an event. "If you believe that how we think about things is how we know them," Scott asserts, "then it is our categories of thought that create knowledge. It then becomes very important to know where those categories come from, how they have been used and by whom, what they permit us to think, and what they rule out of consideration."[2]

What does it mean then to treat something—illness or gender—as a category of historical analysis? In my scholarship as well as my teaching, I try to demonstrate the usefulness of thinking about our categories of analysis by considering, for example, the practice of diagnosis of illness as a performative act, "performative" understood here through the lens of both social interactionist theories, which explore the constitution of the self in the practices of everyday life, and speech act theories of performative utterances, which explore how saying can be doing. Theories of performativity have been utilized to discern, importantly, the how, not the what, of gender—how gender is done rather than, or as well as, what gender is. I am interested here in how such theories can be extended to also discern how illness is done.[3] For example, the utterance "you have _____ [choose your disease here]" does not simply name an existing biological condition; it brings that condition into being. Being diagnosed leads to becoming something new or someone else; it is an estrangement—a kind of differentializing of the self—that can be both painful and productive. I argue that diagnoses reveal not so much *the* or even *a* truth of the self but the self as truth effect of variegated practices, including the practice of diagnosis. One possible effect of an understanding of the self as truth effect of the practice of diagnosis is to provide a measure of relief from the shame and stigma that sometimes attach to experiences of illness as a result of theories of illness causation that link illness with personal failure. Historicizing diagnostic categories works to denaturalize illnesses as stable categories across time and space; as with denaturalizing gender, this process can contribute to changing attitudes and assumptions about the meaning of or associations with particular conditions.

In considering illness as a category of analysis, and diagnosis as a performative act, we can begin to think of illness as operating like gender; and by this I mean, as operating biologically, psychologically, and socially—or biopsychosocially[4]—in particular times and spaces. An example of how I do the work of considering illness as a category of analysis in the classroom is in the way I frame a graduate seminar I teach called "Madness and Civilization, 1960–1980." I describe the seminar as about madness, reason, and time, or about how and why madness emerged as a particular preoccupation at a particular moment in recent history. We read texts written between 1960 and 1980 in order to situate madness in a very specific period of time and because madness and its diagnoses and treatments figured prominently in the social, political, theoretical, and institutional transformations that took place leading up to and after the widespread upheavals of 1968. We trace the multiple figurations of madness in some of the key texts of social and critical theory, as well as in literary and film texts of the period, in order to consider questions about subjectivity, power, and ethics.

It is often forgotten that Foucault's first discussions of sexuality emerged out of—or, perhaps more accurately, in tandem with—his analyses of the historico-ontological categories of madness. In *The History of Madness*, for example, Foucault treats sexuality, along with madness, as one of the domains of experience that "form a homogeneous world in the space of confinement where the meaning of mental alienation as we know it today was born."[5] Madness and sexuality converge again at the end of *The Archaeology of Knowledge*, where he introduces an "archaeological description of 'sexuality'" as one of the "other archaeologies"—yet to be undertaken—that would analyze the multiple discursive practices of sexuality. Such an analysis, Foucault says, "would be carried out not in the direction of the episteme, but in that of what we might call the ethical," indicating that the question of ethics was also important to Foucault's work long before his oft-noted "ethical turn" in the second and third volumes of *The History of Sexuality*.[6] Foucault's discussion of certain forms of sexuality as "directly linked to unreason and certain types of mental illness" can be found in one of the chapters, "The Correctional World," not included in the English translation that became *Madness and Civilization*.[7] Foucault's preoccupation with the history of madness, and its changing figures, was enduring and integral to all of his work and intertwined with his preoccupation with the history of sexuality.

Although Foucault and his work figure prominently in my seminar, the course is not a seminar on Foucault. Rather, inspired by Foucault's call to other scholars not to write about him but to do genealogies, we read his work as a history of the present of the 1960s and 1970s and, as such, as participating in the configuration of the discursive and nondiscursive practices of health and illness at that time, contributing to the extension of politics into domains not previously perceived as domains of political struggle—not just sexual politics but illness politics, too, and the interrelationship between the two. We also ask why, since the 1990s, has critical theory tended to be preoccupied with figures and practices of sexuality but not illness? By doing this, we historicize how illness has been thought with and against gender and sexuality.[8]

Concepts (Intersectionality and Structural Violence)

In "Madness and Civilization, 1960–1980," we focus on a particular historical moment, but we also consider the relationship between sexual and illness politics in that near-past moment and the present and how that past is remembered now. From the opening, when I introduce the course and review the syllabus with students, I encourage students to think about key terms and concepts as tools to help them understand a particular subject and the world more generally. For example, in my "Introduction to Women's, Gender, and Sexuality Studies" class, students are introduced to the key term *intersectionality* by reading critical legal and race theorist Kimberlé Crenshaw's essay in which she coins and defines the term in relation to a study of services provided (and not) at battered women's shelters in minority communities in Los Angeles.[9] Crenshaw shows how certain policies and laws make immigrant women in particular especially vulnerable to spousal violence, and she suggests intervention strategies that take into consideration the burdens of, for example, "poverty, child care responsibilities, and the lack of job skills" for some women.[10]

Crenshaw's concept of intersectionality then becomes a tool to think with throughout the semester—and I hope even beyond the immediate spatial and temporal parameters of the class. For example, in the introductory course in women's, gender, and sexuality studies, the term helps students to understand the intersection of racial and sexual politics in the civil rights movement in a unit focused around a reading of Alice Walker's novel, *Meridian*, published in 1975 and about young people—white and black, men and women—participating in the voter registration efforts in the South in the 1960s. With the recent rise of the Black Lives Matter movement, Walker's novel provides an excellent historical doorway into a discussion of current youth-led social justice activism. I encourage students to compare and contrast the activism portrayed in *Meridian* with contemporary feminist, antiracist, and queer activist movements. We also discuss the main character Meridian's "falling sickness" as a biopsychosocial sign of the political burden she takes on as she "volunteers to suffer" for others[11]—again, illness politics as informed by and inseparable from not only sexual politics but also racial politics.

In all of my classes, I try to give students analytical tools to more fully analyze experiences and events both near to and far from their own lives. I work with theory quite extensively, with both undergraduate and graduate students, because I understand theory as something that emerges out of experiences and events in the real world, abstracts them, and then becomes a prism through which we can view these experiences and events anew. The abstraction that theory performs does not move us beyond the world of "real" experiences and events but becomes a more or less useful explanatory model for describing the world as it is or imagining it otherwise. This is precisely the point of a concept like "intersectionality"—the concept itself provides a prism through which to explore a multiplicity of complex topics, including, for example, how racial, sexual, and illness politics are condensed into a fictional character's falling sickness.

As the *Meridian* example shows, then, intersectionality becomes a useful concept not just in the specific domain in which Crenshaw developed and applied it—laws and policies on domestic violence—but as a more general and mobile tool for understanding how and why particular people are vulnerable in particular situations and for helping come up with some possible remedies for addressing such precarious conditions. As Crenshaw asserts, in the case of battered women, "[T]he physical assault that leads women to these shelters is merely the most immediate manifestation of the subordination they experience."[12] Thinking intersectionally about how certain policies and laws make immigrant women especially vulnerable to spousal violence helps us to consider what anthropologist and doctor Paul Farmer has called "structural violence," his term for those structures that constrain people's choices and make some people more at risk from violence, as well as from infectious diseases like tuberculosis and HIV/AIDS.[13]

I have taught Paul Farmer's work in women's, gender, and sexuality studies classes that deal explicitly with health, such as "Global Science/Women's Health," and in classes in which health is not the main topic, like "Feminist Theories." I always begin discussions of Farmer's work by asking students to consider his interdisciplinary approach to the topic of infectious disease. We discuss his case study method, in which he provides detailed descriptions of the complicated lives of individuals by placing their stories within a context that is both "geographically broad" and "historically deep."[14] Thus, in Farmer's work, a discussion of AIDS in Haiti begins with the building of dams in the central valley of the country that displaced large numbers of people from the land that had sustained them. The point is that one cannot understand the biological experience of HIV/AIDS in Haiti without also accounting for the environmental and social factors that bring people into contact with a virus. Farmer's interdisciplinary methodology is informed by his work as both clinician and anthropologist, and his biopsychosocial analysis combines clinical medicine, social theory, epidemiology, history, ethnography, and political economy. Influenced by liberation theology, Farmer describes his work as a "protest" against the fact that too many people are dying in the developing world from diseases that are treatable. He believes doctors should be advocates for the poor. Although he does not use the word *feminist* all that much, he believes empowering women is the key to better health outcomes for entire communities; and he often ends talks about AIDS by quoting a woman in Cange, Haiti, who told him, "You want to stop HIV in women? Give them jobs."[15] Like intersectionality, the concept of structural violence serves as a linchpin that helps us treat gender and illness together, and illness politics as sexual politics, and vice versa.

In a course like "Global Science/Women's Health," structural violence as linchpin also provides a means to move between scales, a process represented in the course title by the slash linking and separating the transnational event of global science with individual women's experiences of health and illness. Global Science/Women's Health is my more specific reformulation of the structure/agency debates in social theory in relation to both health and gender. We investigate how these macro and micro themes relate to each other through particular case studies. Our first series of case studies looks at various relationships within the institution of medicine: between doctors and patients, patients and nurses, doctors and nurses, etc., as presented in texts like *Wit* (both film and play) and Anne Fadiman's *The Spirit Catches You and You Fall Down*.[16] As we analyze these various relationships, we consider the way knowledge, power, and choice get expressed in and through such relationships. Our second series of case studies expands out from those particular relationships within medicine to larger global structures that affect the health of peoples throughout the world. In this section we explore bioethical issues and the relationship between health and human rights. Some of our organizing questions for the semester include the following: Why are certain treatable diseases not treated in certain parts of the world? What constitutes good healthcare? And how can we better deliver care throughout the world? The course is structured to move from the experience of the ill body in the world to the way global structures affect particular experiences and back again. Methodologically speaking, I want students to grapple with how best to move between different scales—that is, to consider how to situate, formally, an individual's story of health and illness within a larger transnational context.

Methods (Outside In/Inside Out)

I tend to thematize the relationship and movement between bodies and structures in all of my classes. Indeed, I would go so far as to say that this attempt to think bodies and structures together is a key aspect of both my teaching and my scholarship and, again, for me is an important way to link illness politics and sexual politics. As part of this process of thinking bodies and structures together, I look for and deploy various *method-images*—my term for the verbal and visual statements that help articulate through condensation the complexity of an object like illness as phenomenological experience and epidemiological event, as localized virus and global crisis, and as much more in between. As with my scholarship in general, in my teaching, I attempt to account for the often indirect and unstraightforward relationships between very big things (environments, economies, histories, structures, ideologies) and very small things (genes, cells, viruses, conversations, gestures, and feelings) and between very fast things (a flash, an instant, a glimpse, a glance) and very slow things (the interminable, the evolutionary, the gradual, the glacial).

Feminist philosopher Elizabeth Grosz's *Volatile Bodies* is one text that has helped me provide a philosophical grounding—or, in less foundationalist language, a point of departure—for the exploration of questions about the relationship between bodies and structures.[17] I teach *Volatile Bodies* as a model for an open—we might even say promiscuous—approach to feminist theories or theories of sexual difference. In introducing *Volatile Bodies*, I highlight the text's overall structure. The introduction, "Refiguring Bodies," and last chapter, "Sexed Bodies," bookend an argument that arrives at theories of sexual difference in a trajectory that is at once philosophical and political. The chapters in between are divided into two parts—"The Inside Out" and "The Outside In." I have always found that my tongue trips on the definite article *the*, mainly because how I read the structure of Grosz's analysis is less as demonstrating a schematic division between two different kinds of theories of sexual difference and subjectivity than as suggesting different ways of approaching the problem of subjectivity. My reading of Grosz's text is that it is concerned with *how* questions as much as or more than *what* questions, and the definite article is, therefore, contrary to the spirit of an argument that moves between inside out and outside in. Grosz explains that her book is a "kind of experiment in inversion," and this practice of inversion provides me with a useful method-image suggesting a conceptual and methodological strategy of turning things upside down, inside out, and/or outside in. Grosz ends her introduction by asking several key questions: "How, then, is a different analysis of the body to proceed? By what techniques and presumptions is a nondichotomous understanding of the body possible? . . . What criteria and goals should govern a feminist theoretical approach to concepts of the body?"[18] Her inverted approach seeks to avoid dichotomous logic by thinking about subjectivity as embodied and corporeality as psychical. For Grosz, we "must refuse singular models, models which are based on one type of body," and in the chapters that follow, she deploys a both/and model that explores both inside and outside and the interrelationship between inside and outside—that is, inside/out *and* outside/in.

Along with having students locate and define the key terms and method-images an author uses to frame her argument, I also always encourage them to consider the methods used to gather evidence to back up an argument. I want students to think through the multiple ways that knowledge is produced, and when they do their own research projects, I remind them that they too are knowledge producers. In many of my classes, I have students do interviews as one of their main assignments. For example, in my "Cultures of Disability" class, students conduct a one-hour interview with a person with a disability, a healthcare practitioner or educator who works with disabled people, or a person involved with the disability rights movement. Students may interview someone they know or do not know (see handout provided to students at end of chapter). I encourage them to think broadly about the topic of disability and to talk to friends and family about the task. I remind them that, in discussing disability in the class, we touch on almost every aspect of society: medicine, law, public policy, education, the arts. They read Harlan Lane's essay "Constructions of Deafness" and are, therefore, familiar with what Lane calls the "troubled-persons industry," a whole industry that has been "fueled by the disability construction of deafness." He points out the fact that "[a]ll these people and the facilities they command, their clinics, operating rooms, laboratories, classrooms, offices and shops, owe their livelihood or existence to deafness problems."[19] Lane's formulation about the multiple constructions of deafness, and the networks generated by these various constructions, helps students expand their perspective on who they might speak to about disability. I also encourage them to consider all the different experiences of illness and disability we have encountered in our readings, films, and discussions and note as well that there are also many disabling conditions that we have not discussed but would still be interesting to investigate in an interview. Students prepare questions in advance of the interview, which I review with them; they transcribe the interview and they also write a short reaction to the interview process. I find that students are often surprised by the experience of interviewing someone about a particular topic, so I require them to think and write about how the process went for them. They are prompted to consider questions like these: What went well or did not go so well? Did the interviewee talk about things that you expected them to talk about? Was it emotional? Was it different from reading about a topic? Why? Frequently, students express amazement at how much they learned from the interview and how it helped them to relate the course themes to real people in real situations.

If talking to real people in real situations about illness and disability is important, so too is an ability to analyze how illness and disability are portrayed in film and other media. I draw once again on my training, research, and teaching in women's, gender, and sexuality studies to provide tools to analyze ways of seeing illness and questions about what images and stories circulate in different kinds of media. John Berger's discussion of how images embody different ways of seeing men and women in society, what he calls the different social presence of women and men, can be extrapolated to help us interrogate disability and illness representations.[20] The sexual politics of representation provides a useful framework for considering the politics of representation in relation to illness and disability, or what we might call an ableist politics of representation. In my "Cultures of Disability" class, I have students write short reaction papers about how a particular film represents the experience of disability. I introduce our study of illness and disability representation with a brief summary of Berger's analysis of representation as an active process rather than simply a reflection of reality, as well as by introducing the concept of the "male gaze" as articulated in important texts of feminist film theory beginning with Laura Mulvey's classic "Visual Pleasure and Narrative Cinema,"[21] in order to consider whether and how disability films produce an ableist gaze. We explore how the category of disability intersects with other identity categories, including gender, race, class, and sexuality. We discuss how many films about illness and disability demonstrate what disability studies scholar Michael Gill has called *sexual ableism*, a term he glosses as "the system of imbuing sexuality with determinations of qualification to be sexual based on criteria of ability, morality, physicality, appearance, age, race, social acceptability, and gender conformity."[22] The concept of "sexual ableism" suggests the importance of thinking the experiences and events of sexuality and disability together as "especially dense transfer point[s] for relations of power," as Foucault would say.[23]

We watch both documentary and narrative films about illness and disability in class together. We discuss how gender, sexuality, and disability operate together in films like *The Sea Inside* (*Mar Adentro*), directed by Alejandro Amenábar and about the real-life story of Ramón Sampedro, a Spanish quadriplegic who fought for the right to die. The film garnered positive reviews from many critics and won the Academy Award for Best Foreign Language Film in 2005. I have found students generally like and are moved by the film; many of them identify with Ramón's view that, because of his quadriplegia, his life no longer has dignity; and they appreciate his rather bleak description of his predicament, "When you can't escape and you constantly rely on everyone else, you cry by smiling." Many students express sympathy for his wish that he had been killed by the diving accident that paralyzed him and support his passionate pursuit of the right to end his own life. I have students break into small groups to discuss several questions about the film: How do the characters in the film make sense of disability? For example, is it understood as stigmatizing, something to be overcome, a problem, an opportunity, as caused by God's wrath, or as a test from God, etc.? Who are the experts on disability? How is knowledge about disability acquired? Who is the presumed audience for the film: disabled people, non-disabled people, or both? How does identification work in the film? Who is the viewer meant to identify with?

What often becomes apparent is that identification works in an interesting way in this and other films about disability. While students often do identify with Ramón, the film structures this identification around a disidentification with disability formulated as his desire to escape his passivity. The film does offer alternative positions on Ramón's wish to die, yet problematically the disability rights perspective is offered by the unpleasant figure of Padre Francisco, who comes off as a moralistic scold. The scenes with Padre Francisco are played for laughs, but they demonstrate the difficulty of the two sides coming to an understanding. With a flight of stairs between them, an assistant serves as a go-between, running up and down the stairs, physically and emotionally burdened with the difficulty of conveying what each man has to say to the other. The two disabled men eventually jettison the go-between, shouting to each other, and this too suggests the difficulty—perhaps even insurmountability—of communicating their different positions.

Spaces (and Times)

With this image of difficulty in communicating across different spaces in mind, I want to conclude my discussion of ways to treat illness like gender as a multiple and complex object by briefly mentioning my experience teaching film to medical students as part of the then Medicine in Contemporary Society, now Medical Humanities, program at Stony Brook Medical School. Negotiating these multiple classroom genres—from freshman seminars to graduate seminars, from introductory classes to upper-level topics courses, from teaching medical students to teaching women's, gender, and sexuality studies majors—is one of the pleasures of teaching for me. I enjoy the challenge of different pedagogical genres and of modulating my syllabi and pedagogical practices for different kinds of students. Yet I have found that there are some constraints, both structural and in terms of student and institutional expectations, that make it difficult for me to approach teaching health humanities in the medical school in the way I do in women's, gender, and sexuality studies.

Often when we think about what humanities scholars bring to medicine, we think in spatial terms. Humanities scholars bring something—a text, method, interpretation—into medicine from the outside. These texts, methods, and interpretations are meant to expand the view of the medical student or practitioner; they provide a space for certain ways of thinking and feeling that might otherwise get lost in the stark realities of medical education and the clinic. What often remains unthought in this conjuncture between and among ethics, humanities, and medicine are questions about temporality. What if we considered not only those different texts, methods, and interpretations that humanities scholars bring to medicine but also different relationships to time? Or, to put it another way, what if we resisted that tried and true route for dismissing certain questions in medical education and practice—we do not have time—by asking what do humanities scholars have to teach us about time? What if we acted as if there was enough time?

This would require that we refuse the instrumental logic of medical education and practice. I have argued elsewhere for health and medical humanities to challenge rather than help promulgate the instrumentalization of care in medicine,[24] by creating other spaces and temporalities of medicine.[25] Lots of premed students take my classes, and I have been involved in curricular development in women's, gender, and sexuality studies at Stony Brook to create a track for majors in gender, sexuality, and public health. This track is ideal for students interested in further education and career opportunities in medicine and allied health fields. But why not also make it a track for students currently in medical school? Rather than, or along with, having me cross over to the medical school to teach occasional classes to medical students, why not have them come into another space (and time) for treating illness (and gender)—women's, gender, and sexuality studies?

PEDAGOGY EXERCISE SECTION

Cultures of Disability Interview Assignment

CLASS HANDOUT

Students will conduct a one-hour interview with a person with a disability, a healthcare practitioner or educator who works with disabled people, or a person involved with the disability rights movement. Students will transcribe the interview and write a two-page reaction to the interview process. Students must submit a proposal, which will include a brief description of the person to be interviewed, an explanation of why this person will be a good interviewee on the topic of disability, and ten questions for the interview.

Finding someone to interview: You may interview someone you know or do not know. If you do not already have someone in mind, think broadly about the topic of disability, and talk to friends and family about what you have to do. Remember that in discussing disability, we have touched on almost every aspect of society: medicine, law, public policy, education, the arts. In his essay "Constructions of Deafness," Harlan Lane shows us that a whole industry, which he calls the "troubled-persons industry," has been "fueled by the disability construction of deafness." He tells us that, "All these people and the facilities they command, their clinics, operating rooms, laboratories, classrooms, offices and shops, owe their livelihood or existence to deafness problems" (156).

Also think about all the different experiences we have encountered in our readings, films, and discussions: experiences of multiple sclerosis, HIV/AIDS, deafness, chronic fatigue syndrome, spinal cord injury, mental retardation, stroke, blindness. There are also many disabling conditions that we have not (or not yet) discussed but would still be interesting to investigate in an interview: cerebral palsy, Alzheimer's disease, sickle cell anemia, mental illness, cancer.

Arranging and conducting the interview: Interviewing is an excellent method for gathering evidence about a particular subject. It is also a serious endeavor that needs to be approached with care. When you are arranging to do the interview, you will need to get your interviewee's informed consent. This means you need to be sure to explain to the person you plan to interview that this is for a class at Stony Brook University, that you will be tape recording the interview, that you expect it to take about an hour, that you will transcribe the tape and turn it in to your professor to read. No one else will read the interview, and it will only be used as a class assignment and not as a part of a larger research project. Although some people you ask might not want to be interviewed, most students who have done interviews for my classes in the past have found most people ready and willing to talk.

Transcribing the interview: Remember that transcribing an hour of tape takes time. So, do not wait until the last minute to transcribe your interview. You will transcribe the tape word for word, but you do not need to transcribe verbal tics, like "ums" and "uhs." You will want to signal certain other sorts of responses in parentheses, like (laughter) or (long pause) or (crying). Be sure to read over your transcription to correct typos. You will want to use a consistent format throughout to signal who is speaking. For example:

> LD: When were you diagnosed with multiple sclerosis?
> NM: When I was twenty-nine years old.
> LD: How did you discover you had MS?

Your reaction to the interview process: I find that students are often surprised by the experience of interviewing someone about a particular topic. I want you to think and write about how the process went for you. What went well or did not go so well? Did the interviewee talk about things that you expected her or him to talk about? Was it emotional? Was it different from reading about a topic? Why?

Notes

1. Joan W. Scott, *Gender and the Politics of History* (New York: Columbia University Press, 1999), 10.

2. Victoria Hesford and Lisa Diedrich, "On 'The Evidence of Experience' and Its Reverberations: An Interview with Joan W. Scott," *Feminist Theory* 15, no. 2 (2014): 200.

3. I discuss this process in more detail in regard to the disease category hystero-epilepsy in "Illness as Assemblage: The Case of Hystero-epilepsy," *Body & Society* 21, no. 3 (September 2015): 66–90. In regard to social interactionist theories of the self in everyday life, see Erving Goffman, *The Presentation of Self in Everyday Life* (New York: Anchor, 1959); *Asylums: Essays on the Social Situation of Mental Patients and Other Inmates* (New York: Anchor, 1961); and *Stigma: Notes on the Management of Spoiled Identity* (New York: Anchor, 1963). For speech act theories and gender performativity, see Judith Butler, *Excitable Speech: A Politics of the Performative* (New York: Routledge, 1997).

4. *Biopsychosocial* is a term coined by George Engel in his influential article, "The Need for a New Medical Model: A Challenge for Biomedicine," *Science* 196 (1977): 129–36.

5. Michel Foucault, *The History of Madness*, trans. Jonathan Murphy and Jean Khalfa (1961; London and New York: Routledge, 2006), 80. Lynne Huffer's *Mad for Foucault: Rethinking the Foundations of Queer Theory* (New York: Columbia University Press, 2010), places Foucault's preoccupation with madness at the center of the formations of queer theory.

6. Michel Foucault, *The Archaeology of Knowledge and the Discourse on Language*, trans. A. M. Sheridan Smith (New York: Pantheon Books, 1972), 193.

7. Foucault, *History of Madness*, 82.

8. In my book *Indirect Action: Schizophrenia, Epilepsy, AIDS, and the Course of Health Activism* (Minneapolis and London: University of Minnesota Press, 2016), I take up these questions in more detail, exploring what I call the conjunction illness–thought–activism in the period before the emergence of AIDS and AIDS activism.

9. Kimberlé Crenshaw, "Mapping the Margins: Intersectionality, Identity Politics, and Violence against Women of Color," in *An Introduction to Women's Studies: Gender in a Transnational World*, 2nd ed., ed. Inderpal Grewal and Caren Kaplan (New York: McGraw-Hill, 2006), 200–206.

10. Crenshaw, "Mapping the Margins," 201.

11. Alice Walker, *Meridian* (New York: Washington Square Press, 1976), 25.

12. Crenshaw, "Mapping the Margins," 201.

13. Paul Farmer, *Pathologies of Power: Health, Human Rights, and the New War on the Poor* (Berkeley and London: University of California Press, 2003).

14. Ibid., 42.

15. Quoted in Tracy Kidder, *Mountains beyond Mountains: The Quest of Dr. Paul Farmer, a Man Who Would Cure the World* (New York: Random House, 2003), 199.

16. Margaret Edson, *Wit* (New York: Faber and Faber, 1999). The film *Wit* (2001) is directed by Mike Nichols. Anne Fadiman, *The Spirit Catches You and You Fall Down* (Farrar, Straus and Giroux, 1998).

17. Elizabeth Grosz, *Volatile Bodies: Toward a Corporeal Feminism* (Bloomington: Indiana University Press, 1994).

18. Ibid., 21.

19. Harlan Lane, "Constructions of Deafness," in *The Disability Studies Reader*, ed. Lennard J. Davis (New York and London: Routledge, 1997), 156.

20. John Berger, *Ways of Seeing* (1972; London: Penguin Books, 1990).

21. Laura Mulvey, "Visual Pleasure and Narrative Cinema," *Screen* 16, no. 3 (1975): 6–18.

22. Michael Gill, *Already Doing It: Intellectual Disability and Sexual Agency* (Minneapolis and London: University of Minnesota Press, 2015), 3.

23. Michel Foucault, *The History of Sexuality*, vol. 1, *An Introduction*, trans. Robert Hurley (New York: Vintage, 1978), 103.

24. In her ethnography of responses to the epidemics of tuberculosis and suicide among the Inuit in Canada in the twentieth and twenty-first centuries, Lisa Stevenson notes that, "Caring, as it becomes an operationalizable concept—something that can be measured and evaluated, fed through a system of best practices and evidence-based science—simultaneously becomes invested in a certain way of being in time. Caring now occurs on shifts, with most shifts between 9 and 5. It is no longer professional to care after hours. Implicit in the system of care is that the object of care must learn to mime the caregiver's attitudes to time and to care." *Life Beside Itself: Imagining Care in the Canadian Arctic* (Oakland: University of California Press, 2014), 134.

25. For more on compassion as the disciplinary imperative in the medical humanities, as well as a call for doing "critical medical studies," see my essay "Against Compassion: Attending to Histories and Methods in Medical Humanities; Or, Doing Critical Medical Studies," in *Narrative Matters in Medical Contexts across Disciplines*, ed. Franziska Gygax and Miriam Locher (Amsterdam, The Netherlands: John Benjamins Publishing, 2015), 167–82.

Works Cited

Berger, John. *Ways of Seeing*. London: Penguin Books, 1990. First published 1972.

Butler, Judith. *Excitable Speech: A Politics of the Performative*. New York: Routledge, 1997.

Crenshaw, Kimberlé. "Mapping the Margins: Intersectionality, Identity Politics, and Violence against Women of Color." In *An Introduction to Women's Studies: Gender in a Transnational World*, 2nd ed., edited by Inderpal Grewal and Caren Kaplan, 200–206. New York: McGraw-Hill, 2006.

Diedrich, Lisa. "Against Compassion: Attending to Histories and Methods in Medical Humanities; Or, Doing Critical Medical Studies." In *Narrative Matters in Medical Contexts across Disciplines*, edited by Franziska Gygax and Miriam Locher, 167–82. Amsterdam, The Netherlands: John Benjamins Publishing, 2015.

Diedrich, Lisa. "Illness as Assemblage: The Case of Hystero-epilepsy." *Body & Society* 21, no. 3 (September 2015): 66–90.

Diedrich, Lisa. *Indirect Action: Schizophrenia, Epilepsy, AIDS, and the Course of Health Activism*. Minneapolis and London: University of Minnesota Press, 2016.

Edson, Margaret. *Wit*. New York: Faber and Faber, 1999.

Engel, George. "The Need for a New Medical Model: A Challenge for Biomedicine." *Science* 196 (1977): 129–36.

Fadiman, Anne. *The Spirit Catches You and You Fall Down*. New York: Farrar, Straus and Giroux, 1998.

Farmer, Paul. *Pathologies of Power: Health, Human Rights, and the New War on the Poor*. Berkeley and London: University of California Press, 2003.

Foucault, Michel. *The Archaeology of Knowledge and the Discourse on Language*. Translated by A. M. Sheridan Smith. New York: Pantheon Books, 1972.

Foucault, Michel. *The History of Madness*. Translated by Jonathan Murphy and Jean Khalfa. London and New York: Routledge, 2006. First published 1961.

Foucault, Michel. *The History of Sexuality*. Vol. 1, *An Introduction*. Translated by Robert Hurley. New York: Vintage, 1978.

Gill, Michael. *Already Doing It: Intellectual Disability and Sexual Agency*. Minneapolis and London: University of Minnesota Press, 2015.

Goffman, Erving. *Asylums: Essays on the Social Situation of Mental Patients and Other Inmates*. New York: Anchor, 1961.

Goffman, Erving. *Stigma: Notes on the Management of Spoiled Identity*. New York: Anchor, 1963.

Goffman, Erving. *The Presentation of Self in Everyday Life*. New York: Anchor, 1959.

Grosz, Elizabeth. *Volatile Bodies: Toward a Corporeal Feminism*. Bloomington: Indiana University Press, 1994.

Hesford, Victoria, and Lisa Diedrich. "On 'The Evidence of Experience' and Its Reverberations: An Interview with Joan W. Scott." *Feminist Theory* 15, no. 2 (2014): 197–207.

Huffer, Lynne. *Mad for Foucault: Rethinking the Foundations of Queer Theory*. New York: Columbia University Press, 2010.

Kidder, Tracy. *Mountains beyond Mountains: The Quest of Dr. Paul Farmer, a Man Who Would Cure the World*. New York: Random House, 2003.

Lane, Harlan. "Constructions of Deafness." In *The Disability Studies Reader*, edited by Lennard J. Davis, 153–71. New York and London: Routledge, 1997.

Mulvey, Laura. "Visual Pleasure and Narrative Cinema." *Screen* 16, no. 3 (1975): 6–18.

Scott, Joan W. *Gender and the Politics of History*. New York: Columbia University Press, 1999.

Stevenson, Lisa. *Life Beside Itself: Imagining Care in the Canadian Arctic*. Oakland: University of California Press, 2014.

Walker, Alice. *Meridian*. New York: Washington Square Press, 1976.

9

Literacy Beyond the Single Story

TEACHING ABOUT CLASS IN THE HEALTH HUMANITIES

Michael Blackie, Delese Wear, and Joseph Zarconi

> One difficulty in talking about class is that the word means different things to different people. Class is rank, it is tribe, it is culture and taste. It is attitudes and assumptions, a source of identity, a system of exclusion. To some, it is just money. It is an accident of birth that influences the outcome of a life. Some Americans barely notice it; others feel its weight in powerful ways.
>
> Scott and Leonhardt[1]

Class is a confused and confusing concept, especially in the United States. Discuss class in a health humanities classroom or a health professions educational setting and this confusion can lead to heated and unproductive stalemates. Simply put, talking about class can often be distressing to students and educators alike as honest and open conversations become hampered by defensiveness and the discomforts associated with being perceived as negatively biased toward particular groups of people. This chapter presents three interpretive lenses through which to lead productive discussions about class issues related to healthcare in the health humanities classroom in ways that might overcome many of those sensitivities.

Healthcare professionals do not often acknowledge the formative role social class plays in shaping individuals. Health professions education may emphasize to its students the importance of considering a patient's ethnicity, race, or gender in their practices, often through cultural competency initiatives or curricula. Class is, however, a characteristic largely neglected, or it is collapsed into the broader terminology of socioeconomic status. Although a health professional's understanding of a patient's socioeconomic status is essential, we believe that the specificities of class get lost in this more general term. Perhaps because the United States is "a nation whose rhetoric and mythology are predicated on the twin discourses of classlessness and upward mobility,"[2] students and their educators in the health professions often struggle with the category of class as an important determinant of health because it does not square with their personal and familial mythologies.

Indeed, in our own classrooms, we have experienced formative resistance from students at the mere suggestion that their social class may have put them at an advantage over students from less affluent households and communities. They have, they argue, worked hard to get where they are. Upward mobility is seen as attainable by anyone who is willing to put in the effort. When a discussion of class reaches this point, as so often happens, moving it forward productively becomes challenging. To acknowledge the existence of class and its power to structure individuals and communities is not to deny the efforts of medical students who have worked hard to get where they are. Their efforts are, in fact, beside the point.

In what follows, we offer three interpretive lenses through which to guide discussions of class beyond this impasse so that students might come to recognize that achieving upward mobility is not a universal story. The first lens relies heavily on what is known as *attributions for poverty* as they pertain to class and beliefs about upward mobility. The second explores *single-story* thinking and its power to lead to prejudicial judgments regarding class. And the third draws from the critical feminist term *intersectionality* to illustrate the complicated ways in which class, as an identity, intersects with other categories. After describing these three lenses, we turn to the film *Precious*, based on Sapphire's novel *Push*, as a critical text for demonstrating how health humanities and health professions educators can lead productive discussions about class, in general, and about upward mobility, in particular.

Precious tells the story of Claireece Precious Jones, a sixteen-year-old African American woman living in Harlem during the late 1980s. When the film begins, she is pregnant with her second child, both children the product of incest perpetrated by her father. Mary, Precious's mother, is verbally, physically, and sexually violent toward her daughter. Together, Precious and her mother live in squalid public housing. Precious's commitment to becoming literate, despite her mother's ridicule of education in favor of welfare dependence, is the storyline in the film that will be the primary focus of our discussion. This "literacy acquisition narrative," as one insightful scholar calls Precious's quest to live a life markedly different from the one in which she was born,[3] not only documents the negative effects of illiteracy on an individual and a community but also provides health humanities scholars with an opportunity to highlight for their students the costs of their own inability to consider upward mobility beyond the limited scope of the stories they know and tell about it. Indeed, we ultimately argue for the need to address a kind of "illiteracy" in the health professions themselves regarding class.

Attributions for Poverty

Quite often, class is seen as the product of poverty, on the one hand, and as a result of not working hard enough to improve one's station in life, on the other. Those who hold to the latter interpretation draw from a single story of a universal upward mobility. Such a single story's simplicity denies the lived experiences of individuals living in poverty. Physician David Hilfiker bluntly addresses this denial among medical professionals: "Medical students (and most physicians) don't know about the desperation [of the poor] . . . because myths keep affluent people from knowing the burdens under which the poor labor."[4] Such myths are persistent despite the fact that volumes have been written about poverty, illuminating it from multiple disciplines across time, culture, and geography and attempting to answer the perennial questions surrounding causation: why does poverty exist, and why do some people remain in poverty? These explanations are often referred to as *attributions for poverty*,[5] a theoretical framework with tremendous moral and practical implications for how a culture views and treats its members who live in poverty.

What meanings do these explanations have for healthcare providers, in general, and for physicians, in particular? Medical schools certainly do not ignore poverty—the curriculum quite often includes lectures about the social determinants of health as soon as students begin their training. Students learn to take a "social" history; some spend time in free clinics and ambulatory sites caring for economically disadvantaged persons. Often in poor urban neighborhoods, large teaching hospitals offer up poor patients to students' learning and practice. In short, students spend a lot of time with poor patients in clinical settings, but therein lies the problem: students spend this time in settings far removed from the everydayness of living in poverty, observing in the clinical setting the *effects* of poverty in their patients rather than witnessing and comprehending their patients' everyday *experiences* of poverty.

We need to be clear about how we use the terms *poor* and *poverty*. The latter is a term with clear referents. Each year the US government's Health and Human Services Department provides the Annual Update of the HHS Poverty Guidelines, a data-rich document that denotes actual incomes of individuals and families of particular sizes.[6] *Poor*, or specifically, *the poor*, is a far more complex term that involves not just income but the effects of income, including housing, mobility, education, employment, childcare, and food security, along with more intangible effects such as expectations and aspirations. Race, gender, age, and geographic setting also complicate conceptions of "the poor." Because of space restrictions, however, we use generalities even as we recognize the limitations of doing so in this initial discussion of poverty and "the poor."

More than 40 years ago, in his landmark work, *Subordinating the Poor: Welfare and American Beliefs*,[7] sociologist and social theorist Joe Feagin developed an attributions for poverty framework still widely used today. The framework offers two prevailing attributions for poverty. In one, poverty is seen as the result of characteristics of individuals (i.e., their character traits, behaviors, personal efforts, values, and beliefs). In the other, poverty is seen as the result of structures (i.e., lack of community resources, poor schools/infrastructure, low wages, lack of jobs/job training, and other institutional barriers). A third category, infrequently invoked, involves fatalistic beliefs whereby poverty is simply explained by luck, fate, illness, and the like.

The individual characteristics viewpoint often blames the poor for their own poverty, supported by the belief that if only the poor would try harder (e.g., get more education, become more motivated, make better decisions, lose bad habits), they could work their way out of poverty, a view often grounded squarely in the Protestant work ethic.[8] While the research on religiosity and attributions for poverty is scant, Matthew Hunt's study showed that Catholics and Protestants, "due to their dominant religious status in the U.S., were found to be more supportive of individualistic explanations while less dominant religions such as Judaism, displayed more support for structural explanations."[9] Moreover, such beliefs are also tied to political party affiliation in the United States, whereby Republicans are less likely to acknowledge how external structures influence socioeconomic status than Democrats,[10] beliefs that also leak over into explanations for health status.

Structural explanations for poverty or lower social class focus on the cultural and physical environments in which individuals live and how these environments produce stigma. If individuals are not solely responsible for their class status, then, as Jonathan Metzl and Helena Hansen contend, explanations should be sought by looking critically at "the organization of institutions and policies, as well as of neighborhoods and cities"[11] that produce poverty. By looking at structural forces, healthcare professionals can better appreciate how they shape particular lives, despite individuals' best efforts to get ahead. Accordingly, "[M]edical education needs to more systematically train healthcare professionals to think about how such variables as race, class, gender, and ethnicity are shaped both by the interactions of two persons in a room, and by the larger structural contexts in which their interactions take place."[12]

How does all of this relate to medical education? One place to start is with the economic profile of medical students' families in the United States, which remains quite different from that of the mainstream population and markedly different from many of the patients students face in hospital settings. Sixty-four percent of US medical students come from families whose income is $100,000 or more and twenty-two percent from families whose income is $250,000 dollars or more.[13] Notably, fewer than seven percent come from families earning below $25,000. Moreover, most academic medical centers are located in urban settings so that a large majority of students learn medicine on patients with significant social and economic disadvantages and profound health problems that cannot be readily "fixed." It falls, then, to medical education to assist students in developing a fuller understanding of how their own beliefs and biases may be influenced by their wholly different and particular life circumstances, as well as to offer relevant knowledge and skills important to provide care to economically disadvantaged patients from communities that contain little social support and often an abundance of forces that work *against* health and well-being.

While a student at Warren Alpert Medical School of Brown University, Katherine Brooks argued that the medical curriculum is woefully inadequate regarding disparities in health. She refers to it as a *silent curriculum*, one that does not speak directly to the critical health needs of the communities where "Trayvon Martin lost his life, Michael Brown was left to die in the streets of Ferguson, Missouri, and Eric Garner was choked by officers as he repeated 11 times that he could not breathe."[14] Where is a critical examination of these events in the medical curriculum, she wonders, events that characterize the class bias and racism influencing the health of communities? She does not suggest that health disparities are absent in the curriculum—indeed, she writes of being "inundated with lecture PowerPoint slides" on population health, social determinants of health, and other various formats. But that same curriculum rarely focuses on the forces, from individual biases to the innumerable societal, cultural, legal, political, economic, and medical structures, that intersect and greatly influence health outcomes.

Again, David Hilfiker's experience in what he calls poverty medicine is instructive as he urges medical students to "get into a one-to-one relationship with at least one very poor person. I don't care how you do it. It doesn't matter whether it's a helping relationship or what. And have a way to reflect upon it. That is a way to start, then be open to where that leads you."[15] Forming such relationships would, of course, be ideal; but in the absence of experiencing poverty firsthand, narrative inquiry can inch students toward a more abundant and profound understanding of the "burdens of the poor" and of lives so different from their own. The film *Precious*, more specifically Precious's "literacy acquisition narrative," offers a useful example of what healthcare providers and their patients gain when they open themselves to such stories.

Single-Story Thinking

As healthcare professionals and health professions learners explore the stories of patients whose life experiences are substantially different from their own, the narrow narratives they may have constructed to understand such patients can be harmful in their attempts to *care* for them. This is especially true if the narratives they have constructed are what novelist Chimamanda Ngozi Adichie describes as dangerous "single stories." In her TED talk entitled "The Danger of a Single Story,"[16] Adichie describes numerous examples of how we often have single stories of people who are substantially different from ourselves—single stories that are the result of our own limited understanding and knowledge of the complex and varied stories that construct any such individual. Describing her growing up in a middle-class Nigerian family, Adichie relates that they, like many other such families, had live-in domestic help who often came from poor villages nearby. When she was eight, a new houseboy, Fide, arrived, whom her mother described to her as "very poor," telling her that "people like Fide's family have nothing." The Adichie family often sent food and clothing to the boy's family. On a visit to Fide's village, the boy's mother showed Adichie a beautiful basket Fide's brother had made from dyed raffia. Adichie found its beauty startling, confessing that she had never imagined that very poor people like Fide's family could, in fact, create something so beautiful. Since all she had ever heard about them was how poor they were, she had constructed a "single story" of them, a story of poverty and a story that had prevented her from being able to imagine them as artful or creative beings. Further, that story had led her to feel nothing more than "enormous pity" for them.

Adichie goes on to describe a number of ways that she, having arrived in America to attend Drexel University, was imagined by Americans through a single story of Africa and its people—a story of catastrophe that led them to default to the same sort of "well-meaning pity" that she had felt for Fide and his family. Her American college roommate was surprised that Adichie could operate a stove or that she enjoyed music by Mariah Carey and so was not familiar only with the "tribal music" of her homeland. She posits that the single stories that had been constructed about her derived from Western literature, writing that represents "a tradition of telling African stories that depict Africa as a place of negatives, of difference, of darkness."

One of us (J.Z.) has shared with medical students the experience of caring for an older African American man at a local free clinic. Patients who presented at this clinic could only qualify to be seen if they met specific poverty-level conditions, so this man qualified as "poor." His primary concern was his severely elevated blood pressure. In discussing how we would address this concern, I worked especially hard to speak slowly and to use language that a grade school child could understand. At one point during the encounter, well into my discussion about his blood pressure problem, the patient suddenly erupted with laughter, which took me by surprise. Seeing my reaction, he then pointed out, laughing again, some of the words and phrases I had used. "Did you actually say that to me," he asked, "that 'folks like me' thing?" What came next was an articulate and, in fact, scholarly diatribe about how white doctors speak to black patients, citing evidence published in a literature with which he was clearly quite familiar. What I came to learn as he continued to "school" me was that he was a retired college professor who had authored a number of scholarly articles and other texts. Through a number of unfortunate circumstances beyond his control, he found himself without financial resources—he was now "poor." Discovering the intellectual prowess of my free clinic patient was as startling to me as the raffia basket had been to Adichie. And like Adichie, upon reflection, I could not have been more ashamed of myself. Clearly, I had constructed a single story of poor African Americans as uneducated, unsophisticated people whose ignorance would have to be overcome by a talented white physician.

Adichie argues that such single-story thinking has important negative consequences. These stories cause us to "overlook the many other stories" that make a person who she or he is. These stories create stereotypes, and as Adichie points out, "the problem with stereotypes is not that they are untrue, but that they are incomplete. They make one story become the only story." Perhaps the most concerning consequence is that single stories rob people of their dignity. They make "our recognition of our equal humanity difficult," emphasizing our differences rather than our similarities and allowing "no possibility of a connection as human equals." The implications of such failed connections in the healing professions are obvious and profound. Finally, Adichie suggests that when we see others through single stories, we are wielding a kind of power about which we must be fully conscious. She references an Igbo word, *nkali*, which "loosely translates to 'to be greater than another.'" Stories are defined, in her view, "by the principle of nkali: How they are told, who tells them, when they're told, how many stories are told, are really dependent on power."

Raising health professions learners' consciousness about the dangers of single-story thinking, and of their own single stories about people wholly different from themselves, can broaden their way of seeing people they are called to serve. Healthcare professionals learn and propagate single stories about certain types of patients, and the assumptions made from those stories can lead to harm in their care. Efforts to engage learners in meaningful reflection on the dangers of single-story thinking can nurture efforts to see others beyond the confines of such thinking and give them hope for people like Precious, who is much more than simply a poor black woman or a person of a certain class.

Intersectionality

One formidable danger that arises in discussions of class is the tendency to see the characteristic as monolithic—as somehow functioning as a single determinant of the behavior of particular individuals within a group or demographic and as perceived by individuals outside of that group. Class, like other "markers" of identity, intersects with a number of other influential factors, including race, gender, income, and residence, among others. One is never just lower class without also being female or lesbian, African American or white.

Intersectionality describes how race, gender, class, age, and other identities intersect or overlap and how discrimination and bias occur across any number of these identities. For example, knowing that a woman is black tells only one part of the story of the discrimination she faces; one must also consider her sexual identity, her level of education, her socioeconomic status, and her age, among other variables, to understand more broadly the nature of that discrimination. Crenshaw recently commented on intersectionality a quarter century after introducing it:

> Originally articulated on behalf of black women, the term brought to light the invisibility of many constituents within groups that claim them as members, but often fail to represent them. Intersectional erasures are not exclusive to black women. People of color within LGBTQ movements; girls of color in the fight against the school-to-prison pipeline; women within immigration movements; trans women within feminist movements; and people with disabilities fighting police abuse—all face vulnerabilities that reflect the intersections of racism, sexism, class oppression, transphobia, able-ism and more. Intersectionality has given many advocates a way to frame their circumstances and to fight for their visibility and inclusion.[17]

For any health professions learner, understanding the implications of intersectionality in patient care is critically important given the categorical thinking—even single-story thinking—so prevalent across the curriculum. Educators have begun to recognize the value of teaching about intersectionality in health professions education. As Eckstrand and colleagues remind us, "There is value in focusing on singular populations and creating macroscopic frameworks to guide diversity and inclusion initiatives; however, these approaches may not always elucidate the complexities that arise at the intersection between multiple identities and life experiences."[18]

In order to assist students' appreciation of intersectionality, a useful first exercise is to ask them to name the identities that comprise them and the ways these identities intersect. Does each of the identities work in mutually supportive ways, or are there aspects of their lives that are in conflict in particular situations or places? The ultimate goal of this exercise is for students to begin to recognize how their own identities—as medical or nursing students, as Southeast Asian or Midwestern, as bilingual or immigrant, as socially progressive or religiously conservative, for example—intersect in different ways and in different situations depending on circumstances often beyond their immediate control. Ideally, through such an exercise students begin to recognize how "different types of discrimination intersect to oppress people in multiple and simultaneous ways, contributing to social inequality and systemic injustice."[19]

After such an initial exercise, students may be encouraged to discuss how a focus on a single "identity" or story about that identity may lead to oversimplification in terms of how they themselves might be understood. To move the discussion toward an appreciation of the complexities and structural inequalities engendered when identities intersect, students can then be guided through an exercise in which they "ask the other question," a mode of inquiry developed by legal scholar Mari Matsuda:

> When I see something that looks racist, I ask, "Where is the patriarchy in this?" When I see something that looks sexist, I ask, "Where is the heterosexism in this?" When I see something that looks homophobic, I ask, "Where are the class interests in this?"[20]

By asking "the other question," students are invited to see how "identity is experienced not as composed of discrete attributes but as a subjective, even fragmented, set of dynamics."[21]

We recognize that leading such discussions can be tricky because they ask participants to reflect critically on fundamental aspects of their own identities. But this initial work of paying attention to intersectionality, as Crenshaw argues, "highlights the need to account for multiple grounds of identity when considering how the social world is constructed."[22] Such accounting, though, can feel too personal for many students (and educators); and, as a consequence, discussions of these issues can stall or return to defensive posturing on the part of participants. Therefore, after time spent discussing the three approaches, we suggest turning to Lee Daniels's 2009 film *Precious* as a critical text for such analysis.[23] This film offers rich material for sharpening students' appreciation for how attributions for poverty, the dangers of the single story, and the existence of intersectionality inform and shape perceptions of class and upward mobility and hopefully for fostering strategies to overcome these narrow ways of seeing others.

Preliminary Strategies for Discussing *Precious*

Precious is a difficult film to watch, let alone discuss. The history of its reception documents the buttons it pushes. First-time viewers—and a majority of its critics—tend to focus almost exclusively on the film's scenes of violence and poverty—the ugly "truth" about the poor, generally, and African Americans, specifically. Educators should be prepared for strong responses from students. As an example, during a discussion of the film one of our students asked, "Why did you do that to me?" She was responding to having watched a film that left her feeling traumatized and overwhelmed. It is important for educators to anticipate such responses and to know in advance of screening the film that critical responses to *Precious* found it in equal measure "brazenly racist"[24] and "a realistic and therapeutic portrayal."[25] Discussions of *Precious* are likely to oscillate between these two different points of view. Indeed, as African American social critic Darryl Lorenzo Wellington put it, "*Precious* is loaded material, a difficult movie to judge fairly in a society with so many unresolved issues of race and racial stereotypes; poverty and images of poverty; sexism, sexual abuse, and silence."[26]

One way to guide productive discussions, then, is to begin with the very problematic images to which Wellington alludes. Students can be asked to identify two or three scenes in *Precious* that most troubled them, followed by an exploration of why. Students should be encouraged to draw attention to stereotypical representations, to voice their concerns for how Precious, the people in her life, and the world in which she lives are depicted. Only with such initial discussions, we argue, can the critical work of unpacking stereotypes begin, to appreciate how these stereotypes function through single-story thinking and how they intersect with other stereotypes.

Discussing *Precious* Using the Three Interpretive Lenses

After a preliminary discussion of *Precious*, we recommend reviewing with students the three interpretive lenses—attributions for poverty, the dangers of a single story, and intersectionality—before applying them to the film. Although we provide an outline for how to structure discussions, it is only a suggestion. The main objective should be guiding students toward an examination of class and upward mobility through the hard work Precious devotes to learning to read and write.

Despite the tendency to reduce the film to the tribulations of urban life in New York City—a very single-story way of reading it and what more than one critic called "poverty porn"[27]—director Lee Daniels's cinematic treatment of Sapphire's novel insists on the presence of other narratives that compete with such reductive interpretations. Throughout the film, Daniels presents two competing narrative forms: gritty realism and fantasy. Attention paid to the relationship between these two different forms of storytelling highlights Precious's role in structuring each one as her own acquisition of literacy increases, thereby complicating attempts to view class, and even more so poverty, through a single story, like those described by attributions for poverty.

Perhaps because *Precious* depicts the violence experienced by its central character in such a brutally graphic manner, viewers focus much less on the fantasy narrative Daniels deploys in order to tell all of the stories that constitute Precious. Paying attention to these other stories is perhaps the most useful strategy a viewer can employ if one is to see Precious as more than simply the violence that surrounds and befalls her. Indeed, the film presents in brutal unflinching realism the sexual violence and incest, child abuse and neglect, poverty, and corruption plaguing Precious's life. But through Precious's fantasy narratives, Daniels also invites viewers to see that same world through the eyes of a teenager struggling to make sense of life beyond its material reality and, most importantly, imagine a better future for herself and her children.

Students should be encouraged to examine how these two narrative forms are in conflict and therefore resist the reductive nature of single-story readings. Guiding questions for discussion could include the following:

- How do the two narratives provide opposing versions of Precious's life?
- In what ways does the fantasy narrative change as Precious becomes more literate?
- How does her understanding of her situation, as told through the gritty realism form of narrative, begin to change as she learns to express herself in writing?

As one moves through these questions with students, attention can be drawn to how Precious is learning to tell a different story about her life and especially her future. Equally important is to also point out the ever-present social and structural factors threatening to slow, if not stop, that progress.

To explore the powerful nature of Precious's intersecting identities, we suggest introducing into the discussion the following description of Precious by Sapphire, the author of the novel adapted for the film: "I wanted to show that this girl is locked out through literacy. She's locked out by her physical appearance. She's locked out by her class, and she's locked out by her color."[28] As Sapphire makes clear, no single factor or characteristic explains Precious's situation. To simply focus on one of them is to oversimplify the complexities of her lived experience. Indeed, Sapphire draws attention to Precious's weight, gender, color, class, and illiteracy, each one influencing how others see and respond to her.

Conclusion

To attempt to understand more fully the lived experiences of patients like Precious and to work toward promoting their health and well-being, a kind of literacy is needed, a literacy that sees beyond the single story of class to the myriad forces and identities intersecting with it. This engagement asks health professionals to consider the structural factors that influence and often determine the trajectories of patients' lives, often marked by "systemic institutional stigmatization and marginalization."[29] Thus, as health humanities educators we should provide students with the means to look for these structural aspects of patients' stories. This involves both the individual nature of the doctor–patient relationship and all that is gleaned therein, then moving on to examine "the complex relationships between [that patient's] clinical symptoms and social, political, and economic systems."[30]

With both Precious and clinical encounters of all kinds, the ultimate objective is not to draw attention to students' own "illiteracy" regarding unequal playing fields. Rather, it is to demonstrate how "reading" class and upward mobility through these interpretive lenses can make possible more compassionate and realistic perceptions of social status and class.

Notes

1. Janny Scott and David Leonhardt, "Shadowy Lines that Still Divide," *New York Times*, May 15, 2005, accessed August 29, 2016, http://www.nytimes.com/2005/05/15/us/class/shadowy-lines-that-still-divide.html?_r=0.

2. Mary Rizzo, "Teaching Class in the Classroom," *Transformations* 14 (2003): 127–38.

3. Mia Mask, "The Precarious Politics of *Precious*: A Close Reading of a Cinematic Text," *Black Camera: An International Film Journal* 4 (2012): 96–116.

4. David Hilfiker, "From the Victim's Point of View," *Journal of Medical Humanities* 22 (2001): 17–31.

5. Joe R. Feagin, *Subordinating the Poor: Welfare and American Beliefs* (New York: Charles Scribner's Sons, 1975).

6. Health and Human Services Department, "Annual Update of the HHS Poverty Guidelines," *Federal Register*, January 25, 2016, accessed August 29, 2016, https://www.federalregister.gov/articles/2016/01/25/2016-01450/annual-update-of-the-hhs-poverty-guidelines.

7. Feagin, *Subordinating the Poor*.

8. Catherine Cozzarelli, Anna V. Wilkinson, and Michael J. Tagler, "Attitudes toward the Poor and Attributions for Poverty," *Journal of Social Issues* 57 (2001): 201–27.

9. Matthew O. Hunt, "Religion, Race/Ethnicity, and Beliefs about Poverty," *Social Science Quarterly* 83 (2002): 810–31.

10. James R. Kluegal and Eliot R. Smith, *Beliefs about Inequality: Americans' Views of What Is and What Ought to Be* (New York: Aldine de Gruyter, 1986); Linda J. Skitka et al., "Dispositions, Scripts, or Motivated Correction? Understanding Ideological Differences in Explanations for Social Problems," *Journal of Personality and Social Psychology* 83 (2002): 470–87; Sarah E. Gollust, Paula M. Lantz, and Peter A. Ubel, "The Polarizing Effects of News Media Messages about the Social Determinants of Health," *American Journal of Public Health* 89 (2009): 2160–67.

11. Jonathan Metzl and Helena Hansen, "Structural Competency: Theorizing a New Medical Engagement with Stigma and Inequality," *Social Science and Medicine* 103 (2014): 126–33.

12. Ibid.

13. Association of American Medical Colleges, "Matriculating Student Questionnaire," accessed August 29, 2016, https://www.aamc.org/data/msq/.

14. Katherine C. Brooks, "A Silent Curriculum," *JAMA* 313 (2015): 1909–10.

15. David Hilfiker, "Facing Brokenness," *Second Opinion* 11 (1990): 93–101.

16. Chimamanda N. Adichie, "The Danger of a Single Story," TED (video), July 2009, accessed September 18, 2016, http://www.ted.com/talks/lang/eng/chimamanda_adichie_the_danger_of_a_single_story.html.

17. Kimberlé Crenshaw, "Why Intersectionality Can't Wait," *Washington Post*, September 24, 2015, accessed August 29, 2016, https://www.washingtonpost.com/news/in-theory/wp/2015/09/24/why-intersectionality-cant-wait/?utm_term=.e1ed2589465a.

18. Kristen Eckstrand et al., "The Priority of Intersectionality in Academic Medicine," *Academic Medicine* 91 (2016): 904–907.

19. Catherine Butler, "Intersectionality in Family Therapy Training: Inviting Students to Embrace the Complexities of Lived Experience," *Journal of Family Therapy* 37 (2015): 583–89.

20. Mari Matsuda, "Beside My Sister, Facing the Enemy: Legal Theory out of Coalition," *Stanford Law Review* 43 (1991): 1183–92.

21. Cynthia Levine-Rasky, "Intersectionality Theory Applied to Whiteness and Middle-Classness," *Social Identities* 17 (2011): 239–53.

22. Kimberlé Crenshaw, "Mapping the Margins: Intersectionality, Identity Politics, and Violence against Women of Color," *Stanford Law Review* 43 (1991): 1241–99.

23. Lee Daniels (director), *Precious* (Santa Monica, CA: Lionsgate, 2009).

24. Armond White, "Pride and Precious," *Hip-Hop and Politics* (blog), November 19, 2009, accessed August 29, 2016, http://hiphopandpolitics.com/2009/11/19/armond-white-precious-is-the-most-damaging-film-to-the-black-image-since-birth-of-a-nation/.

25. Mask, "Precarious Politics."

26. Darryl Lorenzo Wellington, "Sex, Race, and *Precious*," *Dissent*, March 8, 2010, accessed September 19, 2016, https://www.dissentmagazine.org/online_articles/sex-race-and-precious.

27. Aisha S. Durham, "Precious in the Classroom," *New Black Magazine,* December 12, 2009, accessed September 19, 2016, www.thenewblackmagazine.com/view.aspx?index=2185; Jim Downs, "Are We All Precious?" *Chronicle of Higher Education,* December 13, 2009, accessed September 19, 2016, http://chronicle.com/article/Are-We-All-Precious-/49458/.

28. NPR, "Sapphire's Story: How 'Push' became 'Precious,'" *All Things Considered*, November 6, 2009, accessed September 19, 2016, http://www.npr.org/templates/story/story.php?storyId=120176695.

29. Gollust, Lantz, and Ubel, "The Polarizing Effects."

30. Ibid.

Works Cited

Adichie, Chimamanda N. "The Danger of a Single Story." TED (video), July 2009. Accessed September 18, 2016. http://www.ted.com/talks/lang/eng/chimamanda_adichie_the_danger_of_a_single_story.html.

Association of American Medical Colleges. "Matriculating Student Questionnaire." Accessed August 29, 2016, https://www.aamc.org/data/msq/.

Brooks, Katherine C. "A Silent Curriculum." *JAMA* 313 (2015): 1909–10.

Butler, Catherine. "Intersectionality in Family Therapy Training: Inviting Students to Embrace the Complexities of Lived Experience." *Journal of Family Therapy* 37 (2015): 583–89.

Cozzarelli, Catherine, Anna V. Wilkinson, and Michael J. Tagler. "Attitudes toward the Poor and Attributions for Poverty." *Journal of Social Issues* 57 (2001): 201–27.

Crenshaw, Kimberlé. "Mapping the Margins: Intersectionality, Identity Politics, and Violence against Women of Color." *Stanford Law Review* 43 (1991): 1241–99.

Crenshaw, Kimberlé. "Why Intersectionality Can't Wait." *Washington Post*, September 24, 2015. Accessed August 29, 2016. https://www.washingtonpost.com/news/in-theory/wp/2015/09/24/why-intersectionality-cant-wait/?utm_term=.e1ed2589465a.

Daniels, Lee (director). *Precious*. Santa Monica, CA: Lionsgate, 2009.

Downs, Jim. "Are We All Precious?" *Chronicle of Higher Education*, December 13, 2009. Accessed September 19, 2016. http://chronicle.com/article/Are-We-All-Precious-/49458/.

Durham, Aisha S. "Precious in the Classroom." *New Black Magazine*, December 12, 2009. Accessed September 19, 2016. www.thenewblackmagazine.com/view.aspx?index=2185.

Eckstrand, Kristen, Jennifer Eliason, Tiffani St. Cloud, and Jennifer Potter. "The Priority of Intersectionality in Academic Medicine." *Academic Medicine* 91 (2016): 904–907.

Feagin, Joe R. *Subordinating the Poor: Welfare and American Beliefs*. New York: Charles Scribner's Sons, 1975.

Gollust, Sarah E., Paula M. Lantz, and Peter A. Ubel. "The Polarizing Effects of News Media Messages about the Social Determinants of Health." *American Journal of Public Health* 89 (2009): 2160–67.

Health and Human Services Department. "Annual Update of the HHS Poverty Guidelines." *Federal Register*, January 25, 2016. Accessed August 29, 2016. https://www.federalregister.gov/articles/2016/01/25/2016-01450/annual-update-of-the-hhs-poverty-guidelines.

Hilfiker, David. "Facing Brokenness." *Second Opinion* 11 (1990): 93–101.

Hilfiker, David. "From the Victim's Point of View." *Journal of Medical Humanities* 22 (2001): 17–31.

Hunt, Matthew O. "Religion, Race/Ethnicity, and Beliefs about Poverty." *Social Science Quarterly* 83 (2002): 810–31.

Kluegal, James R., and Eliot R. Smith. *Beliefs about Inequality: Americans' Views of What Is and What Ought to Be*. New York: Aldine de Gruyter, 1986.

Levine-Rasky, Cynthia. "Intersectionality Theory Applied to Whiteness and Middle-Classness." *Social Identities* 17 (2011): 239–53.

Mask, Mia. "The Precarious Politics of *Precious*: A Close Reading of a Cinematic Text." *Black Camera: An International Film Journal* 4 (2012): 96–116.

Matsuda, Maria. "Beside My Sister, Facing the Enemy: Legal Theory out of Coalition." *Stanford Law Review* 43 (1991): 1183–92.

Metzl, Jonathan, and Helena Hansen. "Structural Competency: Theorizing a New Medical Engagement with Stigma and Inequality." *Social Science and Medicine* 103 (2014): 126–33.

NPR. "Sapphire's Story: How 'Push' became 'Precious.'" *All Things Considered*, November 6, 2009. Accessed September 19, 2016. http://www.npr.org/templates/story/story.php?storyId=120176695.

Rizzo, Mary. "Teaching Class in the Classroom." *Transformations* 14 (2003): 127–38.

Scott, Janny, and David Leonhardt. "Shadowy Lines that Still Divide." *New York Times*, May 15, 2005. Accessed August 29, 2016. http://www.nytimes.com/2005/05/15/us/class/shadowy-lines-that-still-divide.html?_r=0.

Skitka, Linda J., Elizabeth Mullen, Griffin Thomas, Susan Hutchinson, and Brian Chamberlin. "Dispositions, Scripts, or Motivated Correction? Understanding

Ideological Differences in Explanations for Social Problems." *Journal of Personality and Social Psychology* 83 (2002): 470–87.

Wellington, Darryl Lorenzo. "Sex, Race, and *Precious*." *Dissent*, March 8, 2010. Accessed September 19, 2016. https://www.dissentmagazine.org/online_articles/sex-race-and-precious.

White, Armond. "Pride and Precious." *Hip Hop and Politics* (blog). November 19, 2009. Accessed August 29, 2016. http://hiphopandpolitics.com/2009/11/19/armond-white-precious-is-the-most-damaging-film-to-the-black-image-since-birth-of-a-nation/.

10

Pedagogy at the Borderlands

WHY HEALTH HUMANITIES NEEDS DIASPORA AND CULTURAL STUDIES

Sayantani DasGupta

> Borders (What's up with that?)
> Politics (What's up with that?)
> Police shots (What's up with that?)
> Identities (What's up with that?)
> Your privilege (What's up with that?)
> Broke people (What's up with that?)
> Boat people (What's up with that?)
> The realness (What's up with that?)
> The new world (What's up with that?)
> Am gonna keep up on all that.
>
> M.I.A. "Borders" (2015)

Activist and scholar Chandra Talpade Mohanty writes, "Education represents both a struggle for meaning and a struggle over power relations . . . questions at stake in the academy are questions of self- and collective knowledge of marginalized peoples and the recovery of alternative, oppositional histories of domination and struggle."[1] Teaching and learning are fundamentally political acts, impacted by what counts as knowledge and who counts as a knowledge-maker. Although the interdisciplinary field(s) of the health humanities has emerged, to some degree, as a challenge to traditional medical epistemologies, diaspora and cultural studies are yet to take a prominent role in health humanities scholarship alongside bioethics, literary studies, disability studies, and other approaches. That being so, this essay will argue that all of health humanities scholarship can be opened up not only by embracing that which is at the margins/pedagogic borderlands but by the health humanities, in the words of educator and feminist critic bell hooks, "choosing the margins as a space of radical openness." In her words,

> Within complex and ever shifting realms of power relations, do we position ourselves on the side of the colonizing mentality? Or do we continue to stand in political resistance with the oppressed, ready to offer our ways of seeing and theorizing, or making culture, towards that revolutionary effort which seeks to create space where there is unlimited access to the pleasure and power of knowing, where transformation is possible? The choice is crucial.[2]

Issues of colonialism, borderlands, diaspora, identity, and home have the potential to deepen all of health and humanities scholarship. Indeed, theorists such as Arthur Frank have argued that it is the *liminal, in-between-ness* of the illness experience that makes meaningless previously held senses of time and space. Illness, disability, indeed any host of embodied changes demand a new story, a new destination and map to life's journey.[3] In her classic *Illness as Metaphor*, Susan Sontag famously framed health and illness with a geographic metaphor, suggesting that travel betwixt the "kingdom of the well" and "that other place" required abandoning one's "good passport" and acknowledging one's status as a "dual citizen."[4] Illness, disabilities, and other identities at the embodied borderlands, then, can be considered akin to a new sort of diaspora, a sort of belonging to nowhere and everywhere that brings with it a unique insight into the human experience.

Yet, we must be cautious not to reduce the postcolonial/diasporic experience to mere metaphor—illness is not "just like" being a refugee, immigrant, cross-border laborer, or the like. Rather, diaspora and cultural studies has the potential to provide a new set of epistemological frameworks for the health humanities. Writer Pico Iyer posits that diasporic identities, in other words, those living outside the traditional nation state categories and now representing the "fifth largest nation on Earth," are creating new cultural vocabularies and hitherto unheard sorts of stories. A diasporic perspective, or scholarship from the borderlands, demands a new relationship to not just knowledge but place and space, our sense of home, and our sense of self. Like the insight arrived at from embodied liminality, diasporic storytellers view the world from a location of permanent dislocation. As Iyer suggests, "[T]he beauty of being surrounded by the foreign is that it slaps you awake, you can't take anything for granted . . . suddenly all your senses are at the setting marked on, suddenly you are aware of all the secret patterns of the world. . . . Home is not just the place you happen to be born. It is the place you become yourself."[5] Teaching health humanities from the borderlands implies embracing marginality even as we seek spaces beyond the oppressive binaries of borders themselves.

This essay will explore why health humanities pedagogy needs diasporic and cultural studies—and how our teaching can help our students, colleagues, and ourselves recover oppositional histories of embodiment and health. To do so, it will use scholar Homi Bhabha's notion of "unhomeliness" and examine what it means to both "unhome" health humanities' expectations of texts as well as "unhome" health humanities' expectations of medical practice itself.

Unhoming Our Texts: Narrative Humility and the Limits of Intelligibility

In fall 2015, I taught for the first time a graduate seminar entitled "Embodied Borderlands: Diasporic Fictions and Narrative Medicine" as part of the health humanities graduate program in which I teach. The heart of the course had been developed, however, over previous years. Two years prior, in response to a request from some of my graduate students to read fictions of the Global South alongside postcolonial theorists, I had set up a group independent study—essentially a faculty and student study group—with three students and myself. I repeated this independent study the following year, with one of the first students this time as a teaching assistant. The ultimate syllabus, therefore, for the 2015 course was developed in conjunction with several students, many of whom are now long graduated but with whom I continue to write and collaborate.[6] I mention these details in order to gesture to the politics of the pedagogical process. Instead of a top-down model of knowledge being deposited into the open mind-vaults of my students, what Paulo Freire would call the "banking model of education," this course was, from its onset, a collaborative set of inquiries between faculty and student co-learners.[7] An attention to power was not just a part of our curricular content but the teaching and learning process itself.

As students and faculty in a narrative-based program, my students and I were quite "at home" in literature. Yet, we began both small groups—and eventually the seminar itself—by examining the "homely" assumptions of literary studies. Iris Murdoch writes in her essay "The Sublime and the Beautiful Revisited" that "a novel must be a house fit for free characters to live in."[8] And as Alice Munro states in the introduction to her 1996 anthology *Selected Stories*,

> a story is not like a road to follow . . . it's more like a house. You go inside and stay there for a while, wandering back and forth and settling where you like and discovering how the room and corridors relate to each other, how the world outside is altered by being viewed from these windows.[9]

Similarly, in *Narrative Medicine: Honoring the Stories of Illness*, Rita Charon writes that "a reader might be considered a guest in the home of the text, eager to see it all and take in its aspects while extending to those who live there gratitude for the welcome."[10]

Yet, cultural studies and postcolonial analyses bring these assumptions regarding the "homeliness" of narrative texts into question. In his essay "The World and the Home," Homi Bhabha asks, "What kind of narrative can house unfree people? Is the novel also a house where the unhomely can live?" Bhabha critiques the metaphor of the house, which has "always been used to talk about the expansive, mimetic nature of the novel," for being "unable to contain the anguish of cultural displacement and diasporic movement."[11] Ultimately, he prefers instead to deem "unhomely" spaces as emblematic of the postcolonial experience. He goes on to say,

> In the stirrings of the unhomely, another world becomes visible. It has less to do with forcible eviction and more to do with the uncanny literary and social effects of enforced social accommodation, or historical migrations and cultural relocations. . . . Although the "unhomely" is a paradigmatic post-colonial experience it has a resonance that can be heard distinctly, if erratically, in fictions that negotiate the powers of cultural difference in a range of historical conditions and social contradictions.[12]

Narrative studies in medicine, at their most simplistic, have been postulated as a way to train doctors and nurses to be skilled close readers who are able to attend to the "text" of a patient in the same way a literary scholar might attend to the text of a novel. In reading a certain type of literature and a certain type of literary theory, students are taught how to enter the "home" of a patient narrative and interpret its architectures. Yet, the students who pushed me for a course in diasporic fictions were seeking not only to read sorts of narratives different from what they had thus far encountered in their studies but to read them in *different ways*, with attention to their historical and social locations and the way that power and privilege determine aesthetics, including whose stories are centered, who speaks and who is spoken for, what is said, and what is silent/silenced. They sought to do this so that they could become the sorts of practitioners who could attend their patients not with any sense of—to use the favored words of traditional medical education—mastery or competence but rather with power-sharing, camaraderie, and humility, recognizing that despite all their studies, literary and otherwise, there would be (perhaps major) aspects of their patients' stories that remained ambiguous, uninterpretable, and "unhomely." A diasporic studies approach to the health humanities suggests, then, that practitioners should abandon the thought of making themselves "at home" in their patients' stories and rather seek to humbly recognize and work on the limits of their own abilities as witnesses and listeners. This attitude toward stories is one I have called "narrative humility,"[13] and in all humility, I turn here to the words of an ex-student who best explained how such an approach to patient stories might work: "Let me give the medical reader this small piece of advice . . . try to understand. Realize you will never understand. Try anyway."[14]

Let me briefly consider here two texts I have read with the students in my diasporic fictions class to explore the impossibility of pinning down the idea of "home": Salman Rushdie's short story "At the Auction of the Ruby Slippers" and Toni Morrison's novella *Home.*[15] Rushdie's sardonic story examines the impossible fabrication of this idea called "home," as represented by *The Wizard of Oz*'s ruby slippers. In a time when "most everyone is sick," the (capitalist overlord-like) "Auctioneers" are sure that the lure of the ruby slippers will tempt people out of their "bunkers." All of humanity clamors to attend the auction of the ruby slippers, drunk on the promise of something called "home": "actors" and "exiles," "deposed monarchs" and "bandit chieftans," "children from nineteenth century Australian paintings," and a creature with a lighted finger who sounds a bit like ET (Steven Spielberg's stranded alien who sought to "phone home"). Rushdie writes,

> "Home" has become such a scattered, damaged, various concept in our present travails. There is so much to yearn for. There are so few rainbows any more. How hard can we expect even a pair of magic shoes to work? They promised to take us *home*, but are metaphors of homeliness comprehensible to them, are abstractions permissible? Are they literalists, or will they permit us to redefine the blessed word?[16]

Taking up Rushdie's suggestion, then, the health humanities might move from taking a literal approach to the idea of "home" (both our patients' actual "homes"/locations and the "home" of the text) to a redefined approach to the word.

If the promise of home is a bill of goods in Rushdie's story, for Morrison, the search for home has even more ominous connotations. Morrison begins her book with the following song (written by herself in a different context, long prior to writing this novella): "Whose house is this? Whose night keeps out the light in here? Say who owns this house? It is not mine. I had another sweeter, brighter. . . . The House is strange. Its shadows lie. Say, tell me, why does its lock fit my key?" What follows is the haunting story of Frank and Cee, siblings each displaced from not only their physical home but any sense of psychic home-place, by violence, war, poverty, and oppression. They are a primordial "Hansel and Gretel," lost children who cannot find that sense of location and self which we commonly call "home." The abusive, spiritually bankrupt house in which they grow up can be read as Morrison's condemnation of the American home built on the racist enslavement, segregation, and abuse of Black men and women. Indeed, the novella opens with Frank and Cee witnessing a lynching without fully being able to comprehend what they see, and ends with them returning to the place of this violence. But Frank and Cee are no simplistic victims. Throughout the novella, Frank carries with him the trauma of the Korean war and his terrible choices to not only witness but participate in violence toward vulnerable others as part of the American war machine. Although it is tempting for a physician-reader to diagnose Frank with post-traumatic stress disorder, Morrison paints his trauma-as-a-veteran as inextricable from the trauma of his and his community's lives. With shifting voices and points of view, Morrison tells the story of Frank's attempts at "coming home" from war and its ultimate impossibility.

The "homefront," however, is just as much of a war for Frank's sister Cee, who is abused by her family and partner, only to eventually find herself employed in the house of a seemingly benign white doctor who practices eugenics, an example of medicine's own racist and violent history toward communities of color. When she is sterilized against her will and becomes gravely ill—mentally, spiritually, and physically—it is the no-nonsense, unsentimental, hard-working women of her community who care for her. Morrison writes, "The women handled sickness as though it were an affront, an illegal, invading braggart who needed whipping. They didn't waste their time or the patient's with sympathy and they met the tears of the suffering with resigned contempt."[17] The women are perhaps the antithesis of what the health humanities might consider "caring healers," berating and hushing and scolding their patient into wellness with their stalwart care. But it is their "demanding love"[18] that is responsible for Cee learning to heal herself, a phenomenon perhaps beyond the understanding of many unfamiliar with the dynamics of marginalized communities. One of the elderly women tells her,

> Look to yourself. You free. Nothing and nobody is obliged to save you but you. Seed your own land. You young and a woman and there's serious limitation in both, but you a person too. Don't let [your grandmother] or some trifling boyfriend and certainly no evil doctor decide who you are. That's slavery. Somewhere inside you is that free person I'm talking about. Locate her and let her do some good in the world.[19]

Like Rushdie's story, which disrupts any previous held, comfortable assumptions the reader might have held about there being "no place like home," Morrison's *Home* is at its heart about unhomeliness—as a text that undermines any readerly attempts at understanding or mastery. Frank repeatedly critiques the author's inability to understand his experience: "You can't imagine it because you weren't there,"[20] he says of the Korean war and of the author's attempt to describe the Louisiana heat. "You can't come up with words that catch it."[21] As Mary Dudziak has observed, the novel is ultimately about the limits of empathy, on the part of the author, the characters, or the readers. Dudziak's conclusion regarding the novella can be read as a warning to health humanities students who look to narrative studies as a way "in" to their patients' lives: "Whether it is a soldier or any other fellow human being, our efforts at understanding must be tempered by the knowledge that true empathy is an impossibility. That we are, in the end, like the character of the author: writing our own narratives, always hampered by what we lack the capacity to see."[22]

Unhoming Our Practices: Medical Colonialism and the Limits of "Helping"

Not only can a study of postcolonial and diasporic texts disrupt our comfortable notions of literary homeliness and patients being ultimately intelligible "texts" for their clinicians to decipher, but it can also shine a light upon postcolonial power relations and the ongoing problems of medicine's global reach. Historically, public health and medicine have been utilized not only to justify the enslavement of peoples of African origin and the genocide of indigenous communities from North America to Australia[23] but to prompt the practices of war and empire-building. In *Imperial Hygiene: A Critical History of Colonialism, Nationalism, and Public Health*, Alison Bashford writes about how imperialists of the nineteenth and twentieth centuries conflated and justified "the power to govern" with "the power to heal." Regarding colonial quarantine practices, she writes, "[S]egregation [was] both hygienic—that is . . . part of public health—and racial—as part of the systems and cultures of race management, including . . . the management of whiteness."[24] Indeed, Victorian ideals of cleanliness were in great part about the management of racial purity. Consider a late nineteenth-century Pears' Soap advertisement featuring a naval commander washing his hands, as his ships import soaps to supplicating dark-skinned "natives." The advertisement reads, "The first step toward lightening the white man's burden is through teaching the virtues of cleanliness. Pears' Soap is a potent factor in brightening the dark corners of the earth as civilization advances."[25] In the words of writer Stassa Edwards,

> If the history of modernity can . . . be written as a triumph of cleanliness over bodily refuse, then so too could the European colonization of Africa and India. The sanitary crusade of the nineteenth century is central to the violent project of empire. Western medicine, with its emphasis on personal hygiene, functioned (and in some arenas still functions) as colonialism's benevolent cover—an acknowledgment that, while empire was about profit at all costs, that it could also conceal this motive slightly by concerning itself with bettering the health of debased bodies.[26]

Medical colonialism hardly stopped, however, at imposed notions of bodily cleanliness. Health humanities teachers need only to turn to Franz Fanon's writings on the subject, including *A Dying Colonialism* (originally published in 1959), in which he describes colonial doctors' roles in the torture of Algerian political prisoners. Tragically, such medical abuses continue into the present day, as revealed by investigations into the CIA torture program.[27]

Blatant abuses as physicians and psychologists being involved in the torture of imprisoned terror suspects notwithstanding, how does modern-day medical colonialism morally justify its interventionist actions to itself? One such strategy in the moral defense of "helping" is undoubtedly the narrative of indigenous absence. I borrow this term from Arthur and Joan Kleinman, who, in discussing the ethics of photographing distant suffering, write that the individual in the photograph

> must be protected, as well as represented, by others. The image of the subaltern conjures up an almost neocolonial ideology of failure, inadequacy, passivity, fatalism and inevitability. Something must be done, and it must be done soon, but from outside the local setting. The authorization of action through an appeal for foreign aid, even foreign intervention, begins with an evocation of indigenous absence, an erasure of local voices and acts.[28]

The narrative of indigenous absence suggests that local individuals, communities, organizations, or governments are either incapable of solving or incompetent to solve local problems and desperately need external help—the nature of which is inevitably determined by those giving the help rather than those receiving it. Despite evidence, for instance, that five decades and billions of dollars of aid to Africa have in fact worsened the cycle of poverty and external dependence,[29] the narrative of indigenous absence continues to justify such paternalistic interventions in both development and health. Originally in a series of tweets critiquing the "Kony 2012" neoliberal debacle, writer Teju Cole named this impetus the "white savior industrial complex." In his words, "The White Savior Industrial Complex is not about justice. It is about having a big emotional experience that validates privilege" and "I deeply respect American sentimentality, the way one respects a wounded hippo. You must keep an eye on it, for you know it is deadly."[30] Similarly, Gayatri Chakravorty Spivak's famous notion of "white men saving brown women from brown men" can be used to understand the ongoing way that notions of "saving oppressed (read: Muslim) women" have served to justify wars in Afghanistan and Iraq, disguising wolf-like foreign policy in seemingly "feminist" sheep's clothing,[31] the assumption being, of course, that Muslim women *need* such saving[32] or, even if they do, that they are not capable of saving themselves.

What is the impact of such understandings on the health humanities? Consider the popularity of overseas medical missions—particularly the short-term medical "voluntour" trips oft frequented by premedical students (who can afford their hefty price tag) in hopes of bolstering their medical school applications. The Global South's profound need for healthcare "help" from the Global North—even ill-trained, ill-prepared, selfie-obsessed, culturally insensitive, short-term "help"—is the underlying belief driving such missions. "At least we are doing something!" is the often indignant reply to any critiques of international health, in general, and short-term medical missions, in particular. Yet, many voluntour students leave the experience distressed, having performed procedures they were not properly trained to do upon patients who had not properly consented. A diasporic/cultural studies health humanities education can give such students the tools to understand the implications of their personal actions, as well as the troubling policies of those organizing their "missions."

A former narrative medicine graduate student of mine came to me with such a sense of disquiet after having gone on several overseas voluntour missions as an undergraduate. She was distressed not only at the culture of white volunteers taking endless "selfies" with brown and black children but at the quick-fix model of her mission's pop-up medical clinics, a model that provided care from ill-trained (and often untrained) undergraduate volunteers, had little to no options for long-term patient relationships or follow-up care, and ultimately undermined the local healthcare economy. This model of untrained volunteers "playing doctor" on communities in the Global South was framed for her with a neoliberal ethos; this was what good-hearted people who wanted to "help" did for the world, without exception, without critique, and without listening to what those they were "helping" in fact desired. After reading and thinking with me for the better part of a year, a time during which we read diasporic and cultural studies scholars together, this student produced and published three essays bringing attention to the bioethics of global medical voluntour missions.[33] She approached these essays with humility, candor, and bravery—critiquing her own actions and assumptions in the process. In one such essay, she describes fumbling through a pelvic exam on a woman in Ghana, a traumatizing experience for both her and the woman:

> Each year, thousands of pre-medical students travel to communities in developing countries, disguised as saviors. What does it mean for students like me to fly around the world "playing doctor"? What impressions are we giving to those we seek to "save" with our improvisational care? The gaze of the woman whose name I never knew followed me home from my trip to Ghana. She forces me to question the quality of care her community receives through medical missions such as the one I took part in; and to ask myself, doesn't she deserve the quality of care I saw [women in the United States] receive? When will we stop practicing on the world's poor?[34]

In another essay examining the phenomenon of privileged voluntours taking and posting selfies with hashtags such as #InstagrammingAfrica, she writes,

> In the end, the Africa we voluntourists photograph isn't a real place at all. It is an imaginary geography whose landscapes are forged by colonialism, as well as a good deal of narcissism. I hope my fellow students think critically about what they are doing and why before they sign up for a short-term global volunteer experience. And if they do go, it is my hope that they

might think with some degree of narrative humility about how to de-center themselves from the Western savior narrative. Most importantly, I hope they leave their iPhones at home.[35]

Cultural studies equips the health humanities to actively critique and challenge neocolonial medical attitudes and actions, promoting partnerships over paternalism, a recognition of community agency rather than any sense of indigenous absence.

Conclusion: Bodies at the Borderlands

Teaching health humanities through a diasporic/cultural studies lens implies recognizing the way that bodies carry the histories of borders, the way that borderlands are drawn on bodies. In "The Homeland, Aztlán/El otro México," Gloria Anzaldúa writes of the psychic and political borders between the United States and Mexico, which split and divide both national and corporeal bodies.

> *1,950 mile-long open wound*
> *dividing a* pueblo, *a culture,*
> *running down the length of my body,*
> *staking fence rods in my flesh,*
> *splits me splits me*[36]

The study of boundaries and borders is perhaps as critical in our current xenophobic, anti-immigrant, Trumpian era as it has ever been. In her *Elsewhere, within Here: Immigration, Refugeeism and the Boundary Event*, feminist scholar and filmmaker Trinh Min-ha writes,

> While the era of colonialism has been officially proclaimed to have practically reached an end, invasion, occupation, disruption and relocation—in other words, colonization by other ways—continue to set the stage for unending aggression and destruction. A state of urgency has become routine. . . . In this quasi-neurotic state of self-induced fear, every immigrant or voyager of color is a potential terrorist.[37]

Given these realities, the need for diasporic/cultural studies–based health humanities teaching is perhaps more ethically imperative than ever. When I began my diasporic fictions seminar in fall 2015, I opened the first class with a video by Sri Lankan British rapper M.I.A. called "Borderlands." Her recent comments about #BlackLivesMatter notwithstanding, this was both an aesthetic and political act. Playing such a video, starring a brown-skinned woman who was herself a refugee (when she was nine, Maya Arulpragasam fled violence in Sri Lanka with her mother and siblings and came to London), was intentionally gesturing to a shift from the pedagogic center to the margins. This was not a class where we would make ourselves at home in certain kinds of written texts by "great Western authors," nor was this a class where we would separate the theoretical or artistic from the global politics or the actual injustices affecting people's lives.

In the video, people by the hundreds behind M.I.A. climb barbed wire fences, cross deserts, and jam into ocean-crossing boats. As these people are specifically all brown men, M.I.A. is undoubtedly making a statement of solidarity here with those who are most often labeled "terrorists" by Western audiences. She confronts the listener with the repetitive question "What's up with that?"—asking the question of pop cultural experiences including "being bae" and "slaying it" but also, damningly, of "love wins." In other words, why does marriage equality rank high as a social justice concern in white Western communities whereas the experience of displaced people of color does not? M.I.A.'s video, like perhaps diasporic/cultural studies in general, demands that we health humanities students and faculty ask ourselves, again and again, whose suffering, whose stories, and whose lives we value. In the words of M.I.A., "Freedom, 'I'dom, 'Me'dom, where's your 'We'dom? This world needs a brand new 'Re' dom." Diasporic/cultural studies perspectives in the health humanities represent, perhaps, such a "re-dom/do" for our fields, bringing the collective, the structural, and the political into focus; approaching our texts and patients with humility and partnership; and ultimately, moving our scholarship to the borderlands, where transformation and revolution are within our reach.

Notes

1. Chandra Talpade Mohanty, *Feminism without Borders: Decolonizing Theory, Practicing Solidarity* (Chapel Hill, NC: Duke University Press, 2003).

2. bell hooks, *Yearning: Race, Gender, and Cultural Politics* (Boston: South End Press, 1999), 203.

3. Arthur W. Frank, *The Wounded Storyteller: Body, Illness, and Ethics* (Chicago: University of Chicago Press, 1995).

4. Susan Sontag, *Illness as Metaphor* (New York: Farrar, Straus and Giroux, 1978).

5. Pico Iyer, "Where Is Home?" TED Global 2013, June 2013, accessed August 8,2016 https://www.ted.com/talks/pico_iyer_where_is_home?language=en.

6. Rebecca K. Tsevat et al., "Bringing Home the Health Humanities: Narrative Humility, Structural Competency, Engaged Pedagogy," *Academic Medicine* 90, no. 11: 1462–65; Kevin J. Gutierrez and Sayantani DasGupta, "The Space That Difference Makes: On Marginality, Social Justice and the Future of the Health Humanities," *Journal of Medical Humanities* 37, no. 4 (2016): 435–48.

7. Paul Freire, *Pedagogy of the Oppressed* (New York: Continuum International Publishing Group, 1970).

8. Iris Murdoch, "The Sublime and Beautiful Revisited," *Yale Review* 49 (1959): 271.

9. Alice Munro, *Selected Stories* (New York: Vintage Books, 1997), 8.

10. Rita Charon, *Narrative Medicine: Honoring the Stories of Illness* (New York: Oxford University Press, 2006), 112.

11. Homi Bhabha, "The World and the Home," *Social Text* no. 31/32 (1992): 142.

12. Ibid., 142–43.

13. Sayantani DasGupta, "Narrative Humility," *The Lancet* 371 (2008): 980–81; and "Narrative Humility," TEDx Sarah Lawrence College, April 2012, https://www.youtube.com/watch?v=gZ3ucjmcZwY

14. C. Sebastian, "My Body, My Self," in *Stories of Illness and Healing: Women Write Their Bodies*, ed. Sayantani DasGupta and Marsha Hurst (Kent, OH: Kent State University Press, 2007), 229.

15. Salman Rushdie, "At the Auction of the Ruby Slippers," in *East West* (New York: Vintage, 1995); Toni Morrison, *Home* (New York: Vintage, 2013).

16. Rushdie, "Auction," 93.

17. Morrison, *Home*, 121.

18. Ibid., 125.

19. Ibid., 126.

20. Ibid., 93.

21. Ibid., 41.

22. Mary Dudziak, "The Limits of Empathy in Toni Morrison's 'Home,'" *OUPblog* (blog), http://blog.oup.com/2012/05/the-limits-of-empathy-in-toni-morrisons-home/.

23. D. Olusoga (director), *Scientific Racism: The Eugenics of Social Darwinism* (London: BBC, 2007).

24. Alison Bashford, *Imperial Hygiene: A Critical History of Colonialism, Nationalism, and Public Health* (New York: Palgrave MacMillan, 2004), 2.

25. Eric Foner, *Give Me Liberty! An American History* (New York: W.W. Norton, 2010), image of Pears' Soap from http://wwnorton.com/college/history/give-me-liberty4/img/ch/17/CH17_05.jpg.

26. Stassa Edwards, "From Miasma to Ebola: The History of Racist Moral Panic over Disease," *Jezebel*, October 14, 2014, http://jezebel.com/from-miasma-to-ebola-the-history-of-racist-moral-panic-1645711030.

27. Physicians for Human Rights, "Physicians for Human Rights Releases Expert Analysis of CIA Report, Calls for Federal Commission to Hold Health Professionals Accountable," December 16, 2014, http://physiciansforhumanrights.org/press/press-releases/physicians-for-human-rights-releases-expert-analysis-of-cia-torture-report-calls-for-federal-commission-to-hold-health-professionals-accountable.html.

28. Arthur Kleinman and Joan Kleinman, "The Appeal of Experience, the Dismay of Images: Cultural Appropriation of Suffering in Our Times," special issue, *Daedalus* 125, no. 1 (1996): 7.

29. See Dambisa Moyo, *Dead Aid: Why Aid Is Not Working and How There Is a Better Way for Africa* (New York: Farrar, Straus and Giroux, 2009).

30. Teju Cole, "The White-Savior Industrial Complex," *Atlantic*, March 21, 2012, http://www.theatlantic.com/international/archive/2012/03/the-white-savior-industrial-complex/254843/.

31. Gayatri Chakravorty Spivak, "History," in *A Critique of Postcolonial Reason: Toward a History of the Vanishing Present* (Cambridge, MA: Harvard University Press, 1999).

32. For a rebuttal, see Leila Abu-Lughod, *Do Muslim Women Need Saving?* (Cambridge, MA: Harvard University Press, 2013).

33. Lauren Kascak, "The Poor Deserve Perfection: The Case against Pre-Health Volunteers in Global Health," *Voices in Bioethics*, July 15, 2014, https://voicesinbioethics.org/2014/07/16/the-poor-deserve-perfection-the-case-against-pre-health-volunteers-in-global-health/; Kascak, "'Wanna Play Doctor?' A Premedical Student Reflects on a Medical Brigade in Ghana," *Intima*, Spring 2014, https://static1.squarespace.com/static/54bc1287e4b09cb81d8d8439/t/554782eee4b0120075049818/1430749934981/Wanna+Play+Doctor%3F.pdf; Kascak and Sayantani DasGupta, "#Instagramming Africa: The Narcissism of Global Voluntourism," *Sociological Images*, December 29, 2014, https://thesocietypages.org/socimages/2014/12/29/instragrammingafrica-the-narcissism-of-global-voluntourism/.

34. Kascak, "'Wanna Play Doctor?'"

35. Kascak and DasGupta, "#Instagramming Africa."

36. Gloria Anzaldúa, *Borderlands: La frontera: The New Mestiza* (San Francisco: Aunt Lute Books, 2007), 24.

37. Trinh T. Minh-Ha, *Elsewhere, within Here: Immigration, Refugeeism and the Boundary Event* (New York: Routledge, 2010), 5.

Works Cited

Abu-Lughod, Lila. *Do Muslim Women Need Saving?* Cambridge, MA: Harvard University Press, 2013.

Anzaldúa, Gloria. *Borderlands: La frontera: The New Mestiza*. San Francisco: Aunt Lute Books, 2007.

Bashford, Alison. *Imperial Hygiene: A Critical History of Colonialism, Nationalism, and Public Health*. New York: Palgrave MacMillan, 2004.

Bhabha, Homi. "The World and the Home." *Social Text* no. 31/32 (1992): 141–53.

Charon, Rita. *Narrative Medicine: Honoring the Stories of Illness*. New York: Oxford University Press, 2006.

Cole, Teju. "The White-Savior Industrial Complex." *The Atlantic*, March 21, 2012. http://www.theatlantic.com/international/archive/2012/03/the-white-savior-industrial-complex/254843/.

DasGupta, Sayantani. "Narrative Humility." *The Lancet* 371, no. 9617 (2008): 980–81.

DasGupta, Sayantani. "Narrative Humility." TEDx Sarah Lawrence College. April 2012. https://www.youtube.com/watch?v=gZ3ucjmcZwY.

Dudziak, Mary. "The Limits of Empathy in Toni Morrison's 'Home.'" *OUPblog* (blog). May 28, 2012. http://blog.oup.com/2012/05/the-limits-of-empathy-in-toni-morrisons-home/.

Edwards, Stassa. "From Miasma to Ebola: The History of Racist Moral Panic over Disease." *Jezebel*, October 14, 2014. http://jezebel.com/from-miasma-to-ebola-the-history-of-racist-moral-panic-1645711030.

Fanon, Frantz. *A Dying Colonialism*. Translated by Haakon Chevalier. New York: Grove Press, 1994.

Foner, Eric. *Give Me Liberty! An American History.* New York: W.W. Norton, 2010. Image of Pears' Soap from http://wwnorton.com/college/history/give-me-liberty4/img/ch/17/CH17_05.jpg.

Frank, Arthur W. *The Wounded Storyteller: Body, Illness, and Ethics*. Chicago: University of Chicago Press, 1995.

Freire, Paolo. *Pedagogy of the Oppressed.* New York: Continuum International Publishing Group, 1970.

Gutierrez, Kevin J., and Sayantani DasGupta. "The Space That Difference Makes: On Marginality, Social Justice and the Future of the Health Humanities." *Journal of Medical Humanities* 37, no. 4 (2016): 435–48.

hooks, bell. *Yearning: Race, Gender, and Cultural Politics.* Boston: South End Press, 1999.

Iyer, Pico. "Where Is Home?" TED Global 2013. June 2013. Accessed August 8, 2016. https://www.ted.com/talks/pico_iyer_where_is_home?language=en.

Kascak, Lauren. "The Poor Deserve Perfection: The Case against Pre-Health Volunteers in Global Health." *Voices in Bioethics*, July 15, 2014. http://www.voicesinbioethics.net/clinical-narratives/2014/07/16/the-poor-deserve-perfection-the-case-against-pre-health-volunteers-in-global-health.

Kascak, Lauren. "'Wanna Play Doctor?' A Premedical Student Reflects on a Medical Brigade in Ghana." *Intima*, Spring 2014. https://static1.squarespace.com/static/54bc1287e4b09cb81d8d8439/t/554782eee4b0120075049818/1430749934981/Wanna+Play+Doctor%3F.pdf.

Kascak, Lauren, and Sayantani DasGupta. "#Instagramming Africa: The Narcissism of Global Voluntourism." *Sociological Images*, December 29, 2014. https://thesocietypages.org/socimages/2014/12/29/instragrammingafrica-the-narcissism-of-global-voluntourism/.

Kleinman, Arthur, and Joan Kleinman. "The Appeal of Experience, the Dismay of Images: Cultural Appropriation of Suffering in Our Times." Special issue, *Daedalus* 125, no. 1 (1996): 1–23.

Minh-ha, Trinh T. *Elsewhere, Within Here: Immigration, Refugeeism and the Boundary Event*. New York: Routledge, 2010.

Mohanty, Chandra Talpade. *Feminism without Borders: Decolonizing Theory, Practicing Solidarity.* Chapel Hill, NC: Duke University Press, 2003.

Morrison, Toni. *Home.* New York: Vintage, 2013.

Moyo, Dambisa. *Dead Aid: Why Aid Is Not Working and How There Is a Better Way for Africa.* New York: Farrar, Straus and Giroux, 2009.

Munro, Alice. *Selected Stories*. New York: Vintage Books, 1997.

Murdoch, Iris. "The Sublime and Beautiful Revisited." *Yale Review* 49 (1959): 247–77.

Olusoga, D. (director). *Scientific Racism: The Eugenics of Social Darwinism.* London: BBC, 2007.

Physicians for Human Rights. "Physicians for Human Rights Releases Expert Analysis of CIA Report, Calls for Federal Commission to Hold Health Professionals Accountable." December 16, 2014. http://physiciansforhumanrights.org/press/press-releases/physicians-for-human-rights-releases-expert-analysis-of-cia-torture-report-calls-for-federal-commission-to-hold-health-professionals-accountable.html.

Rushdie, Salman. "At the Auction of the Ruby Slippers." In *East West*. New York: Vintage, 1995.

Sebastian, C. "My Body, My Self." In *Stories of Illness and Healing: Women Write Their Bodies*, edited by Sayantani DasGupta and Marsha Hurst, 24–29. Kent, OH: Kent State University Press, 2007.

Sontag, Susan. *Illness as Metaphor*. New York: Farrar, Straus and Giroux, 1978.

Spivak, Gayatri Chakravorty. "History." In *A Critique of Postcolonial Reason: Toward a History of the Vanishing Present*. Cambridge, MA: Harvard University Press, 1999.

Tsevat, Rebecca K., Anoushka A. Sinha, Kevin J. Gutierrez, and Sayantani DasGupta. "Bringing Home the Health Humanities: Narrative Humility, Structural Competency, Engaged Pedagogy." *Academic Medicine* 90, no. 11 (2015): 1462–65.

11

Resemblance, Diversity, and Making Age Studies Matter

Andrea Charise

> Let us recognize ourselves in this old man or in that old woman. It must be done if we are to take upon ourselves the entirety of our human state.
>
> Simone de Beauvoir, The Coming of Age (1973)

> Thirty, man. If I'm not dead yet, I'll be old then. Know what I mean?
>
> "Shay," Black male, early twenties (2016)

Introduction

Everyone ages; not everyone grows old. The field of age studies exists to describe the critical study of these interlinking concepts, defined as *age* (the chronological number of years a person has lived), *aging* (the ongoing temporality of the body, including cognitive and physiological changes often associated with post-midlife), and *older age* (a vague, context-dependent designation generally starting at sixty-five years of age). In this chapter, I discuss the relationship between age studies and health humanities primarily with respect to the methods and materials of the arts and humanities. My goal here is to differentiate age studies from other fields (such as gerontology) that emphasize qualitative and some quantitative methodologies associated with the social sciences. Age studies, by contrast, is more concerned with creative and critical representations of the individual experience of age, aging, older age, and intergenerational relationships.

Age studies is a relatively new subfield of the humanities and interpretive social sciences. Like gerontology (which involves the multidisciplinary yet generally health science–based study of aging and older adults), age studies has tended to focus on older age as opposed to a range of age experiences across the life course. Moreover, the field's rootedness in the humanities is evident in what Stephen Katz has described as its "biographical, feminist, and narrative perspectives on self, memory, meaning, and wisdom" and its serious interest in the "imaginative alternative resources and experiences in performative, artistic, fictional, transsexual, poetic, and futuristic fields."[1] In the twenty-first century, age studies also encompasses cognate concerns inspired by new cultural processes that have redefined aging and later life in response to issues including late capitalism, globalization, cosmetic and body technologies, consumer marketing, and age-based hierarchies.

The purpose of this chapter, and that of age studies more broadly, is threefold:

- To demonstrate how the arts and humanities provide valuable insights into the individual experience of aging and growing older, by means of data and forms of knowledge that are not primarily quantitative or clinical
- To bridge gaps between clinical, theoretical, creative, and embodied modes of learning about age
- To balance, even disrupt, largely pessimistic portrayals of aging and older age both in the personal sphere and in the public, especially those generated by apocalyptic visions of an aging population

Yet this chapter is also a critical response to how age studies has generally been practiced over the past four decades. As I have argued elsewhere,[2] to ensure the long life of this important field, research and education in age studies—like health humanities more generally—must mindfully engage the specificities of locale (i.e., where such work is practiced), beginning by confronting its ideological centeredness in upper-middle-class, white, Western experience.

Age Studies and/as Health Humanities

I stopped dyeing my hair when I was in my late twenties. I could not, in all conscience, research, teach, or advocate for age studies while concealing my body's clearest manifestation of growing older: its whitening. After all, our age—whether chronological, biological, apparent, implied, or imagined—constitutes a significant part of our identity, on par with other aspects such as gender, race, or sexuality. As with these aspects of identity, older age often carries a stigma in the popular consciousness. It was psychiatrist and gerontologist Robert Butler who, in 1969, first coined the term *ageism*—discrimination against people based on the perception that they are old or elderly.[3] Even health professionals are not immune from such long-standing prejudices, which have resulted in the systemic maltreatment of older persons in a range of healthcare environments.[4] In the medical (and public) setting, people in older age are regularly subjected to devaluations of their worth, dignity, and personhood.

In addition to more aesthetically oriented topics such as later-life creativity, age studies converges with the interdisciplinary mandate of health humanities: for example, in the use of arts as a therapeutic or health-supporting practice for older persons. Age studies further lays bare how ideological valuations of age—especially in conjunction with cognitive and/or physical impairments—underpin broader paradigms of health-related policy, decision-making, education, and clinical practice, in terms of healthcare resource allocation (including for long-term care and institutionalized living); the management of chronic illnesses; debates concerning euthanasia and assisted suicide; the individual and societal burden (perceived and real) of age-related dementias; and formal and informal caregiving. As well, dire pronouncements often predict the specter of medical and economic catastrophe as the result of an aging population (a phenomenon Margaret Cruikshank calls *apocalyptic demography*).[5]

Thus, crucial age studies concepts also constitute important points of reference for educators, practitioners, students, and activists in the health humanities. These concepts include not just ageism but also the stages-of-life model of aging,[6] the ideology of decline,[7] aging as an arena of invisibility and hypervisibility,[8] the pedagogy of mortification,[9] neuroculture and personhood,[10] "successful" aging,[11] and assisted living and intergenerational relations.[12] I will reference these points later in this chapter.

However, despite obvious intersections with major subfields of health humanities (such as bioethics) and cross-pollinating perspectives from the critical studies of disability, race, and gender, age studies still appears to lack the urgency and activist draw of its intersectional counterparts. One reason might be the fact that, unlike other binarized axes of identity and privilege—dyads such as black:white, female:male, or disabled:able-bodied, for example—old:young lacks a status obviously privileged by the structures of ideological power. On the one hand, the designation of "old" is saturated with connotations of lack and diminution: physical frailty, illness, confusion, dementia, and decline contrast with (often ableist) connotations of youth such as health, vitality, and energy. Yet the old may also be perceived as hoarders of wealth; as overdue retirees who prevent the advance of youthful potential; as "bed blockers" (older patients who cannot be discharged from hospital, having nowhere to go); and, in their pension demands, as economic burdens (both individual and societal). Aging, of course, is a luxury: its very possibility indicates the existence of effective yet expensive social services and healthcare. In the binary pair that gives rise to age studies, who loses and who wins is neither clear nor constant—especially in comparison with the historical patterns of oppression that have delineated other profoundly "othered" bodies.

Such ideological baggage about the body's temporal nature gives rise to the need for age studies and highlights the opportunities presented by this field to the broader concerns of health humanities. Without specific attention to the interlinked concepts of age, aging, and older age, health humanities risks merely reproducing the age biases that saturate Western culture. The immutable fact of aging generates a unique opportunity for individuals to explore, even mobilize, their common experience (even if this experience is deeply contingent upon other facets of identity). Sociologist Anne Karpf, among others, has suggested that ageism is, at root, a prejudice against our own future selves[13]; and French philosopher Simone de Beauvoir, in 1973, wrote that we must "recognize ourselves in this old man or in that old woman."[14] If that is the case, age studies might be said to offer a rich and self-invested form of empathy training—a pedagogical outcome often suggested as the raison d'être of health humanities.[15]

The Problem of "Relatability"

On a practical level, the issue that age studies continues to face—especially as it is taught to undergraduates—is one of *relevance*: how can young people be convinced that aging, especially older age, is relevant to their lives? This is a question I'm asked often—by family and friends, colleagues and department chairs, journalists and health professionals. The powerful Western resistance to aging can make this field seem fatally off-putting, particularly when coupled with the relative paucity of critical discussion on how to actually teach age studies.[16] Yet in my experience as a researcher, educator, and activist, the matter of whether late teens and twenty-somethings can relate to the study of aging has always puzzled administrators far more than students themselves. The supposed "alienation" of intellectually engaging with older age can be easily mitigated by effective modeling and pedagogy. The alienation of age studies springs, rather, from its default positioning of white Western experience and the limitation of its spheres of concern to medicalized anxieties about and the institutionalized setting of aging, a liability that this field shares more broadly with health humanities.

I should know—I fit that profile exactly. I am a white settler Canadian of English–Irish heritage who lives, works, and teaches in Toronto on the former traditional territory of the Haudenosaunee and Mississaugas of the New Credit First Nation. I enter my health humanities classroom with the additional privileges of working as a tenure-track professor at Canada's largest research university. While I am not the first to point out the whiteness of age studies, the field has done little to reshape itself in response—though, granted, this task is made more challenging by the lack of textbooks that would support that aim.[17] My own transformation of practice developed out of my launching of Canada's first baccalaureate health humanities program, at the University of Toronto Scarborough. This mid-sized campus (approximately eleven thousand undergraduates) is located in the northeastern part of Toronto—an area with higher-than-average numbers of at-risk populations such as recent immigrants, racialized communities, and low-income households.

Two moments in my teaching of a senior-level seminar, "Aging and the Arts," stand out for the way they required me to confront my own default assumptions regarding age studies.

- During a discussion of what "growing old" meant to my conventionally aged undergraduates (*Sixty-five! Eighty! Wrinkles! Gray hair! Not going out!*), "Shay," a Black man in his early twenties, offered up "thirty." When I asked him to say more, Shay's answer was raw and clear. Racial disparities in health mean that life expectancy for Black men and women across North America is significantly lower than for other populations; in the case of specific cancers (prostate and cervical, for example), these differences are profound. Shay then turned to the highly publicized deaths of young Black men at the hands of police. What does age signify if a twelve-year-old boy is shot for supposedly looking like a gun-wielding adult—as was Tamir Rice? For Shay, and for many others like him, merely being a young Black man posed a significant obstacle to growing old. "Thirty, man. If I'm not dead yet, I'll be old then. Know what I mean?"
- During a discussion of Michael Ignatieff's 1993 novel *Scar Tissue* (a searing portrayal of dementia, disability, and institutionalized care), several students shared their experiences of working in care homes for older people. When I asked how they felt about the possibility of each of us ending up in a similar situation, they had little reason to identify with this dread. "Noor," a young Pakistani woman, set me straight. She, and her fellow students of South Asian heritage, shared a culture of large multigenerational households. In contrast to a major concern of contemporary age studies, which views dementia and the nursing home as primary scenes of abject and traumatic incarceration, they had no personal or cultural affiliation with the concept of a nursing home, negative or otherwise—it was just a volunteering opportunity. "Honestly? I see a nursing home as a place where white people put their relatives when they're old. It's just not where my people go."

These two vignettes illustrate the need for a more expansive arena of practice for age studies. For Shay, "old age" was something very different from a comforting vision of serene retirement (as for other prominent figures in the Black Lives Matter movement, such as Evelyn Reynolds, who asserts that "[a]ging while Black is an act of survival").[18] For Noor, a medicalized institutional setting was something she felt protected from by a culture of intergenerational cohabitation. How, then, can educators ensure that age studies reflects—or at least resembles—the lived experiences of its learners? How to adapt, diversify, even decolonize age studies and make it a field with which my students can most meaningfully engage? What conditions might create new insights and resources, especially for learners currently underrepresented in the field? And how much sameness is required, and how much difference can be tolerated, in the learning of a subject that is inescapably embodied?

The solution, I argue, is not simply "more" diversity. As Sara Ahmed has shown, *diversity* is often a vacuous term in the academic context, one that merely re-establishes whiteness at the center of a system of diverse others.[19] Like the concept of empathy (something close to a "god term" in health humanities), diversity is often a fantasy of the frictionless incorporation of vastly different bodies and experiences. (Of course, age too is an aspect of diversity.) Admirable as de Beauvoir's ethical principle of recognition may be, the empathy training approach to age studies might in fact lead to students colonizing the experience of others in the name of identification. This is true both of the older population the field focuses on and of the differences between the subject itself and the varied inheritances of its learners. If age studies is to thrive, its educators need a practice that can address wide gaps between its core concepts and the plurality of students' lived experiences and inherited stories about aging. It is vital to nurture such a sense of resemblance with the lives and communities of learners. (A question I never hear: *How old should a person be to teach age studies?*)

Remixing Age Studies

Teaching students whose racial, religious, and cultural backgrounds differ profoundly from my own has nevertheless demonstrated the enduring applicability of several core age studies concepts. For example, many, if not most, conventionally aged undergraduates are not only anxious about their own aging but gripped by visions of cognitive and physical decline. The practice of questioning their assumptions—that aging is equivalent to decline—is at once simple and revelatory; as is pointing out that ageism is a powerful mode of *othering*, along the more familiar lines of, say, racism or sexism. My pedagogical approach, which I term *remixing*, means identifying the elements of age studies that are especially resonant for my students and finding ways to place those elements in new relationships with my students' embedded knowledge and values around aging. Lawrence Lessig has described the contemporary phenomenon of *remix culture* as the combining of existing creative materials to produce new and often original work.[20] Remixing changes the conventional flow of intellectual authority or information from professor to learner. My remixing of age studies makes learners the agents of their own windows into aging and older age, rather than passive receptacles for "more" texts, essays, and content.

In what follows, I describe three "layers" of effort in the teaching process. I begin by inviting students to mix various media forms of a standard age studies text, *King Lear*. The next layer opens the way to experience a multidirectional exchange of information using a shared creative text. Finally, I present my vision of a truly creative health humanities classroom: first we read, then we make.

LAYER 1: GLOBAL *KING LEAR*

Learning objectives:

- To alert learners to ageism and its manifestations in creative texts
- To seek out textured stories and representations of aging from a range of textual sources and cultural traditions
- To use the methods of the arts and humanities to answer the question, What does it mean to grow old?

In my "Aging and the Arts" seminar, my first attempt to help students "relate" to old age began with Shakespeare's *King Lear*. My aim was to show how a four hundred–year-old play about an old man could be substantially translated across different times, cultures, and textual forms. The tale of Lear, abandoned and misused by his adult children, has also resonated profoundly in other artistic traditions—as I showed by assembling a collection of versions and adaptations of the play for my students to explore. These included a 2007 filmed version of the play, directed by Trevor Nunn and starring Ian McKellen as Lear[21]; film adaptations such as Akira Kurosawa's 1985 film *Ran*[22]; a graphic novel by Ian Pollock[23]; and the short documentary *South Korea: Suicide Nation*.[24] The graphic novel *King Lear*, in particular, allowed students to visualize elder abuse, intergenerational conflict, male friendship, elder suicide, homelessness, cognitive impairment, and the pedagogy of mortification—a number of themes elaborated on in the course anthology, *Figuring Age*.[25]

The students who were most engaged by the story's issues found what seemed to me a novel way of accessing the play: they watched the filmed performance online while reading the text. (That was a moment of real generational difference for me: when I asked how they were able to pay attention to two or three sensory inputs at once, my students were incredulous. *You just do it!*). Printed text, visual, audio, performance: they had effectively remixed the suggested resources to create something that was, for them, more immersive, accessible, and compelling than any one form alone. As well as layering these multimedia forms, my students offered additional interpretations of the story from their own geographical and cultural traditions—including Rohinton Mistry's 2003 Indo-Canadian novel *Family Matters*[26] and Bollywood productions *The Last Lear* (2007)[27] and *Baghban* (2003).[28] My students effectively assembled their own learning corpus, mapping their intertextual experiences to arrive—via their own paths—at a more personal understanding of *King Lear*'s value as a touchstone for age studies concerns.

I still use Shakespeare's *King Lear* (1608 quarto edition)[29] as the foundational text for that seminar, but I now encourage such multimodal practices of experiencing texts and such remixing and multiple perspectives from day one. Because I am not teaching a conventional literature class, students are free to choose from any of the diverse media forms that appeal to them. They are also free to integrate their own personal, cultural, ethnic, and racial experience to their apprehensions of what it means to grow old. My remixing of age studies has now evolved to include the critical–creative work of making, following my realization that valuable texts could be shared, challenged, and re-created by my students, in response to critical prompts generated by compelling age studies materials.

LAYER 2: ASSEMBLING STORIES OF AGING

Learning objectives:

- To explore how the universalizing experience of bodily aging intersects with multiple facets of personal identity
- To bridge the gap between clinical, theoretical, creative, and embodied modes of learning about aging

To explore the creative possibilities of remixing, my students and I turn to the art form known as *assemblage*. As the name implies, this is a form of sculpture—a kind of three-dimensional collage—that uses "found" materials (*objets trouvés*). As a pedagogical principle, assemblage is an appealing classroom activity. It has both range and accessibility: its components may include text, visuals, textiles, postcards, photographs, packaging, or any other materials; and students do not need to be accomplished artists to make an interesting and relevant assemblage. In the context of age studies, the purpose of assemblage—both a creative and a pedagogical principle—is to focus learners on the concept of aging itself, an experience that involves the constant remixing of our identity, capabilities, privileges, and ideas of the self (in terms of coherence, autonomy, continence, fluency, and so on). As a critical and artistic principle, assemblage offers a valuable expansion of the limits of conventional teaching of age studies, especially its static homogeneity in terms of representation as well as in form.

I now begin my seminar by discussing Betye Saar, the nonagenarian African American assemblage artist whose sixty-year career offers an excellent introduction to standard age studies concepts like late-life creativity, reminiscence, and the stages-of-life model of aging.[30] Students are encouraged to watch Saar's 2014 lecture "Fade: The Art of Aging," which begins with Saar's reflection on one of her best-known early assemblages, *Black Girl's Window* (1969).[31] A productive counterpoint to Saar's work is that of French photocollagist Gilbert Garcin, whose creations meditate on universal topics such as masculinity, artistic and intellectual strength and impotence, and resistively narrative portraits of the aging body.[32] Both of these older artists make fine starting points for discussing aging and creative practices as they intersect with other axes of identity (supplementary critical readings include essays by Audre Lorde, Tamara Baker, and Lynne Segal).

We then focus on a specific example of the representation of aging through creative assemblage. Especially for students less familiar with the epistemological values and methods of the arts and humanities, modeling this remixing of texts is crucial to transforming old age from something that they perceive as "out there"—that is, only a problem for public health, economists, or demographers—to identifiable as an aspect of individual experience. Two texts deserve special mention: anthropologist Dana Walrath's autobiographical memoir *Aliceheimer's: Alzheimer's through the Looking Glass* (2016)[33] and Jane Aiko Komori's webcomic *Embodied Futures: A Comic about Aging Together* (2016).[34]

Walrath's *Aliceheimer's*—a powerful and humorous memoir of caring for her mother, Alice, and a strongly recommended example of a critical and creative representation of Alzheimer's—uses assemblage to complement the memoir's intertextual engagement with Lewis Carroll's *Alice's Adventures in Wonderland*. However, in light of cost and length (I have in mind here the economies of undergraduate budgets as well as reading workloads), I usually focus on *Embodied Futures*, which is readily available for free online. Komori is a Canadian undergraduate of Japanese heritage, and this diasporic identity profoundly shapes the way her work explores a nonwhite, non-Western, queer experience of older age in the Canadian urban setting. Moreover, as a conventionally aged university student, her perspective resembles that of my own students. The comic's attractive yet readable assemblage aesthetic makes this work ideal for two reasons: it catalyzes discussion of the ways art can illustrate crucial concepts in age studies, and it jump-starts my students' own imagination of their own stories of aging. Next, I discuss some of the topics generated by the form and content of *Embodied Futures* as a means of laying the groundwork for my students' critical–creative practice of age studies assemblage.

The Conversation

In the first panel, a young character—probably Komori herself—speaks with her grandmother on the phone. The entire comic takes place within the framework of this phone call, with the two figures—the older woman and the younger woman—placed on opposite sides of the text. This visual device frames the intergenerational conversation with two distinct yet interwoven perspectives. Each clearly feels a deep affection for the other; and readers learn how each woman regards the other's age identity, with admiration and anxieties traveling both ways ("You know, I look at you kids, and I [wonder] what your world will be like after I'm gone."/"But Grandma, what about *you*?"). The bulk of the text is filled with references to the other characters in their lives, particularly the queer support group the grandmother belongs to. The text is less a conventional narrative than a fluid, open-ended meditation on the meaning of aging, sexuality, and health-related disparities.

I open the discussion about *Embodied Futures* with several prompting questions designed to generate dialogue and to provide students with possible content for their own assemblages of aging. I ask them, for instance, if they themselves have ever had a conversation about aging—and if so, with whom?

- Have they ever discussed either their own future aging or someone else's or a shared experience? How might such conversations be made possible?
- What might they do to encourage intergenerational conversations?
- What resources and concepts—such as relationships, technologies, texts, or activities—might help? Some that I suggest are reminiscence (Butler, Woodward), filial obligation and social isolation (Kobayashi), and queer aging and kinship (Segal).

Layers of (In)Visibility

We then discuss Komori's visual strategy for the comic. A typed narrator's "voiceover"—literally, since the text is rendered as strips of paper overlaid on the pages—gives context to cut-out illustrations of characters and their speech bubbles. These all form a foreground to the background composed of what appear to be photographs and postcards depicting a range of landscapes (presumably from the North American West Coast but also a few starscapes—a curious backdrop for a conversation about aging). These multiple layers give extra dimensions to the conversations shown, many of which describe the "invisibilizing" tendencies of contemporary Western culture ("Because of the way older people are invisibilized, funding and dialogue with broader communities is always a challenge service providers face").

Yet a paradox of this layering technique—voices, images, experiences, and texts—is that each layer effectively obscures what is underneath it. The complexity of a subject like aging (or, more generally, the individual experience of health and illness in the health humanities context) may mean that layering—that is, to honor complexity—also tends to obscure details.

When I discuss issues of visibility, health, and age with my students, topics that I raise include the following:

- How do the health needs of younger people differ from those of older persons? Are there cases where they might overlap? Do the labels "young" and "old" amplify or mute the concerns of other age cohorts?
- In what ways does age intersect, complement, or challenge other aspects of identity, including race, gender, class, or sexuality?

- What concepts or resources are most relevant to the discussion? Some that I suggest include aging and ambivalence (Baars), "pedagogy of mortification" (Woodward), narratives of aging (Gullette), age and race (Lorde, Baker), and late life and the language of "burden" (Charise 2012).

Sites of Learning about Aging

Komori's comic highlights the cultural and generational differences in sites where aging is learned and supported, ranging from religious organizations to queer communities to Indigenous (First Nations) practices and traditions. The relative significance of these sites changes over time, as is pointed out in the comic ("Institutions like Japanese cultural centres and churches, which provide social hubs, were much more popular with my grandparents' generation"). In the classroom, I ask students about their own sites of learning about aging:

- Where did learning about aging take place? How does their relationship to places—geographical, domestic, institutional, medical, and community—prepare them for the idea of aging? Those spaces may be both present and past, concrete and virtual, public and private. Where might other sites of learning exist?
- Are intergenerational relationships or spaces available to them? Where are they located? If they do not have access to those encounters, why not? What are the obstacles to intergenerational encounters, and how might they be mitigated?
- In terms of concepts and resources, I recommend the ACT (Aging + Communications + Technology) Project, intergenerational interaction, and Anne Basting's *Forget Memory*.[35]

Addressing Accessibility

Embodied Futures also gives students the opportunity to discuss aging's intersection with disability. As one character says, "Addressing accessibility across generations benefits all of us, not just older people." Yet such age-related differences in accessibility may, ironically, affect the creative forms used to discuss the subject: how likely is it that Komori's Web-based comic might be read by older audiences, for example? Classroom discussions about aging and disability might involve my asking students the following questions:

- How do, or should, principles of accessible (or universal) design in healthcare settings take into account the specific needs of older people? How do studies of disability intersect with, or diverge from, the issue of older age?
- In terms of presenting health information to an older demographic, how might age affect the most effective format? Would paper-based

brochures be more acceptable to older people than digital content, for example? What about three or four decades from now?

- Some concepts and resources that are relevant to this topic include the intersection of aging and disability and universal design.[36]

Tradition, Futurity, and Temporality

As a character in *Embodied Futures* points out, our future-obsessed culture often "tends to forget those people already living in the future that we all have to look forward to." Both the content and the aesthetic style of the comic invite readers to consider people's relationship to various types of temporality: chronological, embodied, environmental, national. We might all usefully consider our relationships to times past and future; I invite my own students to consider such issues with questions like the following:

- Is there something from the past that they value? How do they engage with the past through objects or concepts that are old, retro, obsolete, antique? What might people who are older or younger than them value that they do not?
- What are the timelines that structure their life and/or health identity? How do they feel about the relative importance of ages such as 18, 21, 30, 40, 65, 80, 100, and where do Western chronologies diverge from other cultural life-staging practices? How do they account for the age of land and the environment or the effects of migration and national identity (e.g., the implied temporalized language of Indigenous peoples as First Nations or of immigrants as "new" Canadians) on healthcare access and experience?
- Some concepts and resources for this topic include aging and discourses of technological obsolescence, discourses of futurity, and transcultural care.[37]

To conclude, Komori's *Embodied Futures* offers students opportunities to discuss and generate ideas that may shape their own aging. Articulating assumptions about what it means to grow old can shine a spotlight on what has been described as "epistemologies of ignorance"[38] as they influence the study of age and aging across the life course.

LAYER 3: FROM THINKING TO MAKING

Learning objectives:

- To diversify the kinds of stories and methods of representation used to illuminate experiences of aging
- To expand the critical study of aging within the academic context and beyond, by engaging with larger public and creative communities

Komori's webcomic, and other assemblage-inspired texts, can provide a valuable catalyst for fruitful discussion; and educators may wish to prompt students to use this discussion to make a tangible record of their thinking on this topic. As physician and short story author Jay Baruch writes in his recent article "Doctors as Makers," the "maker" movement has emerged to empower individuals to move from being passive users of information to its active creators.[39] Baruch describes how clinical practitioners might benefit from engaging in creative thinking and doing, as a means of "responding and making meaning from ill-defined or unusual problems." Perhaps, Baruch speculates, such health professional student-makers will now "ask different types of questions, engage in conversations, seek compassionate solutions"—doing this "not because they are striving to be more *empathic* but because they are trying to be more *creative*" (my italics). It's not much of a leap from that creative response to adapting the concept to the cultural phenomenon of aging. The outcome of the creative and critical thoughts about age studies, generated by classroom discussion, need not be restricted to the usual output form of an essay. Surely, it is also possible to make such learning and thought tangible by forging new knowledge about aging.

Thus, over the course of the semester we imagine how we might each assemble the pieces of our own stories of aging. Concepts I ask them to consider include examining what objects, words, stories, and images help them to think about their own aging, in terms of their own individual cultural, racial, artistic, political, and personal resources. Using our course texts as touchstones, they mingle ideas as various as Saar's images, key terms drawn from the *Figuring Age* anthology, cut-ups of medical journal articles on aging and pharmaceutical advertisements, and the punk amateur DIY aesthetic of zines. (Often, these are drawn from their own cultural communities—for example, as in *AQSAzine*'s "Ancestors + Descendants" issue [2011], whose mandate was to challenge "the monolithic narratives of Islam and Muslims in mainstream Western media").[40] I encourage students to share links, via a course Google doc, to collage and/or assemblage artists of all ages whose topic is aging.

In fact, I have coined a term for this particular approach: *resemblage*—a portmanteau word that mingles *resemblance, assemblage*, and *age*. As an age studies initiative, The Resemblage Project asks each student in the course to seek out "found materials" concerning the universal yet unique aspects of "this old man or that old woman," materials inspired by assemblage, collage, zine, DIY, and maker culture. I encourage weirdness and creativity at all stages of the task. The very act of assembling such jagged contours and incomplete relationships inculcates the kind of humility that bypasses the separation of youth and age, of learner and educator. (Some students with the technical ability like to digitize their project. In my view this can diminish the tactile pleasures and possibilities of the work, yet a fully digital assemblage can also be a valid means of artistic expression if this skill set is already in place or adequately supported by instructor or library resources.) These materials are curated on the project's website, www.resemblageproject.org. This mode of pedagogy, integrating knowledge creation and activism, gives age studies the opportunity to break down the rigid stratifications that often separate critical, creative, research, and relational work in health—thus asserting an inventive epistemology of accessibility and inclusion at the center of health humanities.

Conclusion: Making Age Studies Matter

One limitation of age studies, as it is currently taught, is the fact that the field focuses predominantly on white, Western, and female experience. Unusually, age studies is saturated by a deeply feminist ethos—which makes it an important exemplar for the health humanities. However, these default settings of race, geography, and gender may clash with the experiences of an increasingly diverse student body. As an educator, I teach what I know (and judge to be valuable age studies competencies). But I am also compelled to confront the gaps in my personal knowledge—lacunae that arise from my own age as well as my lack of lived experience with facets of identity that are not mine to live and breathe. My hope for The Resemblage Project is that, through its beginnings as a pedagogical strategy, it has the potential to generate new materials for age studies practitioners. By emphasizing creativity as a concrete expression of complex modes of thinking, the creative ethos of resemblage encourages critically embodied considerations of age and aging, while responding to valuable critiques of empathy as the foundation of teaching and learning of health humanities.

PEDAGOGY EXERCISE SECTION

The Resemblage Project: Instructions and Practical Tips

ONGOING PROMPT

Throughout this course we will imagine, separately and together, what each of us might assemble as important pieces of our own, individual stories of aging. To prepare for this ongoing task, begin by asking yourself, What are the objects, words, stories, and images that help you think about your own aging?

Draw deeply from the resources that inspire you: cultural, racial, artistic, political, personal.

PRACTICAL TIPS

At the beginning of the course, give each student an extra-large ziplock bag for collecting the component pieces of their assemblage. Assignments and notes, along with other found materials, can go in here—no limits. Encourage weirdness and creativity. Keep your own bag as well, and bring it to class every week to model the accumulation and layered thinking process (obviously, you are going to make one too).

Encourage students to scan and/or print copies of precious things (like photos) and to photocopy excerpts from books so that books remain intact and, if course-related, can be sold again.

Basic budget items include extra-large ziplock bags, tape (clear, matte, and decorated if you can), glue (ideally glue-stick, fabric, and heavy-duty like Gorilla Glue—watch the fumes), and scissors (a one-time start-up expense). Depending on numbers, budget is between $50 and $100 per year.

Recommended but optional are backings for assemblage (like foam boards sold at major stationery supply stores; 10" × 12" is a good start, but too big a surface can be overwhelming; go smaller to start).

Digitizing a project reduces costs almost to nil but assumes facility with basic digital image manipulation and assembly; the tactile pleasures and possibilities of the work are diminished, but fully digital assemblage can fit the bill if supported by curriculum and learners' skill level.

Teaching grants, if available at your institution, might help cover expenses, especially if presented as a research-creation and/or experiential learning initiative.

Notes

1. Stephen Katz, "What Is Age Studies?" *Age, Culture, Humanities* 1, no. 1 (2014): 17–23.

2. Andrea Charise, "Site, Sector, Scope: Mapping the Epistemological Landscape of Health Humanities," *Journal of Medical Humanities* 38, no. 4 (2017): 431–44.

3. Robert Butler, "Age-ism: Another Form of Bigotry," *Gerontologist* 9, no. 4, pt. 1 (1969): 243.

4. Nathan Stall, "Time to End Ageism in Medical Education," *Canadian Medical Association Journal* 184, no. 6 (2012): 728.

5. Margaret Cruikshank, *Learning to Be Old: Gender, Culture, and Aging* (Lanham, MD: Rowman and Littlefield, 2009), 27.

6. Thomas R. Cole, *The Journey of Life: A Cultural History of Aging in America* (New York: Cambridge University Press, 1992).

7. Margaret Morganaroth Gullette, *Agewise: Fighting the New Ageism in America* (Chicago: University of Chicago Press, 2011).

8. Kathleen Woodward, ed., *Figuring Age: Women, Bodies, Generations* (Bloomington: Indiana University Press, 1999).

9. Ibid.

10. Simon J. Williams, Paul Higgs, and Stephen Katz, "Neuroculture, Active Ageing and the 'Older Brain': Problems, Promises and Prospects," *Sociology of Health & Illness* 34, no. 1 (2012): 64.

11. John Rowe and Robert L. Kahn, "Successful Aging," *Gerontologist* 37, no. 4 (1997): 433.

12. Anne Basting, *Forget Memory: Creating Better Lives for People with Dementia* (Baltimore: Johns Hopkins University Press, 2009).

13. Anne Karpf, "The Liberation of Growing Old," *New York Times*, January 3, 2015, accessed October 28, 2017, https://www.nytimes.com/2015/01/04/opinion/sunday/the-liberation-of-growing-old.html.

14. Simone de Beauvoir, *The Coming of Age*, trans. Peter O'Brien (New York: W. W. Norton, 1996).

15. Therese Jones, Delese Wear, and Lester D. Friedman, eds., *Health Humanities Reader* (New Brunswick, NJ: Rutgers University Press, 2014), 3.

16. Important exceptions are Leni Marshall, "Teaching Ripening: Including Age when Teaching the Body," *Transformations: The Journal of Inclusive Scholarship and Pedagogy* 19, no. 2 (2008): 55–80; and Erin Gentry Lamb, "'Polyester Pants and Orthopedic Shoes': Introducing Age Studies to Traditional Undergraduates," *Age, Culture, Humanities* 1, no. 1 (2014): 223–38.

17. Important contributions are Tamara Baker, "The Importance of Aging Studies: Understanding the Influence of Diversity and Culture," *Age, Culture, Humanities* 1, no. 1 (2014): 39–41; Sally Chivers, *The Silvering Screen: Old Age and Disability in Cinema* (Toronto: University of Toronto Press, 2011); and Aimi Hamraie, "Inclusive Design: Cultivating Accountability toward the Intersections of Race, Aging, and Disability," *Age, Culture, Humanities* 2, no. 1 (2015): 337–46.

18. Evelyn Reynolds, "In America, Aging while Black Takes Solidarity, Activism and Magic," *Huffington Post*, February 15, 2017, accessed October 28, 2017, https://www.huffingtonpost.com/entry/aging-while-black-activism_us_58a477efe4b094a129f106eb.

19. Sara Ahmed, *On Being Included: Racism and Diversity in Institutional Life* (Durham, NC: Duke University Press, 2012), 33.

20. See Lawrence Lessig, *Remix: Making Art and Commerce Thrive in the Hybrid Economy* (New York: Penguin, 2008).

21. Trevor Nunn (director), *King Lear* (PBS, 2007).

22. Akira Kurosawa (director), *Ran* (Tokyo: Nippon Herald Films, 1985).

23. William Shakespeare, *King Lear*, illus. Ian Pollock (New York: Black Dog, 1984).

24. Veronique Mauduy (director), *South Korea: Suicide Nation* (Doha, Qatar: Al-Jazeera English, 2015).

25. Woodward, *Figuring Age*.

26. Rohinton Mistry, *Family Matters* (Toronto: McClelland and Stewart, 2003).

27. Rituparno Ghosh (director), *The Last Lear* (Mumbai, India: Planman Motion Pictures, 2007).

28. Ravi Chopra (director), *Baghban* (Mumbai, India: B. R. Films, 2003).

29. William Shakespeare, *The History of King Lear*, ed. Stanley Wells (Oxford: Oxford University Press, 2008).

30. Betye Saar, "Fade: The Art of Aging," lecture delivered at UCLA Department of Art Lecture Series, February 27, 2014, https://www.youtube.com/watch?v=aHusqpfkjz4.

31. Gilbert Garcin, "Photographies," n.d., http:// www.gilbert-garcin.com.

32. Butler, "Age-ism"; Woodward, *Figuring Age*; Cole, *The Journey of Life*.

33. Dana Walrath, *Aliceheimer's: Alzheimer's through the Looking Glass* (University Park, PA: Penn State University Press, 2016).

34. Jane Aiko Komori, "Embodied Futures: A Comic about Aging Together," *GUTS Feminist Magazine*, May 9, 2016, http://gutsmagazine.ca/a-comic-about-aging/.

35. For intergenerational interaction, see Peter Whitehouse and Danny George, *The Myth of Alzheimer's* (New York: St Martin's, 2008).

36. For aging and disability, see Chivers, *The Silvering Screen*; Lamb, "'Polyester Pants'"; for universal design, see Hamraie, "Inclusive."

37. For technological obsolescence, see Teresa Mangum, "Longing for Life Extension: Science Fiction and Late Life," *Journal of Aging and Identity* 7, no. 2 (2002): 69–82; for discourses of futurity, see Cynthia Port, "No Future? Aging, Temporality, History, and Reverse Chronologies," *Occasion: Interdisciplinary Studies in the Humanities* 4 (2012): 1–16; for transcultural care, see Rudiger Kunow, "Another Kind of Intimacy: Care as Transnational and Transcultural Relationship," *Age, Culture, Humanities* 2, no. 1 (2015): 329–35.

38. See Shannon Sullivan and Nancy Tuana, eds., *Race and Epistemologies of Ignorance* (Albany: State University of New York Press, 2007).

39. Jay Baruch, "Doctors as Makers," *Academic Medicine* 92, no. 1 (2017): 40.

40. *AQSAzine* Online, accessed December 17, 2017, http://zeedesigns.wixsite.com/aqsazineonline.

Works Cited

Ageing + Communication + Technologies (ACT) Project. Accessed February 21, 2017. Actproject.ca.

Ahmed, Sara. *On Being Included: Racism and Diversity in Institutional Life*. Durham, NC: Duke University Press, 2012.

AQSAzine Online. Accessed December 17, 2017.http://zeedesigns.wixsite.com/aqsazineonline.

Baars, Jan. "Aging and the Exploration of Lived Ambivalence." *Age, Culture, Humanities* 1, no. 1 (2014): 43–46.

Baker, Tamara. "The Importance of Aging Studies: Understanding the Influence of Diversity and Culture." *Age, Culture, Humanities* 1, no. 1 (2014): 39–41.

Baruch, Jay. "Doctors as Makers." *Academic Medicine* 92, no. 1 (2017): 40–44.

Basting, Anne. *Forget Memory: Creating Better Lives for People with Dementia*. Baltimore: Johns Hopkins University Press, 2009.

Butler, Robert. "Age-ism: Another Form of Bigotry." *Gerontologist* 9, no. 4, pt. 1 (1969): 243–46.

Charise, Andrea. "'Let the Reader Think of the Burden': Old Age and the Crisis of Capacity." *Occasion: Interdisciplinary Studies in the Humanities* 4 (2012): 1–16.

Charise, Andrea. "Site, Sector, Scope: Mapping the Epistemological Landscape of Health Humanities." *Journal of Medical Humanities* 38, no. 4 (2017): 431–44.

Chivers, Sally. *The Silvering Screen: Old Age and Disability in Cinema*. Toronto: University of Toronto Press, 2011.

Chopra, Ravi (director). *Baghban*. Mumbai, India: B.R. Films, 2003.

Cole, Thomas R. *The Journey of Life: A Cultural History of Aging in America*. New York: Cambridge University Press, 1992.

Cruikshank, Margaret. *Learning to Be Old: Gender, Culture, and Aging*. Lanham, MD: Rowman and Littlefield, 2009.

De Beauvoir, Simone. *The Coming of Age*. Translated by Peter O'Brien. New York: W. W. Norton, 1996.

Garcin, Gilbert. "Photographies." Accessed February 21, 2017. http://www.gilbert-garcin.com/.

Ghosh, Rituparno (director). *The Last Lear*. Mumbai, India: Planman Motion Pictures, 2007.

Gullette, Margaret Morganaroth. *Agewise: Fighting the New Ageism in America*. Chicago: University of Chicago Press, 2011.

Hamraie, Aimi. "Inclusive Design: Cultivating Accountability toward the Intersections of Race, Aging, and Disability." *Age, Culture, Humanities* 2, no. 1 (2015): 337–46.

Ignatieff, Michael. *Scar Tissue*. New York: Penguin, 1993.

Jones, Therese, Delese Wear, and Lester D. Friedman, eds. *Health Humanities Reader*. New Brunswick, NJ: Rutgers University Press, 2014.

Karpf, Anne. "The Liberation of Growing Old." *New York Times*, January 3, 2015. Accessed February 12, 2015. https://www.nytimes.com/2015/01/04/opinion/sunday/the-liberation-of-growing-old.html.

Katz, Stephen. "What Is Age Studies?" *Age, Culture, Humanities* 1, no. 1 (2014): 17–23.

Kobayashi, Karen. "Do Intersections of Diversity Matter? An Exploration of the Relationship between Identity Markers and Health for Mid- to Later-Life Canadians." *Canadian Ethnic Studies* 85, no. 3 (2003): 85.

Komori, Jane Aiko. "Embodied Futures: A Comic about Aging Together." *GUTS Feminist Magazine*, May 9, 2016. http://gutsmagazine.ca/a-comic-about-aging/.

Kunow, Rudiger. "Another Kind of Intimacy: Care as Transnational and Transcultural Relationship." *Age, Culture, Humanities* 2, no. 1 (2015): 329–35.

Kurosawa, Akira (director). *Ran*. Tokyo: Nippon Herald Films, 1985.

Lamb, Erin Gentry. "Age and/as Disability: A Call for Conversation." *Age, Culture, Humanities* 2, no. 1 (2015): 313–22.

Lamb, Erin Gentry. "'Polyester Pants and Orthopedic Shoes': Introducing Age Studies to Traditional Undergraduates." *Age, Culture, Humanities* 1, no. 1 (2014): 223–38.

Lessig, Lawrence. *Remix: Making Art and Commerce Thrive in the Hybrid Economy*. New York: Penguin, 2008.

Lorde, Audre. "Age, Race, Class and Sex: Women Redefining Difference." In *Sister Outsider: Essays and Speeches*, 114–23. (Freedom, CA: Crossing Press, 1984).

Mangum, Teresa. "Longing for Life Extension: Science Fiction and Late Life." *Journal of Aging and Identity* 7, no. 2 (2002): 69–82.

Marshall, Leni. "Teaching Ripening: Including Age when Teaching the Body." *Transformations: The Journal of Inclusive Scholarship and Pedagogy* 19, no. 2 (2008): 55–80.

Mauduy, Veronique (director). *South Korea: Suicide Nation*. Doha, Qatar: Al-Jazeera English, 2015.

Mistry, Rohinton. *Family Matters*. Toronto: McClelland and Stewart, 2003.

Nunn, Trevor (director). *King Lear*. PBS, 2007.

Port, Cynthia. "No Future? Aging, Temporality, History, and Reverse Chronologies." *Occasion: Interdisciplinary Studies in the Humanities* 4 (2012): 1–16.

Reynolds, Evelyn. "In America, Aging while Black Takes Solidarity, Activism and Magic." *Huffington Post*, February 15, 2017.

Rowe, John, and Robert L. Kahn. "Successful Aging." *Gerontologist* 37, no. 4 (1997): 433–40.

Saar, Betye. "Fade: The Art of Aging." Lecture delivered at UCLA Department of Art Lecture Series. February 27, 2014. https://www.youtube.com/watch?v=aHusqpfkjz4.

Segal, Lynne. *Out of Time: The Pleasures and the Perils of Ageing*. Introduction by Elaine Showalter. Brooklyn, NY: Verso, 2013.

Shakespeare, William. *King Lear*. Illustrated by Ian Pollock. New York: Black Dog, 1984.

Shakespeare, William. *The History of King Lear*, edited by Stanley Wells. Oxford: Oxford University Press, 2008.

Stall, Nathan. "Time to End Ageism in Medical Education." *Canadian Medical Association Journal* 184, no. 6 (2012): 728.

Sullivan, Shannon, and Nancy Tuana, eds. *Race and Epistemologies of Ignorance*. Albany: State University of New York Press, 2007.

Walrath, Dana. *Aliceheimer's: Alzheimer's through the Looking Glass*. University Park, PA: Penn State University Press, 2016.

Whitehouse, Peter, and Danny George. *The Myth of Alzheimer's*. New York: St Martin's, 2008.

Williams, Simon J., Paul Higgs, and Stephen Katz. "Neuroculture, Active Ageing and the 'Older Brain': Problems, Promises and Prospects." *Sociology of Health & Illness* 34, no. 1 (2012): 64–78.

Woodward, Kathleen, ed. *Figuring Age: Women, Bodies, Generations*. Bloomington: Indiana University Press, 1999.

12

Who's Teaching Whom? Disability and Deaf Studies Approaches to the Health Humanities

Rebecca Garden

Medical humanities has long promoted its ability to teach empathy. The focus of health humanities increasingly extends beyond the individual encounter of patient and provider to the broader social and structural context and is concerned with social justice as well as empathy. Education that addresses social justice must take into account differences and disparities in health and healthcare due to disparities in access. This essay will address some disciplinary and theoretical understandings of the relationship between health humanities and disability studies. It will then engage in a more practical discussion of teaching disability studies and creating access in the classroom for disabled and otherwise marginalized co-educators.

The field of health humanities offers a unique opportunity for immersing students in analyses of the ethical, social, cultural, political, and historical dimensions of health and healthcare—the structural and social determinants of health most expansively defined.[1] Health humanities "texts" (whether fiction, film, blogs, photography, or autobiographical narratives, to name a few) that represent this context are dense with the particulars and nuances of relationships, identities, histories, landscapes and cityscapes, economies, policies, and politics. Thus, even a one-page narrative like that by Tony Gramaglia taken from a collection published during the AIDS crisis in the United States in the 1980s and 1990s draws students so deeply into an experience—of suffering, the fear of death, and the loss of self-determination, as well as resilience and humor in a hospital ward—that they are haunted by its intensity.[2] Students learn from Gramaglia's narrative not only the history of a plague worsened by anti-gay discrimination but also the subtle hospital politics that exact sympathetic performances from patients who cannot rely on justice alone for their care: Gramaglia's narrator says, "I am the good patient in the bed. I can make doctors laugh. I can make the nurses love me" (196). In this kind of health humanities text, questions of individual encounters between patients and providers are inextricably bound to broader social issues, such as homophobia and health disparities, and to the principle of justice, as well as autonomy.

Increasingly, health humanities scholarship is addressing the inequalities in society beyond the clinic, as well as the inequities within. Thus, the field is strongly positioned to educate students in the health professions not only about the people who seek healthcare but also about the "conditions in the environments in which people are born, live, learn, work, play, worship, and age"[3] and other structural forces that shape health inequities. The field of disability studies has long analyzed the structural impacts on embodiment and health, providing a way of discussing social determinants without reducing them to "risk factors" and other epidemiological understandings that can reinforce rather than deconstruct differences associated with disparities.[4]

Health humanities scholarship in general represents varying degrees and depths of critical approaches to power, culture, and language in medicine, as well as embodiment and identity. In the past, when the field was known primarily as *medical humanities*, scholars often neglected the social context of illness, reducing the critical analysis of a literary text to a discussion of interpersonal factors in the "patient–provider relationship," often based on the assumption that reading or writing about patients develops empathy[5] and/or provides "self-care" for overtaxed medical students and physicians, as respite from the rigors of "hard" science gained through a refined discussion of the "soft" humanities.[6] Disability studies scholar Diane Price Herndl, in an essay published in 2005, identified the way that what was more or less the "first wave" of medical humanities did not challenge but rather reinforced physician authority and the medical model of disability (and, by extension, chronic illness). This conception of disability ignores the way that social arrangements and practices disable, and it reiterates, rather than deconstructs, the distinction between the normal and the pathological. It medicalizes embodied differences and thus privileges medical authority. As Price Herndl points out, this kind of medical humanities scholarship underwrites the constructs that contribute to discrimination and bias in medicine while simultaneously advocating for disempowered patients and attempting to humanize medicine through the humanities.[7]

While Price Herndl's critique applied to much of medical humanities scholarship at the time (and is still relevant today), it overlooked the scholarship that—then and now—critiques not only the medicalization of difference but also the assumption that the humanities somehow automatically engenders empathy and that the humanities can essentially "humanize medicine," a persistent cliché of the field.[8] This *health* humanities criticism advocates a pedagogy of discomfort through a critique of institutions and social systems and practices[9] and rejects the instrumentalization of representations of difference and suffering as occasions for health professions students to exercise their sympathy. Scholars like Delese Wear have long critiqued this investment in the humanities' purportedly "humanizing" effect and the concomitant neglect of the structural dimensions of health and healthcare.[10] Wear and other health humanities scholars have moved the field beyond an exclusive focus on individual experiences of illness to analyses of the institutions, policies, and social practices that determine that experience.

The structural analyses that are fundamental to disability studies can help health humanities scholars to unpack the social forces that discriminate against and disable non-normative embodiments. The medical model, as bioethicist Adrienne Asch observes, contributes to a false assumption that "if a disabled person experiences isolation, powerlessness, poverty, unemployment or low social status, these are the inevitable consequences of biological limitation," as opposed to social limitation: society's refusal to create full access to participation for all embodiments.[11] (I will note here that I follow Asch in her usage of *disabled person* as a way of locating disability in social forces, rather than embodiment.) The social model approach to disability recognizes that structural inequalities have been biologized, individualized, and naturalized in the same way that discriminatory practices related to racialization, ethnicity, gender, and sexuality have been naturalized. By revealing disabling policies, programs, and practices, disability studies provides a critical paradigm for a socially engaged health humanities.

Educating health professions students about the social model of disability helps them to comprehend inequalities so deeply embedded in our social systems and structures that they are imperceptible to those who do not experience the barriers. Students may grasp relatively easily how the lack of a ramp creates a barrier to a wheelchair user's ability to vote or how the absence of a height-adjustable exam table or mammography machine can lead to disparities in preventive healthcare for those who cannot stand. This helps them to understand how disability is intertwined with other marginalized identities and embodiments.[12] These (sometimes literally) concrete examples of the social model of disability introduce students to more abstract analyses of other structural harms—such as unequal access to safe and accessible housing, to good education, and to transportation—that cause health disparities. I explain to students how disability is both a cause and an effect of low socioeconomic status. Disabled people experience lower educational levels, lower incomes, and higher unemployment than nondisabled people. Analyses that consider not only income but also material hardship—such as inadequate housing, unmet need for medical care, food insecurity, and difficulty paying bills—find that "at least 40% of all groups of people with disabilities at any given time experienced material hardship."[13] These disadvantages feed into the disparities that disabled people experience in healthcare, such as lower rates of screening and more difficulty accessing services, compared to nondisabled people.[14]

In lectures that establish fundamental concepts, I link the social model of disability to the increasingly familiar concept of structural violence. I discuss the World Health Organization's perspective that "the *social model* . . . views [disability] mainly as a socially created problem and . . . a matter of the full integration of individuals into society. Disability is not an attribute of an individual, but rather a complex collection of conditions, many of which are created by the social environment."[15] I then discuss the definition of structural violence as "preventable harm or damage to persons . . . where there is no actor committing the violence. . . . Such violence emerges from the unequal distribution of power and resources. . . . [It is] built into the structure(s)."[16] Because many students are already familiar with Paul Farmer, I review his and his colleagues' definition of *structural violence* as the "avoidable impairment of fundamental human needs or . . . the impairment of human life, which undermines people's ability to meet their own needs."[17] By juxtaposing the social model of disability and structural violence, students better comprehend how inequalities in resources cause illness and injury and that inequality disables.

Inequalities in power that contribute to structural violence and disability include healthcare providers' tendency to pathologize what might be understood as human variation and their inability or refusal to recognize patients' expertise (which is also a fundamental tenet of *cultural humility*).[18] Disability studies scholars and activists reject the ways that embodied differences are medicalized—defined and managed by medical authority rather than by disabled people themselves. They reveal the ways that medical culture objectifies those who are non-normatively embodied and excludes them from access not only to clinic space but also to healthcare education and practice. Disability and deaf studies scholarship identifies discriminatory medical cultural systems and practices and generates solutions.[19] I assign my students readings by Eli Clare and Kenny Fries, among others, for perspectives from those who reject pathologization and control by medical authority, even while some, like Fries, choose to have medical interventions and work collaboratively with clinicians who respect their authority and expertise.[20] Like many disability studies narrative texts, those of Clare and Fries integrate critical analysis with first-person narrative accounts.

Narrative and literature studies provide critical tools for the contextualization and historicization of health and healthcare.[21] Narrative is a genre and methodology central to health humanities and "narrative medicine" because it represents the perspectives of people who seek healthcare while also critiquing discrimination and disparities in healthcare. Environmental illness and disability narratives provide a rich resource for understanding social determinants of health.[22] In addition to Clare and Fries, scholars and activists such as Stephen Kuusisto, Simi Linton, Nancy Mairs, and Dawn Prince-Hughes use narrative as a mode of self-representation that merges autobiography and analysis.[23] These texts represent an individual perspective and yet resist individualization.

Through this social model lens, students recognize the disabling nature of social structures, whether biased and stigmatizing language; discrimination in housing, food sovereignty, education, incarceration, and employment; or other biases that underwrite disparities in healthcare.

As an educator who identifies as nondisabled, I carefully frame my teaching of disability as inevitably participating in the objectification of disabled people. When I refer to disabled people as "they" and "them," I am continuing a long history of othering. I acknowledge the problem and yet persist in teaching disability, given the lack of attention paid to the issues faced by the world's largest minority.[24] I may provide a model for allyship for nondisabled students who, like me, must immerse themselves in the study of disability and can only imagine the barriers, bias, and discrimination experienced by identities far more marginalized than mine. First-person accounts help to address the problem of representation by giving forms of "voice"—words, images, and signs—to the embodied experience of disability. However, embodiment is central to disability studies' exploration of the richness and benefits of human variation. Agency—as expressed in the disability rights slogan "Nothing about us without us"—is central to disability justice. Thus, inclusiveness in teaching, as well as in students' experience of education, is fundamental to teaching disability studies in the health humanities.

A Case Study in Inclusive Co-Education: Disability Studies and Community Educators

When I teach disability and deaf issues, I invite deaf and disabled scholars to lecture with me or to lead their own sessions in lecture courses and seminars. Thanks to my institution's proximity to Syracuse University, home to a robust disability studies program and a wide range of disability studies scholars, I was able to invite Professor Michael Schwartz, a Deaf (culturally deaf and signing) law professor with a Ph.D. in disability studies, to co-teach a course called "Culture, Communication, and Ethics in Healthcare: Deaf and Disability Studies Approaches." (Over the years, I have had experts guest lecture at single sessions but not for an entire course.)

This elective seminar is part of the Consortium for Culture and Medicine, an interinstitutional collaboration with Syracuse University and Le Moyne College.[25] The Consortium incorporates undergraduate and graduate students from the two liberal arts and sciences colleges into classes with students from Upstate Medical University, primarily nursing and some medical students. The students in my fall 2015 course were an ideal mix. The Syracuse University students were majors or graduate students in public health, disability studies, law, audiology, psychology, and collaborative design (which is itself founded in narrative methodologies). They were joined by Upstate undergraduate nursing and advanced practice nursing students. Teaching across these differences in training, education, and experience involves facilitating peer expertise and education. Through course readings and videos and through my "mini-lectures," the students were immersed in deaf and disability studies theory and narrative and in basic oral history interviewing skills.

I also wanted to immerse the students in experiences that would open up the way that they think about communication and difference to include intersectionality. Thus, in addition to co-teaching with a deaf colleague who communicates through sign, I brought three "community educators" into the classroom for three separate sessions of discussion and engagement through in-depth interviews and dialogue. The community educators were Micah Fialka-Feldman, a disability self-advocate who works to raise awareness about access for people with intellectual disability;[26] Mable Wilson, a community gardener and food justice activist who lobbies for better healthcare access for people with physical and mental disability; and Monu Chhetri, a deaf Bhutanese Nepali New American who provides communication access for other deaf Bhutanese Nepali people and has particular expertise in the healthcare setting.

One of the objectives for the course was for students to be able to understand and identify disability-based disparities and discrimination. Professor Schwartz's dissertation investigates the experiences of deaf people in Syracuse regarding access to healthcare.[27] He has interviewed many deaf people about their experiences of communication barriers when seeking healthcare in Syracuse and through his role as the director of the Disability Rights Law Clinic. I wanted the students to not only read about but also have experience communicating with deaf and disabled people with different social backgrounds and at least basic knowledge about access strategies to enable that communication. Co-teaching with Professor Schwartz was fundamental to educating about access. Professor Schwartz is deaf, and thus I needed to negotiate the arrangements for those of us who did not know American Sign Language (ASL) to have access to him and his expertise. Creating mutual access involved arranging for ASL interpreters and for open captioning, which in our case applied to teleconferencing with a person who was off-site. So each week one of Upstate's audiovisual technicians would set up the room with a teleconference microphone, teleconferencing software, and a free-standing monitor that would display a website with the typed transcription of everything that was said in the classroom, as well as relevant sounds, like laughter. This typed text would scroll in real time on the screen.

At the beginning of every class my students would arrive while the audiovisual technician and Professor Schwartz discussed the best positioning of captioning setup. Professor Schwartz also worked with the ASL interpreters so that there were clear sightlines with the screen. Students not only witnessed but also soon participated in these arrangements, learning how to check the captioning to make sure that their voices were loud and distinct enough to register and how to spell out proper nouns or clarify medical terms, as needed. All of this increased access for everyone present, of every ability. We had a transcription of every class discussion, which we could later use in our writing or other projects. Further, many of us benefitted from having a visual text of what was spoken during class to track or return to, whether because of cognitive, learning, or hearing differences. I want to note here that emphasizing the way that access measures like open captioning benefit those who do not identify as disabled or typically experience barriers, as well as disabled people, can play into bias toward access that provides "added value" and against other types of access, like Braille or sign language interpreters, where there is little of benefit to normates.

Keeping these ethical dimensions of access in mind, my students learned to consult the people who require access about what works best for them and to manage arrangements accordingly. They learned that while Professor Schwartz prefers to switch between reading captioning and having interpreters sign and voice for him, Monu Chhetri prefers working exclusively with interpreters. Ms. Chhetri is from Bhutan and spent many years in a refugee camp in Nepal, and while she and I can communicate by handwriting notes to each other in English, it is a limited form of communication. Ms. Chhetri needs interpreters for full access, and when I have planning meetings with her or bring her to our school to do presentations, I ask her which interpreters she prefers because she should work with people who she knows will provide the best access for her. When Professor Schwartz and I work alone together or go to lunch, I don't need an interpreter because he voices and I can speak well enough for him to lip read. However, he may choose to have an interpreter with other colleagues.

My students learned about all of these nuances of communication access through the arrangements that we made in the classroom, and they learned that both ethics and the data regarding what constitutes effective communication stipulate that the person most affected by barriers should be consulted about his or her preferred mode of access.[28] Through the stories that Professor Schwartz and Ms. Chhetri told, my students learned about many instances in which deaf people did not have good communication access or did not have any at all—including Ms. Chhetri herself when newly arrived from a camp in Nepal. The housing and services, including healthcare, provided in the refugee camp she had lived in were rudimentary. She had had so little experience with technology that she was confused and frightened by the bathrooms in the airport when she finally made her way from Nepal to the United States. Soon after she arrived, Ms. Chhetri became ill and went to the hospital emergency room. Without consulting her, hospital staff assumed that providing a video conference with an interpreter via a laptop would be sufficient communication. It was not. Ms. Chhetri was confused by the video display of an off-site sign language interpreter, and the interpreter did not know Nepalese sign language or the Syracuse dialect of ASL that Ms. Chhetri was just beginning to learn. The technology itself created a barrier rather than enabling communication. After training to become a medical interpreter herself, Ms. Chhetri encountered physicians who refused to hire interpreters because they believed that the rudimentary sign language they learned in high school was sufficient for effective communication about medical concerns or because they did not want to cover the expense of interpreting.

There is a significant number of deaf Bhutanese Nepali refugees in Syracuse (possibly as many as fifty),[29] and Ms. Chhetri quickly became an organizer in her community, teaching ASL to other deaf refugees and organizing weekly meetings in her home, where deaf refugees can share resources and work collectively. Friends tell her about hospitals refusing deaf access. In one case, a deaf mother brought her hearing five-year-old daughter to the emergency room. The hospital called in a spoken-language Nepali interpreter. The physician and the nurse used the interpreter to speak directly to the little girl, and the mother was completely excluded from communication. For my students, this example is a straightforward illustration of the social model of disability. When there is communication access (whether because everyone signs fluently or because there is an interpreter), there is no disability: deafness is cultural, not pathological. The lack or refusal of access is the barrier, the pathology that contributes to disparities in care. The lack of access disables and causes "preventable harm or damage" or impairment through structural violence.

What emerged as the students interviewed the community educators was the way that structures matter. Through their interviews, the team of students working with Micah Fialka-Feldman learned that, in part due to the arrangements of public insurance for people with intellectual disability, Mr. Fialka-Feldman lives independently through interdependence with an excellent staff. His team learned about the legal battle with the first college he attended when they refused to allow him to live independently in the dorms. He won that battle. Students also learned how he then attended Syracuse University's Inclusive U program, where he took a full schedule of courses, participated in many of the same activities and college rites that they did, and walked across a stage to receive his Inclusive U certificate. Mr. Fialka-Feldman uses technology not only in his work as a teaching assistant for two classes at Syracuse University but also for full communication access with his healthcare providers, advising them in best practices: he prefers to bring a friend or staff member to take notes and requests printed materials and email follow-up to visits so that he has time to review everything that providers have shared with him. Mr. Fialka-Feldman also taught us about how he advocates for disabled people with healthcare providers, making sure that they know to communicate directly with the patient, not *through* family members, staff, or others who might accompany the patient.

Small teams of students were assigned to different community educators, but from our large group discussions we all learned how differently disability is structured for different embodiments and identities. We learned from Ms. Chhetri about refugees who struggle with trauma-related mental and physical health problems and receive inadequate care and social support. Those who can learn English and navigate technology and systems can thrive. Those who do not may suffer, often in isolation and substandard conditions. Our third educator, Mable Wilson, is a black lesbian in her sixties who speaks openly about her past substance abuse issues and her experiences of bipolar disorder, physical disability, and chronic illness. She lives in public housing that lies just across the elevated interstate from the hospital, where shootings and other forms of community violence are frequent. Her public support is so inadequate that she regularly runs out of food at the end of each month. Ms. Wilson cares for two young grandchildren while her daughter works and occasionally for her grandson who has a severe chronic illness. Ms. Wilson told the students that she thinks her grandson's illness was caused by early exposure to lead paint. Students learned that lead poisoning is a health problem for children in Syracuse[30] and that "extreme poverty" afflicts many in our city. Of the hundred most populous cities in the United States, Syracuse has the highest concentration of African Americans and Latinx living in extreme poverty and the fifth highest number of whites.[31] Students learned how Ms. Wilson's socioeconomic status shapes her experiences of healthcare and how she spends long periods of time on the phone on hold just trying to book an appointment (and how her friends with cellphones with prepaid minutes use up those minutes before ever hearing a human voice). They learned that Ms. Wilson was prescribed muscle relaxants but not physical therapy for chronic back pain, that she was told to lose weight and to get exercise, and that her providers then recommended bariatric surgery, yet her providers did not discuss her situation: she lives without a car in housing where drug dealing and gang violence discourage outdoor activity, where the nearest supermarket is over a mile and a half away. She was offered a nicotine patch to help her stop smoking but not offered help with case management for her dangerously stressful life.

Ms. Wilson taught us the ways that disability, race, and socioeconomic status interconnect. The students learned that classroom access for community educators includes childcare, transportation, and sometimes meals. We learned together about the degree to which embedded advantages and disadvantages enable or disable, improving students' "structural competency." Jonathan Metzl and Dorothy Roberts have argued that healthcare providers need structural competency, the ability to identify and work with not only cultural and racialized differences but also "health care . . . delivery systems, zoning laws, local politics, urban and rural infrastructures, and structural racisms."[32] Disability studies is a field rich with narratives and theory that analyze the impact of these structural factors on health and well-being, particularly the role of healthcare. Courses that make these concerns explicit and that make those most affected central to and, whenever possible, leaders of the educational process can help deepen students' understandings of how they might work more effectively toward more equitable healthcare.

Access Basics

Ideally, access is created collectively across embodiments and identities.[33] A primarily inaccessible university, campus, and classroom block the potential for this model. Thus, nondisabled educators and scholars must negotiate access arrangements with and for disabled colleagues and students. Nondisabled educators who invite disabled educators to co-teach accrue social and cultural capital.[34] This can come at the cost of requiring disabled people invited into the classroom to have to educate around access. Nondisabled educators should do their homework first, learning as much as they can about disability access to be able to share in the labor of making the arrangements for those who will be co-teaching. Because technologies and theories of access are continuously evolving, this means doing research to find the most current information. What follows is a very general outline of where to begin that research and collaborative work.

FUNDING

Providing access means negotiating different resources including funding, which relates to questions about the financial costs of access in the healthcare setting. (Course materials can include models of crowd-sourcing access, such as models of crowd-sourcing the writing of captions for videos on the Web.) I received support through our Upstate Foundation for deaf and disability access and to pay the community educators stipends. However, given that this was one-time support for what was essentially a demonstration course, I need to find other sources for future iterations of the course. I continuously advocate for budget lines to support disability access for faculty and community educators.

ACCESSIBLE COURSE MATERIALS

Not everyone can read course texts and blogs and view videos normatively, so you will want to provide multiple options for accessing course materials, including blogs, PowerPoints, PDFs, and videos. If you have deaf participants, you need captioned videos and voiceovers. If you have blind participants, you need alt text for blog images (WordPress makes this relatively easy) and screen reader–accessible PDFs, or you must cut and paste the content of PDFs into a Word document and clean them up to be readable by a computer screen reader. Software applications are improving at making it easy to create accessible materials, and there are many resources available on the Web to guide this process. Assign your students materials that demonstrate access that is integrated into the conceptualization of the material itself. For example, Kevin Gotkin's documentary video "The Rupture Sometimes" makes description of the visual elements of the video and captioning an integral part of the documentary, smoothly integrating them into each segment, in which disabled scholars describe their own embodiment and how it has shaped their ontology and epistemology.[35]

ENGAGE STUDENTS IN ARRANGING FOR ACCESS

Describe to students the process you go through to secure and maintain an accessible classroom. Assign duties to them whenever possible. Ask students to arrive a few minutes early and confirm that the automatic door opener on the building is working and to follow up with activating it if it is not. Have them make maps of access on campus, including gender-neutral as well as wheelchair-accessible bathrooms and other intersectional aspects of disability.

EXPLICITLY RELATE ACCESS IN THE CLASSROOM TO THE HEALTHCARE SETTING

Provide resources for students to understand the access barriers that deaf and disabled people encounter in healthcare, the disparities that result, and ways to arrange for access. You can use resources for providing access in the healthcare setting in your class to explain access for the students and assist them in arranging for classroom access.

FINDING ACCESS GUIDES

You can focus on the types of access most needed for your students, instructors, visitors, and community educators; or you can select one or two types of access to review and arrange as an exercise. Organizations like the National Association of the Deaf (https://nad.org/issues/health-care/position-statement-health-care-access-deaf-patients) provide detailed statements and resources. The Disability Rights Education and Defense Fund provides training modules on disability access for healthcare providers on its website (http://dredf.org/2014/11/28/improving-access-health-care-people-disabilities/). Institutions that demonstrate strong commitments to disability often have access resources on their websites. For example, Syracuse University's Disability Cultural Center provides an inclusive event planning guide on its website (http://sudcc.syr.edu/resources/event-guide.html). You can search the Web for resources like guides on captioning videos, and platforms like YouTube offer specific guides. Many organizations, like the Modern Language Association, the American Sociological Association, and the American Public Health Association, offer guidelines for accessible meetings and presentations that can help you to begin to create access in the classroom. These are generally good for getting started but do not provide full access. They also reinforce individualized notions of access rather than advocating for collective access, so you will wish to emphasize the difference.[36]

COMMUNICATION ACCESS

Check with your community educators about their preferred modes of communication, beginning with scheduling a planning meeting. While most educators rely on email to arrange for guest participants and to communicate with students, many people prefer texting or a phone call or an in-person visit to make arrangements. I bring printed materials as an additional source of information and as an aid to memory for all participants, doing the best I can to draft the materials to be effective for each recipient's learning style. Make sure your students understand this process. Ask them to relate it to the healthcare setting.

LANGUAGE ACCESS

In some cases you will need to hire foreign-language or ASL interpreters. Make sure that students understand that interpreters are providing access to those in the classroom who are not fluent in sign or the foreign language. Ask the sign or foreign-language user if he or she has a preference of interpreting agencies, individuals, or styles/dialects.

ACCESS AND DOCUMENTATION

Real-time transcription or open captioning (sometimes called CART, or Communication Access Realtime Translation) provides a different kind of access for deaf people and others. A transcriptionist, in person or listening in via a teleconference connection, types up a transcript of what is spoken and other relevant sounds, which scrolls onto a screen, either a computer monitor or projection screen, in real time. The text of the transcribed discussion can be projected in large type for good visibility, and if the screen is large enough, the total amount of text projected includes the text of what has been recently transcribed. Therefore, real-time transcription provides access not only to deaf or hard-of-hearing people but also to those whose attention may wander as they listen since it is possible to look back at what was said previously and review it. The transcription is saved as a document in its entirety, providing a full and complete transcript of the discussion that can be used to caption videos that are made of the discussion or for further analysis.

Provide interpreters and transcriptionists with advance copies of talks or at least an outline of what will be discussed or presented. Make sure they are aware of proper names, jargon, and other terms that might be hard for them to catch initially and provide them with the accurate spelling. Some interpreters may wish to have resources on topics in advance so that they can prepare conceptually as well as linguistically. Speak clearly, and spell words as needed.

WHEELCHAIR AND MOBILITY ACCESSIBILITY

When co-teaching with wheelchair users, I learned how spaces that meet Americans with Disabilities Act (ADA) requirements are still inaccessible. I sometimes teach classes in my office building, which has a gated entrance to the parking lot; and I have to use my ID to swipe in someone who needs to park close to the building entrance. Otherwise, my office building is accessible, especially since the chair of my department lobbied for automatic door openers, which are not required by the ADA. When I invited a colleague, Bill Peace, who uses a wheelchair, to lecture with me in the main auditorium for the medical school, I called a facilities person and learned that there is wheelchair-accessible parking in the lot behind the building and that he could gain access without an employee ID by speaking to a security guard via intercom. Bill suggested (wryly, as I later realized) that we sort of "walk through" the process together prior to the event. He picked me up in his car, and we drove to the parking lot, where one of the "accessible" spaces was flush with a wall on the right side of the car, which meant that he would not be able to set up his wheelchair and get out, and the other space was blocked by a delivery van. At his suggestion, I walked over to the intercom and pushed the button to ring for security. There was no answer, even after trying repeatedly. If I had simply assured him that there was accessible parking, as I was told, he would have been stranded at the beginning of the lecture and thus excluded. It may have been interpreted that his impairment prevented him from being present for the lecture, rather than the lack of access impairing his ability to attend the lecture. We decided that I would drop him off in front of the building, but we still did an overview of the lecture space.

FRAGRANCE AND CHEMICAL SENSITIVITY

Make students aware that scents, even subtle ones, can cause discomfort and illness for those who are sensitive to them.[37] Ask them to avoid scented body and laundering products before meeting with the group. You can find recommendations for unscented products online and provide those to students. If students cannot avoid using scents, seat them in a group as far away from those with sensitivities as the space will allow.

LIGHTING

Some people are sensitive to LED and fluorescent lighting, which includes projectors as well as room lighting. Thus, arrangements intended to create access, like open captioning and slides projected onto a screen, may cause debilitating illness to others. Work with all involved to negotiate access needs.

BLINDNESS

Students say their names ("This is Alex" or "Alex here") before comments or questions, as they would in a telephone conference call. People may ask students to sit in the same places each week so as to differentiate voices and associate them with identities. Students can learn to describe images on slides and ways of making digital environments accessible to blind people, including the basics for creating digital documents that are screen reader accessible.

NARRATIVE DIMENSIONS OF ACCESS

Many times access arrangements involve working with overworked and perhaps even undervalued staff on campuses. When you approach technicians with a set of logistics unfamiliar to them, share the conceptual goal of access and engage them as experts in creating access arrangements through collaboration and creativity. Our audiovisual technicians became part of the course, working with students, community members, and faculty, not invisibly behind the scenes but as resources for problem-solving. I have gotten to know audiovisual staff more personally and intellectually, including those who have a personal connection to disability. These relationships have built over the years and created more of a sense of community for me at my institution.

PEDAGOGY EXERCISE SECTION

Classroom Exercise

This exercise gives students an opportunity to talk to each other before engaging in a class discussion led by the instructor. Students either read this excerpt in advance or read it out loud in class. Divide the students into pairs, and give them time (at least ten minutes) to discuss the questions before having a large group discussion. The questions engage the students in thinking about embodiment in an intersectional way, where disability and sexuality are dimensions of a constellation of social and cultural textures, including urban and rural differences. Clare describes the way that belonging depends in part on social context and on language. The excerpt gives students an opportunity to think about the ways that their experiences of place and culture intersect with their embodiment, inviting them to connect with the difference that Clare describes.

Talking about "Home"

EXCERPT FROM ELI CLARE, *EXILE AND PRIDE: DISABILITY, QUEERNESS, AND LIBERATION*

> Home starts here in my body, in all that lies imbedded beneath my skin. My disabled body: born prematurely in the backwoods of Oregon, I was first diagnosed as "mentally retarded," and then later as having CP [cerebral palsy]. I grew up to the words *cripple, retard, monkey, defect,* took all the staring into me and learned to shut it out. . . .
>
> My white body: the only person of color in my hometown was an African American boy adopted by a white family. I grew up to persistent rumors of a lynching tree way back in the hills, of the sheriff running people out of the county. For a long time after moving to the city, college scholarship in hand, all I could do was gawk at the multitude of humans: homeless people, their shopping carts and bedrolls, Black people, Chinese people, Chicanos, drag queens and punks, vets down on Portland's Burnside Avenue, white men in their wool suits, limos shined to sparkle. I watched them all, sucking in the thick weave of Spanish, Cantonese, street talk, formal English. This is how I became aware of my whiteness.
>
> My queer body: I spent my childhood, a tomboy not sure of my girlness, queer without a name for my queerness. I cut firewood on clearcuts, swam in the river, ran the beaches at Battle Rock and Cape Blanco. When I found dykes, fell in love for the first time, came into a political queer community, I felt as if I had found home again.

The body as home, but only if it is understood that bodies are never singular, but rather haunted, strengthened, underscored by countless other bodies. My alcoholic, Libertarian father and his father the gravedigger from whom my father learned his violence. I still dream about them sometimes, ugly dreams that leave me panting with fear in the middle of the night. One day I will be done with them. The white, working-class loggers, fishermen, and ranchers I grew up among: Les Smith, John Black, Walt Maya. Their ways of dressing, moving, talking helped shape my sense of self. Today when I hear queer activists say the word *redneck* like a cuss word, I think of those men, backs of their necks turning red in the summertime from long days of work outside, felling trees, pulling fishnets, baling hay. I think of my butchness, grounded there, overlaid by a queer urban sensibility. A body of white, rural, working-class values. I still feel an allegiance to this body even as I reject the virulent racism, the unexamined destruction of forest and river.

How could I possibly call my body home without the bodies of trees that repeatedly provided me refuge? Without queer bodies? Without crip bodies? Without transgender and transsexual bodies? Without the history of disabled people who worked as freaks in the freak show, displaying their bodies: Charles Stratton posed as General Tom Thumb, Hiram and Barney Davis billed as the "Wild Men from Borneo"? The answer is simple. I couldn't.

The body as home, but only if it is understood that place and community and culture burrow deep into our bones. . . . The body as home, but only if it is understood that language too lives under the skin. I think of the words *crip, queer, freak, redneck*. None of these are easy words. They mark the jagged edge between self-hatred and pride, the chasm between how the dominant culture views marginalized peoples and how we view ourselves, the razor between finding home, finding our bodies, and living in exile, living on the metaphoric mountain. Whatever our relationships with these words—whether we embrace them or hate them, feel them draw blood as they hit our skin or find them entirely fitting, refuse to say them or simply feel uncomfortable in their presence—we deal with their power every day. I hear these words all the time. They are whispered in the mirror as I dress to go out, as I straighten my tie and shrug into my suit jacket; on the streets as folks gawk at my trembling hands, stare trying to figure out whether I'm a woman or a man; in half the rhetoric I hear from environmentalists and queer activists, rhetoric where working-class people get cast as clods and bigots. At the same time, I use some, but not all, of these words to call out my pride, to strengthen my resistance, to place myself within community. *Crip, queer, freak, redneck* burrowed into my body.

The body as home, but only if it is understood that bodies can be stolen, fed lies and poison, torn away from us. They rise up around me—bodies stolen by hunger, war, breast cancer, AIDS, rape; the daily grind of factory sweatshop, cannery, sawmill; the lynching rope; the freezing streets; the nursing home and prison. . . .

The body as home, but only if it is understood that the stolen body can be reclaimed. The bodies irrevocably taken from us: we can memorialize them in quilts, granite walls, candlelight vigils; remember and mourn them; use their deaths to strengthen our will. And as for the lies and false images, we need to name them, transform them, create something entirely new in their place, some thing that comes close and finally true to the bone, entering our bodies as liberation, joy, fury, hope, a will to refigure the world. The body as home. (10–13)

Questions for discussion:

- How does Clare describe "place and community and culture" as shaping his body and personality?
- How does Clare's embodiment—physicality and personality—help him to "fit in" with his hometown and/or make him an outsider?
- What is "home" to Clare?
- In what ways are "place and community and culture" embedded in your body and/or personality? (Think about a place where you lived that has shaped your physicality and your personality in some way.)
- How does language shape Clare's experience of being home—in a place and in his body?

Notes

1. Rebecca Garden, "Who Speaks for Whom? Health Humanities and the Ethics of Representation," *Medical Humanities* 41, no. 2 (2015): 77–80; Garden, "Social Studies: The Humanities, Narrative, and the Social Context of the Patient–Professional Relationship," in *The Health and Humanities Reader*, ed. Therese Jones, Delese Wear, and Lester Friedman (New Brunswick, NJ: Rutgers University Press, 2014), 127–37.

2. Tony Gramaglia, "Okay, So I'm in This Bed," in *From a Burning House: The AIDS Project LA Writers Workshop Collection*, ed. Irene Borger (New York: Washington Square Press, 1996), 196–97.

3. Office of Disease Prevention and Health Promotion, "Social Determinants of Health," Healthy People 2020, last modified March 8, 2018, https://www.healthypeople.gov/2020/topics-objectives/topic/social-determinants-of-health.

4. Jennifer Tsai et al., "Race Matters? Examining and Rethinking Race Portrayal in Preclinical Medical Education," *Academic Medicine* 91, no. 7 (2016): 916–20.

5. For a more thorough critique of this narrow focus of medical humanities, see, e.g., Susan Merrill Squier, "Beyond Nescience: The Intersectional Insights of Health Humanities," *Perspectives in Biology and Medicine* 50, no. 3 (2007): 334–47; Garden, "Social Studies."

6. See, for example, Catherine Belling, "Toward a Harder Humanities in Medicine," *Atrium* 3 (Fall 2006): 1–5.

7. With even-handed rigor, Herndl critiques disability studies scholars for neglecting the materiality of impairment and criticizing medicine without nuance. Diane Price Herndl, "Disease versus Disability: The Medical Humanities and Disability Studies," *PMLA* 120, no. 2 (March 2005): 593–98.

8. For a detailed critique of this approach, see, e.g., Olivia Banner, *Communicative Biocapitalism: The Voice of the Patient in Digital Health and the Health Humanities* (Ann Arbor: University of Michigan Press, 2017).

9. Delese Wear and Julie M. Aultman, "The Limits of Narrative: Medical Student Resistance to Confronting Inequality and Oppression in Literature and Beyond," *Medical Education* 39, no. 10 (2005): 1056–65.

10. Delese Wear and Mark G. Kuczewski, "The Professionalism Movement: Can We Pause?" *American Journal of Bioethics* 4, no. 2 (2004): 1–10.

11. Adrienne Asch, "Disability, Bioethics, and Human Rights," in *The Handbook of Disability Studies*, ed. Gary L. Albrecht, Katherine Seelman, and Michael Bury (Thousand Oaks, CA: SAGE Publications, 2001), 300.

12. Mia Mingus, "Reflections on an Opening: Disability Justice and Creating Collective Access in Detroit," *Leaving Evidence* (blog), August 23, 2010, https://leavingevidence.wordpress.com/2010/08/23/reflections-on-an-opening-disability-justice-and-creating-collective-access-in-detroit/.

13. Julia A. Rivera Drew, "Disability, Poverty, and Material Hardship since the Passage of the ADA," *Disability Studies Quarterly* 35, no. 3 (2015): http://dsq-sds.org/article/view/4947.

14. Lisa I. Iezzoni, "Eliminating Health and Health Care Disparities among the Growing Population of People with Disabilities," *Health Affairs* 30, no. 10 (2011): 1947–54.

15. World Health Organization, *International Classification of Functioning, Disability and Health* (Geneva, Switzerland: World Health Organization, 2001).

16. Kathleen Mass Weigert, "Structural Violence," in *Encyclopedia of Violence, Peace, and Conflict*, vol. 3, *Po–Z* (San Diego, CA: Academic Press 1999), 431.

17. Paul E. Farmer et al., "Structural Violence and Clinical Medicine," *PLoS Medicine* 3, no. 10 (2006): e449.

18. Melanie Tervalon and Jann Murray-Garcia, "Cultural Humility versus Cultural Competence: A Critical Distinction in Defining Physician Training Outcomes in Multicultural Education," *Journal of Health Care for the Poor and Underserved* 9, no. 2 (1998): 117–25.

19. See, for example, Simi Linton, *Claiming Disability: Knowledge and Identity* (New York: New York University Press, 1998); Shelley Lynn Tremain, *Foucault and the Government of Disability* (Ann Arbor: University of Michigan Press, 2010); Tom Shakespeare, Lisa I. Iezzoni, and Nora E. Groce, "Disability and the Training of Health Professionals," *The Lancet* 374, no. 9704 (2009): 1815–16; Jackie Leach Scully, *Disability Bioethics: Moral Bodies, Moral Difference* (Lanham, MD: Rowman & Littlefield, 2008); Carol A. Padden and Tom L. Humphries, *Inside Deaf Culture* (Cambridge, MA: Harvard University Press, 2006); Erik Parens and Adrienne Asch, eds., *Prenatal Testing and Disability Rights* (Washington, DC: Georgetown University Press, 2000); Jim Ferris, *The Hospital Poems* (Charlotte, NC: Main Street Rag, 2004). For an online resource of video interviews, see Disability Rights Education and Defense Fund, "Healthcare Stories," accessed March 9, 2018, https://dredf.org/healthcare-stories/.

20. See, for example, Eli Clare, *Exile & Pride: Disability, Queerness and Liberation* (Cambridge, MA: South End Press, 2009); Kenny Fries, *The History of My Shoes and the Evolution of Darwin's Theory* (New York; Berkeley, CA: Da Capo Press, 2007).

21. See, for example, Suzanne Bost, *Encarnación: Illness and Body Politics in Chicana Feminist Literature* (New York: Fordham University Press, 2010); Janis M. Caldwell, *Literature and Medicine in Nineteenth-Century Britain: From Mary Shelley to George Eliot* (Cambridge: Cambridge University Press, 2004); Rebecca Garden, "Disability and Narrative: New Directions for Medicine and the Medical Humanities," *Medical Humanities* 36, no. 2 (2010): 70–74; Garden, "Language, Identity, and Belonging: Deaf Cultural and Narrative Perspectives," *Journal of Clinical Ethics* 21, no. 2 (2010): 159–62; Garden and Hyon Joo Yoo Murphree, "Class and Ethnicity in the Global Market for Organs: The Case of Korean Cinema," *Journal of Medical Humanities* 28, no. 4 (2007): 213–29; Meegan Kennedy, *Revising the Clinic: Vision and Representation in Victorian Medical Narrative and the Novel* (Columbus: Ohio State University Press, 2010); Ann F. Stanford, *Bodies in a Broken World: Women Novelists of Color and the Politics of Medicine* (Chapel Hill: University of North Carolina Press, 2003); Andrea Stone, *Black Well-Being: Health and Selfhood in Antebellum Black Literature* (Gainesville: University of Florida Press, 2016); Erika Wright, *Reading for Health: Medical Narratives and the Nineteenth-Century Novel* (Columbus: Ohio State University Press, 2016).

22. See, for example, Susanne Antonetta, *Body Toxic: An Environmental Memoir* (Berkeley, CA: Counterpoint Press, 2002); Bernice L. Hausman, "Contamination and Contagion: Environmental Toxins, HIV/AIDS, and the Problem of the Maternal Body," *Hypatia* 21, no. 1 (2006): 137–56; Laurie Clements Lambeth, "Lucia Perillo. I've Heard the Vultures Singing: Field Notes on Poetry, Illness, and Nature," *Disability Studies Quarterly*

27, no. 4 (2007): http://dsq-sds.org/article/view/61; Leslie Marmon Silko, *Ceremony* (New York: Penguin Books, 2006); Sandra Steingraber, *Living Downstream: An Ecologist's Personal Investigation of Cancer and the Environment* (Cambridge, MA: Da Capo Press, 2010); Terry Tempest Williams, *Refuge: An Unnatural History of Family and Place* (New York: Vintage Books, 1992).

23. See, for example, Stephen Kuusisto, *Planet of the Blind* (New York: Dial Press, 1998); Simi Linton, *My Body Politic: A Memoir* (Ann Arbor: University of Michigan Press, 2006); Nancy Mairs, *Waist-High in the World: A Life among the Nondisabled* (Boston: Beacon Press, 1997); Dawn Prince-Hughes, *Songs of the Gorilla Nation: My Journey through Autism* (New York: Harmony Books, 2004).

24. United Nations International Convention on the Rights of Persons with Disabilities, "Some Facts about Persons with Disabilities," August 2006, https://nashia.org/pdf/fact_sheet_disability_rights_treaty.pdf.

25. See Consortium for Culture and Medicine, SUNY Upstate Medical University, http://upstate.edu/ccm/.

26. See Micah Fialka-Feldman, *Through the Same Door* (blog), http://www.throughthesamedoor.com/blog/.

27. Michael A. Schwartz, "Communication in the Doctor's Office: Deaf Patients Talk about Their Physicians" (Ph.D. diss., Syracuse University, 2006).

28. Michael Schwartz, "Deaf Patients, Doctors, and the Law: Compelling a Conversation about Communication," *Florida State University Law Review* 35, no. 4 (2008): 947–1002.

29. Samantha Mendoza, "Deaf Refugees in Syracuse Work to Overcome Unique Challenges," NewsHouse, September 7, 2016, http://www.thenewshouse.com/story/deaf-refugees-syracuse-work-overcome-unique-challenges.

30. James T. Mulder, "Docs Say Syracuse Getting Bum Rap over Lead Poisoning," Syracuse.com, September 29, 2016, http://www.syracuse.com/health/index.ssf/2016/09/docs_say_syracuse_getting_bum_rap_over_lead_poisoning.html.

31. Paul Jargowsky, "Architecture of Segregation: Civil Unrest, the Concentration of Poverty, and Public Policy," The Century Foundation, August 7, 2015, https://tcf.org/content/report/architecture-of-segregation/.

32. Jonathan M. Metzl and Dorothy E. Roberts, "Structural Competency Meets Structural Racism: Race, Politics, and the Structure of Medical Knowledge," *Virtual Mentor* 16, no. 9 (2014): 674.

33. Aimi Hamraie, "Designing Collective Access: A Feminist Disability Theory of Universal Design," *Disability Studies Quarterly* 33, no. 4 (2013): http://dsq-sds.org/article/view/3871/3411.

34. Alyson Patsavas, "Disabilities Studies Gains Cultural Capital? And Now What?" *Feminist Wire*, November 22, 2013, http://www.thefeministwire.com/2013/11/disabilities-studies-gains-cultural-capital-and-now-what/.

35. Kevin Gotkin, "The Rupture Sometimes," YouTube Video, 27:44, September 19, 2012, http://www.youtube.com/watch?v=3YkWsk1tXLw&feature=youtube_gdata_player.

36. Aimi Hamraie, "Designing Collective Access."

37. Adrian Ballou, "Get Mad When Folks Ask You to Be Scent-Free? Here Are 8 Things to Consider," *Everyday Feminism*, July 25, 2015, accessed March 9, 2018, http://everydayfeminism.com/2015/07/being-scent-free/.

Works Cited

Antonetta, Susanne. *Body Toxic: An Environmental Memoir*. Berkeley, CA: Counterpoint Press, 2002.

Asch, Adrienne. "Disability, Bioethics, and Human Rights." In *The Handbook of Disability Studies*, edited by Gary L. Albrecht, Katherine Seelman, and Michael Bury, 297–326. Thousand Oaks, CA: SAGE Publications, 2001.

Ballou, Adrian. "Get Mad When Folks Ask You to Be Scent-Free? Here Are 8 Things to Consider." *Everyday Feminism*, July 25, 2015. Accessed March 9, 2018. http://everydayfeminism.com/2015/07/being-scent-free/.

Banner, Olivia. *Communicative Biocapitalism: The Voice of the Patient in Digital Health and the Health Humanities*. Ann Arbor: University of Michigan Press, 2017.

Belling, Catherine. "Toward a Harder Humanities in Medicine." *Atrium* 3 (Fall 2006): 1–5.

Bost, Suzanne. *Encarnación: Illness and Body Politics in Chicana Feminist Literature*. New York: Fordham University Press, 2010.

Caldwell, Janis M. *Literature and Medicine in Nineteenth-Century Britain: From Mary Shelley to George Eliot*. Cambridge: Cambridge University Press, 2004.

Clare, Eli. *Exile & Pride: Disability, Queerness and Liberation*. Cambridge, MA: South End Press, 2009.

Consortium for Culture and Medicine. SUNY Upstate Medical University. http://upstate.edu/ccm/.

Disability Rights Education and Defense Fund. "Healthcare Stories." Accessed March 9, 2018. http://dredf.org/healthcare-stories/.

Drew, Julia A. Rivera. "Disability, Poverty, and Material Hardship since the Passage of the ADA." *Disability Studies Quarterly* 35, no. 3 (September 2, 2015): http://dsq-sds.org/article/view/4947.

Farmer, Paul E., Bruce Nizeye, Sara Stulac, and Salmaan Keshavjee. "Structural Violence and Clinical Medicine." *PLoS Medicine* 3, no. 10 (2006): e449.

Ferris, Jim. *The Hospital Poems*. Charlotte, NC: Main Street Rag, 2004.

Fialka-Feldman, Micah. *Through the Same Door* (blog). http://www.throughthesamedoor.com/blog/.

Fries, Kenny. *The History of My Shoes and the Evolution of Darwin's Theory*. New York; Berkeley, CA: Da Capo Press, 2007.

Garden, Rebecca. "Disability and Narrative: New Directions for Medicine and the Medical Humanities." *Medical Humanities* 36, no. 2 (2010): 70–74.

Garden, Rebecca. "Language, Identity, and Belonging: Deaf Cultural and Narrative Perspectives." *Journal of Clinical Ethics* 21, no. 2 (2010): 159–62.

Garden, Rebecca. "Social Studies: The Humanities, Narrative, and the Social Context of the Patient–Professional Relationship." In *The Health and Humanities Reader*, edited by Therese Jones, Delese Wear, and Lester Friedman, 127–37. New Brunswick, NJ: Rutgers University Press, 2014.

Garden, Rebecca. "Who Speaks for Whom? Health Humanities and the Ethics of Representation." *Medical Humanities* 41, no. 2 (2015): 77–80.

Garden, Rebecca, and Hyon Joo Yoo Murphree. "Class and Ethnicity in the Global Market for Organs: The Case of Korean Cinema." *Journal of Medical Humanities* 28, no. 4 (2007): 213–29.

Gotkin, Kevin. "The Rupture Sometimes." YouTube Video, 27:44, September 19, 2012. http://www.youtube.com/watch?v=3YkWsk1tXLw&feature=youtube_gdata_player.

Gramaglia, Tony. "Okay, So I'm in This Bed." In *From a Burning House: The AIDS Project LA Writers Workshop Collection*, edited by Irene Borger, 196–97. New York: Washington Square Press, 1996.

Hamraie, Aimi. "Designing Collective Access: A Feminist Disability Theory of Universal Design." *Disability Studies Quarterly* 33, no. 4 (2013): http://dsq-sds.org/article/view/3871/3411.

Hausman, Bernice L. "Contamination and Contagion: Environmental Toxins, HIV/AIDS, and the Problem of the Maternal Body." *Hypatia* 21, no. 1 (2006): 137–56.

Herndl, Diane Price. "Disease versus Disability: The Medical Humanities and Disability Studies." *PMLA* 120, no. 2 (2005): 593–98.

Iezzoni, Lisa I. "Eliminating Health and Health Care Disparities among the Growing Population of People with Disabilities." *Health Affairs* 30, no. 10 (2011): 1947–54.

Jargowsky, Paul. "Architecture of Segregation: Civil Unrest, the Concentration of Poverty, and Public Policy." The Century Foundation, August 7, 2015. https://tcf.org/content/report/architecture-of-segregation/.

Kennedy, Meegan. *Revising the Clinic: Vision and Representation in Victorian Medical Narrative and the Novel*. Columbus: Ohio State University Press, 2010.

Kuusisto, Stephen. *Planet of the Blind*. New York: Dial Press, 1998.

Lambeth, Laurie Clements. "Lucia Perillo. I've Heard the Vultures Singing: Field Notes on Poetry, Illness, and Nature." *Disability Studies Quarterly* 27, no. 4 (2007): http://dsq-sds.org/article/view/61.

Linton, Simi. *Claiming Disability: Knowledge and Identity*. New York: New York University Press, 1998.

Linton, Simi. *My Body Politic: A Memoir*. Ann Arbor: University of Michigan Press, 2006.

Mairs, Nancy. *Waist-High in the World: A Life among the Nondisabled*. Boston: Beacon Press, 1997.

Mendoza, Samantha. "Deaf Refugees in Syracuse Work to Overcome Unique Challenges." NewsHouse, September 7, 2016. https://ww2.thenewshouse.com/story/deaf-refugees-syracuse-work-overcome-unique-challenges.

Metzl, Jonathan M., and Dorothy E. Roberts. "Structural Competency Meets Structural Racism: Race, Politics, and the Structure of Medical Knowledge." *Virtual Mentor* 16, no. 9 (2014): 674–90.

Mingus, Mia. "Reflections on an Opening: Disability Justice and Creating Collective Access in Detroit." *Leaving Evidence* (blog). August 23, 2010. https://leavingevidence.wordpress.com/2010/08/23/reflections-on-an-opening-disability-justice-and-creating-collective-access-in-detroit/.

Mulder, James T. "Docs Say Syracuse Getting Bum Rap over Lead Poisoning." Syracuse.com, September 29, 2016. http://www.syracuse.com/health/index.ssf/2016/09/docs_say_syracuse_getting_bum_rap_over_lead_poisoning.html.

Office of Disease Prevention and Health Promotion. "Social Determinants of Health." Healthy People 2020. Modified March 8, 2018. https://www.healthypeople.gov/2020/topics-objectives/topic/social-determinants-of-health.

Padden, Carol A., and Tom L. Humphries. *Inside Deaf Culture*. Cambridge, MA.: Harvard University Press, 2006.

Parens, Erik, and Adrienne Asch, eds. *Prenatal Testing and Disability Rights*. Washington, DC: Georgetown University Press, 2000.

Patsavas, Alyson. "Disabilities Studies Gains Cultural Capital? And Now What?" *Feminist Wire*, November 22, 2013. http://www.thefeministwire.com/2013/11/disabilities-studies-gains-cultural-capital-and-now-what/.

Prince-Hughes, Dawn. *Songs of the Gorilla Nation: My Journey through Autism*. New York: Harmony Books, 2004.

Schwartz, Michael A. "Communication in the Doctor's Office: Deaf Patients Talk about Their Physicians." PhD diss., Syracuse University, 2006.

Schwartz, Michael A. "Deaf Patients, Doctors, and the Law: Compelling a Conversation about Communication." *Florida State University Law Review* 35, no. 4 (2008): 947–1002.

Scully, Jackie Leach. *Disability Bioethics: Moral Bodies, Moral Difference*. Lanham, MD: Rowman & Littlefield, 2008.

Shakespeare, Tom, Lisa I. Iezzoni, and Nora E. Groce. "Disability and the Training of Health Professionals." *The Lancet* 374, no. 9704 (2009): 1815–16.

Silko, Leslie Marmon. *Ceremony*. New York: Penguin Books, 2006.

Squier, Susan Merrill. "Beyond Nescience: The Intersectional Insights of Health Humanities." *Perspectives in Biology and Medicine* 50, no. 3 (2007): 334–47.

Stanford, Ann F. *Bodies in a Broken World: Women Novelists of Color and the Politics of Medicine*. Chapel Hill: University of North Carolina Press, 2003.

Steingraber, Sandra. *Living Downstream: An Ecologist's Personal Investigation of Cancer and the Environment*. Cambridge, MA: Da Capo Press, 2010.

Stone, Andrea. *Black Well-Being: Health and Selfhood in Antebellum Black Literature*. Gainesville: University of Florida Press, 2016.

Tervalon, Melanie, and Jann Murray-Garcia. "Cultural Humility versus Cultural Competence: A Critical Distinction in Defining Physician Training Outcomes in Multicultural Education." *Journal of Health Care for the Poor and Underserved* 9, no. 2 (1998): 117–25.

Tremain, Shelley Lynn. *Foucault and the Government of Disability*. Ann Arbor: University of Michigan Press, 2010.

Tsai, Jennifer, Laura Ucik, Nell Baldwin, Christopher Hasslinger, and Paul George. "Race Matters? Examining and Rethinking Race Portrayal in Preclinical Medical Education." *Academic Medicine* 91, no. 7 (2016): 916–20.

United Nations International Convention on the Rights of Persons with Disabilities. "Some Facts about Persons with Disabilities." August 2006. https://nashia.org/pdf/fact_sheet_disability_rights_treaty.pdf.

Wear, Delese, and Julie M. Aultman. "The Limits of Narrative: Medical Student Resistance to Confronting Inequality and Oppression in Literature and Beyond." *Medical Education* 39, no. 10 (2005): 1056–65.

Wear, Delese, and Mark G. Kuczewski. "The Professionalism Movement: Can We Pause?" *American Journal of Bioethics* 4, no. 2 (2004): 1–10.

Weigert, Kathleen Mass. "Structural Violence." In *Encyclopedia of Violence, Peace, and Conflict*. Vol. 3, *Po–Z*, edited by Lester Kurtz, 431–40. San Diego, CA: Academic Press, 1999.

Williams, Terry Tempest. *Refuge: An Unnatural History of Family and Place*. New York: Vintage Books, 1992.

World Health Organization. *International Classification of Functioning, Disability and Health*. Geneva, Switzerland: World Health Organization, 2001.

Wright, Erika. *Reading for Health: Medical Narratives and the Nineteenth-Century Novel*. Columbus: Ohio State University Press, 2016.

13

Introducing Climate Change to Medical Students

A HUMANITIES APPROACH

David Kline, Thomas R. Cole, and Susan Pacheco

There is no greater threat to the future of the planet and the health of humanity than anthropogenic climate change. Increased intensity and frequency of heatwaves, floods, and droughts; the melting of arctic ice, rising sea levels, and ocean acidification; and extreme weather events: these are caused by the ever-increasing release of carbon dioxide and other greenhouse gases into the atmosphere.[1] Despite the ever-growing threat of ecological, public health, and medical problems caused by climate change, very few medical schools in the United States have included it as a significant aspect of their curricula.

This issue presses on humanities teachers as well: what can *we* contribute to the education of health professionals (and their patients) whose lives and work will increasingly be affected by a changing global climate? The humanities, in our view, can (1) recover a more robust approach to bioethics and (2) serve as a bridge between students' biomedical training and their own spiritual and ethical convictions. As a test case, we examine a course we recently taught on climate change, health, and the humanities to students at the McGovern Medical School at the University of Texas Health Science Center in Houston.

Rationale for the Course

Climate change is the present and the future. It already affects human health, locally and globally, through "multiple direct and indirect pathways."[2] A warming climate means increases in allergic and respiratory disorders[3]; increases in injuries and premature deaths related to extreme weather events[4]; and increases in and new forms of vector-borne, waterborne, and foodborne infectious diseases.[5] Warmer global temperatures, for example, lead to the expansion of mosquito-friendly habitats and therefore increased incidences of malaria, Zika virus, dengue fever, and West Nile virus. More frequent and severe droughts, tornadoes, wildfires, hurricanes, and other extreme weather events also lead to increased injuries, deaths, and significant mental health problems.[6]

Despite this rapidly encroaching reality, our fear is that neither organized medicine nor local and regional medical groups will take strong public positions and actions until a great deal more preventable damage has been done. Even after fifty-four inches of rain fell in some parts of Houston during Hurricane Harvey in August 2017, the leadership of the Texas Medical Center—the largest medical complex in the world—failed to draw attention to the relationship between Hurricane Harvey and climate change. While the Texas Medical Center rightly focuses on "adaptation" (e.g., improving infrastructure to protect buildings and medical equipment), little attention is paid to the possibilities of "mitigation" (efforts to reduce or prevent emission of greenhouse gases), which range from the generation and use of power to temperature control to transportation of patients and supplies to medical waste.[7]

Despite strong scientific consensus and highly visible informational materials at the Centers for Disease Control and the World Health Organization,[8] we find very little effort to use the humanities to generate awareness or educate students about the relationship between climate change and health.[9]

Teaching climate change within a medical school presents its own unique challenges and opportunities. In a context where specialization and technical training are emphasized above all else, it is difficult to know how to help students connect the vast issue of climate change and their imagined professional future. In our experience, students feel overwhelmed and at a loss for what to do. It is difficult for them to feel that climate change is relevant to how they study medicine, how they will treat patients, how they see their public roles and responsibilities as medical experts. Furthermore, the issue of making a substantial difference seems so far out of the reach of the individual's ability that students often feel there is nothing to do but ignore the issue and go about their normal business.

The humanities are well equipped to help students move beyond this stance and gain a deeper perspective on their own identities and ethical responsibilities. With its traditional frames of philosophy, art, literature, religion, history, and language, the humanities have always helped human beings explore and understand the world and their own sense of self within it. These two themes—self-understanding and personal/professional responsibility (or, in other terms, identity and ethical responsibility)—constitute the core of what we explore with students in small group conversations. Using scientific reports and texts from public health, theology, ethics, and fiction, we provide medical students with intellectual resources to reflect on their personal and professional responses to climate change.

The Humanities, Climate Change, and the Framework of a New Bioethics

Presenting the issues of climate change and health through a humanities lens, however, does not mean that scientific perspectives are excluded. In fact, it is vital to cultivate frameworks and perspectives in which the sciences and humanities speak to each other even to the point where the science–humanities distinction blurs. For this reason, we have been drawn—in some ways against the grain of the medical and health humanities literatures—toward the framework of bioethics for addressing the conjuncture of medicine and anthropogenic climate change. This may not be an obvious framework at first glance, for *bioethics* is usually not the first term that comes to mind when reflecting on ecological issues, not least climate change. However, looking back to the term's original coinage, it becomes clear that there are valuable resources within the history of bioethics that connect both the humanities and the biological sciences directly to climate change.

The third edition of the *Encyclopedia of Bioethics* defines the discipline as "the systematic study of the moral dimensions—including moral vision, decisions, conduct, and policies—of the life sciences and health care, employing a variety of ethical methodologies in an interdisciplinary setting."[10] It also notes that the term *bioethics* was coined by biologists in the 1970s in order to promote attention to two urgent issues: "(1) the responsibility to maintain the generative ecology of the planet, upon which life and human life depends; and (2) the future implications of rapid advances in the life sciences with regard to potential modifications of a malleable human nature."[11]

As it developed, however, bioethics diverged from its original connection to global ecology. It became associated with (and often indistinguishable from) medical ethics and the ethics of biomedical science, housing itself primarily within philosophy departments and medical schools. Dominating the field's attention are problems such as healthcare aims, the definition of death, patient rights, the cessation of treatments, the meaning of illness, the distribution of healthcare resources, and biotechnological intervention and manipulation. While these are certainly important problems that deserve sustained and serious attention, confining bioethics within this biomedical institutional framework has diverted its attention away from its original ecological concern. Bioethics can no longer afford to bracket the ecological questions that animated the field in the first place. Climate change calls bioethics not only to include climate-related concerns within its normative purview but to return to its original concern with the generative ecology of the planet.

Recovering biologist Van Rensselaer Potter's original vision of bioethics helps such a return. In *Bioethics: A Bridge to the Future*, published in 1971, Potter defines bioethics as a new field meant to incorporate "ecological concepts and values into medicine and health."[12] He imagines this new discipline as providing a bridge between the sciences and the humanities, "two cultures that seem unable to speak to each other."[13] The problem for Potter is that these two "cultures" understand themselves as distinct and not directly related. Reminiscent of C. P. Snow's diagnosis of a "gulf of mutual incomprehension" between literary intellectuals and scientists,[14] Potter laments the assumption that the natural sciences, most importantly biology, are dissociated from human values. This distinction does not leave much room for integration or collaboration. When there are attempts at integration, discussions often seem stunted and unable to get past each respective side's particular vocabularies and modes of thinking. In response to this failure—which he connects to a general pessimism regarding humanity's ability to address its most pressing concerns in the contemporary age—Potter developed the idea of "bioethics."

The conviction that human values and biology are inseparable emerges from Potter's cybernetics-influenced understanding of knowledge and wisdom as biologically conditioned tools for human beings' *survival*. The notion of survival—the capacity to *go on* living in a given environment—often evokes negative feelings because it is associated with reducing life down to a bare minimum. People do not want to just survive; they want to flourish. It is easy to dismiss the question of survival when it is taken for granted, as has been the case until recently. Yet, dismissing survival in order to affirm flourishing misses the forest for the trees. Flourishing is impossible without survival. In the age of anthropocentric climate change, flourishing may become an obsolete notion because survival itself has become precarious. For this reason, thinking about human survival ecologically is crucial. Thinking about survival, as Potter insisted, involves reconceiving human values in ecological terms.

Human values are just as much of a biological mechanism of survival as is the instinct to procreate. This is because human values play a specific role in the ability to navigate and adapt to complex environments. They are part of evolutionary developments that "guide an organism when the limits of intellect[ual] problem-solving are met."[15] In this sense, emphasizing the connection between human values and survival is essential for facing an uncertain future: "understanding the 'is' of the natural environment leads to value judgments of the 'ought' for the human species, that is, to an ecological bioethic."[16] Linking this program to the humanities, human values developed under the categories ethics, philosophy, literature, religion, and theology are *ecologically* linked to the broader environment. Human values do not transcend the natural world. The categories that give our lives meaning are conditioned by and developed within the ecological limits imposed upon us. Anthropogenic climate change is a sign that human values and the categories that inform them have lost sight of their ecological grounding.

The loss of ecologically grounded human values connects to the Enlightenment view of progress that understands science as the handmaiden of human empowerment. This perspective still dominates scientific thinking today but is weakening as the reality of climate change sets in. The Enlightenment view operates on the assumption that scientific knowledge allows human beings to remove themselves from nature and treat the world as what the philosopher Martin Heidegger calls "standing reserve." The earth and everything in it becomes raw material only to be stored and used up toward humanity's determined ends. Technological knowledge has so enveloped the human imagination that nature is perceived only through "calculation" and "orderable as a system of information."[17] Within such an imaginative framework, a sense of ecological wholeness is lost. Enlightenment is about empowerment and control of nature, not symbiosis with it.

As the philosopher David Wood points out, we are in a cultural and historical moment where these ideas have lost their optimistic and hopeful valence. People are skeptical of progress. Enlightenment rationality and its ability to subdue and control nature has been disconnected from old ideas of perfecting the human condition. There is "increasing recognition of obstacles to [progress]: unintended consequences, blowback, autoimmune response, resistance, uneven development and so on. They don't just reflect temporary set backs—two steps forward, one step back—but structural or systematic impediments to the realization of our ends."[18] As Potter reminds us, "our ends" are only possible because we survive long enough to meet them. In the contemporary age, the bleak attitude toward progress reflects the sense of human survival's precarious state. Climate change is threatening the very category of human survival and therefore demands that we adapt and change our trajectory. The implications are clear: either change or face extinction.

If this is the case, where does the individual begin? Where does the medical student at the very beginning of a career begin to incorporate climate change into his or her vision of the future? What does it mean to think about the future in a way that does not simply slip into nihilism or despair? Is hope possible? Is there anything for individuals to do? Though the question of large-scale climate action is out of the individual's hands, this does not mean that individual action is meaningless or pointless. Individual action is more about personal transformation than systemic change. Changing our lives and practices for an ideal happens because we change our ideas of who we are. When we seek remedies for the world's systemic problems as individuals, we are working on ourselves much more than actually mitigating the problems. Medical professionals pursuing individual (and even collective) actions in light of an environmental ideal may not make a substantial impact on the climate. But these actions do provide symbolic and existential meaning for the individuals and communities pursuing them. As Wood notes, this is what Heidegger referred to as "preparing the way." We cannot be sure that what we are doing will make a difference, but we can act *as if* it might make a difference.

These symbolic and existential actions also point to what Wood, along with Jacques Derrida and Che Guevara, refers to as "thinking the impossible." As Guevara famously put it, "Be realistic: demand the impossible."[19] The "impossible" refers to changes in the status quo. It refers to the impossibility of changes in our habits, values, and priorities, the impossibility of an American economy not based on perverse incentives.[20] Yet, thinking the "impossible" might actually be the only basis of hope: "[M]any such changes are indeed unpalatable if we think that business-as-usual is an option. But once we are convinced that it is not, we might be willing to change."[21]

Potter's vision of bioethics and Wood's call for symbolic reflection and action can help link students' individual lives and sense of professional responsibility to an ecological paradigm. When room is made for these ideas within the medical school environment, students will be better equipped to enter a world of caregivers and patients that is being affected by climate change.

With Potter's productive synthesis of the humanities and scientific perspectives in mind, we developed a class on climate change and human health from an enlarged bioethical perspective. The class is structured around a specific arc meant to enable students to journey through climate change's technical, existential, and ethical registers. The arc is meant to help medical students decipher and negotiate their personal and professional relationship to climate change. It is divided into three general sections that provide different approaches and perspectives to climate change, ranging from the presentation of scientific data to religiously informed reflection.

Course Description

We present a summary of the course we have developed. We encourage readers teaching humanities in medical and the health professional schools to use this as a guide in developing their own courses.

FACTS, FIGURES, AND WHAT TO DO

The first two sessions are meant to expose students to the basic facts of anthropogenic climate change in clear, concise, nontechnical language. We present its implications for human health, current responses at the levels of policy and politics, and potential courses of action for everyday individual lives. For example, in order to give students an easily graspable understanding of the basic science and broad implications of climate change, we read selections from Robert Hensen's *A Thinking Person's Guide to Climate Change.*[22] Popular-level readings like this allow students to gain a competent understanding of the issue and approach more technical documents such as the Intergovernmental Panel on Climate Change[23] report with confidence. For climate change's connection to human health, we use selections from the edited volume *Climate Change and Public Health*.[24] These first two sessions can be a difficult experience. Often, students encounter the facts of climate change and are left feeling helpless. The issue of climate change is so enormous and catastrophic in its scope that students feel overwhelmed and demoralized and find it difficult to make real connections with their own individual lives at both the personal and the professional levels. Being exposed to the facts of a warming planet often makes thinking about a tangible or effective course of action impossible.[25] This is where the humanities enter the picture.

BIOETHICAL AND HUMANISTIC PERSPECTIVES

The middle section of the course includes class sessions on bioethical, religious, ethical, and aesthetic perspectives on climate change. Using Potter's *Bioethics: A Bridge to the Future* as a guide, we begin by introducing a bioethical perspective that emphasizes the cultivation of human values as an ecological imperative.[26] We then consider various theological and religious responses to the issue, including Christian, Islamic, Hindu, Jewish, and Buddhist.[27] Students are encouraged to think critically about their own religious (or non-religious) perspectives and how these influence their view and experience of climate change. We discuss various ethical perspectives of climate change, focusing on the ethics of human healthcare in a changing global climate. For example, we read a wide variety of ethical perspectives from *Moral Ground: Ethical Action for a Planet in Peril*, from the religiously inspired vision of care for Creation advocated by figures such as John Paul II to Peter Singer's utilitarian vision of fairly dividing human access to diminishing natural resources.[28] We present fictional depictions of climate change and examine how art and imagination can help us cope and respond to a changing world.[29] And we direct them to recent historical and literary perspectives on the age of the Anthropocene.[30]

The primary goal of the middle section is to get students to "sit with" the issue of climate change and connect it to their deepest spiritual, ethical, and moral convictions. We find that by reading through these humanistic lenses, students are able to come to terms with the overwhelming nature of the issue and begin to "think the impossible" and what responsible, ethical, and spiritually nourishing action might look like in their own limited contexts, both as individuals and as members of the medical profession.

RESPONSIBILITY AND TAKING ACTION

The final section of the course brings students back to the concrete questions of personal and professional responsibility and practical action. After "sitting with" climate change through bioethical and humanistic perspectives, approaching the concrete and practical takes on a much more vibrant and holistic relation to students' lives. We discuss medical professionals' roles as experts in human health and how such expertise might be applied to advocacy for climate change awareness and action. For example, we discuss the Code of Ethics of the American Medical Association within the specific framework of climate change.[31] In light of students' own self-understanding, we focus on their roles as public health advocates and how medical professionals are in a unique position to educate and inform the public about climate change's impact on human health. We also discuss what it means to be ethical agents within a professional setting and possible challenges and decisions that students might face in a future determined by a changing global climate.[32]

Finally, we arrive at the last session in which students answer a question we ask them on the first day of class: what one thing do you wish to accomplish or contribute in relation to climate change? By this time students have a basic working knowledge of the facts of climate change and what is being done to fight it. They have reflected bioethically, religiously, morally, and aesthetically on the issue and have been challenged to connect it to their own spiritual, moral, and imaginative perspectives. They have reflected on their own roles as health professionals in a changing global climate and have committed to practical actions geared toward reducing their carbon footprints. By the time students have worked through these different perspectives and approaches in readings and class discussions, we think that they are better equipped to think critically and practically about climate change.

PEDAGOGY EXERCISE SECTION

Exercise: Climate Change and *The Physician Charter*

Toward the end of the twentieth century, physician leaders in the United States and Europe became increasingly concerned that commercialization, for-profit insurance companies, bureaucratic payment mechanisms, specialization, increasingly technical testing and medical procedures, and electronic medical records were crowding out ethical values and standards of professionalism in medicine. As a result, the American Board of Internal Medicine Foundation, the American College of Physicians Foundation, and the European Federation of Internal Medicine came together and produced a seminal document: "Medical Professionalism and the New Millennium: A Physician Charter."[33]

The core principles and commitments of the charter are as follows:

Fundamental Principles

- Principle of primacy of patient welfare
- Principle of patient autonomy
- Principle of social justice

Professional Responsibilities

- Commitment to professional competence
- Commitment to honesty with patients
- Commitment to patient confidentiality
- Commitment to maintaining appropriate relations with patients
- Commitment to improving quality of care
- Commitment to a just distribution of finite resources
- Commitment to scientific knowledge
- Commitment to maintaining trust by managing conflicts of interest
- Commitment to professional responsibilities

Read "The Physician Charter" carefully, and think about its ethical implications for medical education, public health, and healthcare as they relate to climate change. Does "The Physician Charter" obligate physicians to work for climate change mitigation or adaptation? Which principles relate to the impact of climate change on poor and vulnerable populations? What actions, policies, and healthcare practices follow from the commitments to managing a just distribution of finite resources?

Pick one commitment and write a two-page essay explaining (1) how it relates to climate change and (2) what specific action, policy, or practice might be taken to fulfill that commitment.

Notes

1. Intergovernmental Panel on Climate Change, *Climate Change 2014: Impacts, Adaptation, and Vulnerability. Part A: Global and Sectoral Aspects. Contribution of Working Group II to the Fifth Assessment Report of the Intergovernmental Panel on Climate Change*, ed. Christopher B. Field et al. (Cambridge and New York: Cambridge University Press, 2014). A fourth assessment was recently published: US Global Change Research Program, *Climate Science Special Report: Fourth National Climate Assessment*, Vol. 1, ed. Donald J. Wuebbles et al. (Washington, DC: US Global Change Research Program, 2017).

2. Barry Levy and Jonathan A. Patz, eds., *Climate Change and Public Health* (New York: Oxford University Press, 2015), 25.

3. Kirk R. Smith et al., "Human Health: Impacts, Adaptation, and Co-Benefits," in *Climate Change 2014*, 709–54.

4. Ibid., 717 ff.

5. Ibid., 722 ff.

6. Ibid., 732 ff.

7. Myles E. Tieszen, "A Quantitative, Qualitative, and Critical Assessment of Surgical Waste," *JAMA* 267, no. 20 (1992): 2765–68.

8. Centers for Disease Control and Prevention, "Climate and Health," last updated October 19, 2016, accessed November 27, 2017, https://www.cdc.gov/climateandhealth/default.htm; World Health Organization, "Climate Change and Human Health," accessed November 27, 2017, http://www.who.int/globalchange/summary/en/index10.html.

9. In September 2017, the Harvard University Center for the Environment sponsored the conference Medical Humanities, Social Sciences, and the Environment, http://environment.harvard.edu/events/2017-09-29-160000-2017-09-29-210000/medical-humanities-social-sciences-and-environment.

10. Stephen G. Post, ed., "Introduction," in *Encyclopedia of Bioethics*, vol. 1, 3rd ed. (New York: Macmillan Reference, 2004), xi–xv.

11. Ibid.

12. Peter J. Whitehouse, "The Rebirth of Bioethics: Extending the Original Formulations of Van Rensselaer Potter," *American Journal of Bioethics* 3, no. 4 (2003): W26,

13. Van Rensselaer Potter, *Bioethics: Bridge to the Future* (Englewood Cliffs, NJ: Prentice Hall, 1971), vii.

14. C. P. Snow, *The Two Cultures* (Cambridge: Cambridge University Press, 1998), 4.

15. Whitehouse, "Rebirth of Bioethics."

16. Van Rensselaer Potter, *Global Bioethics: Building on the Leopold Legacy* (Englewood Cliffs, NJ: Prentice Hall, 1983), 59.

17. Martin Heidegger, *The Question Concerning Technology and Other Essays* (New York: Harper and Row, 1977), 23.

18. Zan Boag, "The End of Progress," *New Philosopher*, February 18, 2015, accessed May 23, 2016, http://www.newphilosopher.com/articles/the-end-of-progress/.

19. Quoted in ibid.

20. Ibid.

21. Ibid.

22. Robert Henson, *The Thinking Person's Guide to Climate Change* (Washington, DC: American Meteorological Society, 2014).

23. Intergovernmental Panel on Climate Change, *Climate Change 2014*.

24. Levy and Patz, *Climate Change*.

25. One of our students, Sarah, captures this struggle in a written reflection on the course: "While this is a concept I will continually work through, this class taught me much about climate change's effects on health, a relevant topic to discuss amongst my peers. Shockingly, when I asked a random group of fellow medical students if they considered a climate change course necessary to our curriculum the majority said no. However, when I asked them about their opinion on the 2015 Paris Climate Deal, they all had no knowledge on the subject. Thus, them not wanting a course on climate change has nothing to do with their lack of good intentions, rather it is based on their lack of knowledge. How can we expect those to care about these worldly issues when they do not even know their magnitude?"

26. Potter, *Bioethics*.

27. Robin Globus Veldman, Andrew Szasz, and Randolph Haluza-Delay, eds., *How the World's Religions Are Responding to Climate Change: Social Scientific Investigations* (London: Routledge, 2013); Sallie McFague, *A New Climate for Theology: God, the World, and Global Warming* (Minneapolis, MN: Augsburg Fortress, 2008).

28. Kathleen Dean and Michael P. Nelson, eds., *Moral Ground: Ethical Action for a Planet in Peril* (San Antonio, TX: Trinity University Press, 2011); also see Stephen M. Gardiner et al., eds., *Climate Ethics: Essential Readings* (New York: Oxford University Press, 2010).

29. Naomi Oreskes and Erik M. Conway, *The Collapse of Western Civilization: A View from the Future* (New York: Columbia University Press, 2014); Barbara Kingsolver, *Flight Behavior* (New York: Harper Collins, 2012).

30. Jeremy Davies, *The Birth of the Anthropocene* (Berkeley: University of California Press, 2016); J. R. McNeill and Peter Engelke, *The Great Acceleration: An Environmental History of the Anthropocene since 1945* (Cambridge, MA: Harvard University Press, 2014); Kate Rigby, *Dancing with Disaster* (Charlottesville: University of Virginia Press, 2015).

31. American Medical Association, "AMA Code of Medical Ethics," accessed June 7, 2016, http://www.ama-assn.org/ama/pub/physician-resources/medical-ethics/code-medical-ethics.page. Also see ABIM Foundation, ACP-ASIM Foundation, and European Federation of Internal Medicine, "Medical Professionalism in the New Millennium: A Physician Charter," *European Journal of Internal Medicine* 13, no. 3 (May 2002): 215–19; Van Rensaeler Potter, "Bioethical Creed for Individuals," in *Global Bioethics: Building on the Leopold Legacy* (East Lansing: Michigan State University Press, 1988), 193–96.

32. K. Patrick, "Physicians and Climate Change Policy: We Are Powerful Agents of Change," *Canadian Medical Association Journal* 187, no. 5 (2015).

33. American Board of Internal Medicine, "The Physician Charter," 2002, accessed November 27, 2017, http://abimfoundation.org/what-we-do/physician-charter.

Works Cited

ABIM Foundation, ACP-ASIM Foundation, and European Federation of Internal Medicine. "Medical Professionalism in the New Millennium A Physician Charter." *European Journal of Internal Medicine* 13, no. 3 (May 2002): 215–19.

American Board of Internal Medicine Foundation. "The Physician Charter." 2002. Accessed November 27, 2017. http://abimfoundation.org/what-we-do/physician-charter.

American Medical Association. "AMA Code of Medical Ethics." Accessed June 7, 2016. https://www.ama-assn.org/delivering-care/ama-code-medical-ethics?

Boag, Zan. "The End of Progress." *New Philosopher*, February 18, 2015. Accessed May 23, 2016. http://www.newphilosopher.com/articles/the-end-of-progress/.

Centers for Disease Control and Prevention. "Climate and Health." Last updated October 19, 2016. Accessed November 27, 2017. https://www.cdc.gov/climateandhealth/default.htm.

Davies, Jeremy. *The Birth of the Anthropocene*. Berkeley: University of California Press, 2016.

Dean, Kathleen, and Michael P. Nelson, eds. *Moral Ground: Ethical Action for a Planet in Peril*. San Antonio, TX: Trinity University Press, 2011.

Gardiner, Stephen M., Simon Caney, Dale Jamieson, and Henry Shue, eds. *Climate Ethics: Essential Readings*. New York: Oxford University Press, 2010.

Harvard University Center for the Environment. "Medical Humanities, Social Sciences, and the Environment." http://environment.harvard.edu/events/2017-09-29-160000-2017-09-29-210000/medical-humanities-social-sciences-and-environment.

Heidegger, Martin. *The Question Concerning Technology and Other Essays*. New York: Harper and Row, 1977.

Henson, Robert. *The Thinking Person's Guide to Climate Change*. Washington, DC: American Meteorological Society, 2014.

Intergovernmental Panel on Climate Change. *Climate Change 2014: Impacts, Adaptation, and Vulnerability. Part A: Global and Sectoral Aspects. Contribution of Working Group II to the Fifth Assessment Report of the Intergovernmental Panel on Climate Change*, edited by Christopher B. Field, Vicente R. Barros, David Jon Dokken, Katharine J. Mach, Michael D. Mastrandrea, T. Eren Bilir, Monalisa Chatterjee, et al. Cambridge and New York: Cambridge University Press, 2014.

Kingsolver, Barbara. *Flight Behavior*. New York: Harper Collins, 2012.

Levy, Barry, and Jonathan A. Patz, eds. *Climate Change and Public Health*. New York: Oxford University Press, 2015.

McFague, Sallie. *A New Climate for Theology: God, the World, and Global Warming*. Minneapolis, MN: Augsburg Fortress, 2008.

McNeill, J. R., and Peter Engelke. *The Great Acceleration: An Environmental History of the Anthropocene since 1945*. Cambridge, MA: Harvard University Press, 2014.

Oreskes, Naomi, and Erik M. Conway. *The Collapse of Western Civilization: A View from the Future*. New York: Columbia University Press, 2014.

Patrick, K. "Physicians and Climate Change Policy: We Are Powerful Agents of Change." *Canadian Medical Association Journal* 187, no. 5 (2015): 307.

Post, Stephen G., ed. "Introduction." In *Encyclopedia of Bioethics*. Vol. 1, 3rd ed., xi–xv. New York: Macmillan Reference, 2004.

Potter, Van Rensselaer. "Bioethical Creed for Individuals." In *Global Bioethics: Building on the Leopold Legacy*, 193–96. East Lansing: Michigan State University Press, 1988.

Potter, Van Rensselaer. *Bioethics: Bridge to the Future*. Englewood Cliffs, NJ: Prentice Hall, 1971.

Potter, Van Rensselaer. *Global Bioethics: Building on the Leopold Legacy*. Englewood Cliffs, NJ: Prentice Hall, 1983.

Rigby, Kate. *Dancing with Disaster*. Charlottesville: University of Virginia Press, 2015.

Smith, Kirk R., Alistair Woodward, Diarmid Campbell-Lendrum, Dave D. Chadee, Yasushi Honda, Qiyong Liu, Jane M. Olwoch, Boris Revich, and Rainer Sauerborn. "Human Health: Impacts, Adaptation, and Co-Benefits." In *Climate Change 2014: Impacts, Adaptation, and Vulnerability. Part A: Global and Sectoral Aspects. Contribution of Working Group II to the Fifth Assessment Report of the Intergovernmental Panel of Climate Change*, edited by Christopher B. Field, Vicente R. Barros, David Jon Dokken, Katharine J. Mach, Michael D. Mastrandrea, T. Eren Bilir, Monalisa Chatterjee, et al., 709–54. Cambridge and New York: Cambridge University Press, 2014.

Snow, C. P. *The Two Cultures*. Cambridge: Cambridge University Press, 1998.

Tieszen, Myles E. "A Quantitative, Qualitative, and Critical Assessment of Surgical Waste." *JAMA* 267, no. 20 (1992): 2765–68.

US Global Change Research Program. *Climate Science Special Report: Fourth National Climate Assessment*, Vol. 1, edited by Donald J. Wuebbles, David W. Fahey, Kathy A. Hibbard, David J. Dokken, Brooke C. Stewart, and Thomas K. Maycock. Washington, DC: US Global Change Research Program, 2017.

Veldman, Robin Globus, Andrew Szasz, and Randolph Haluza-Delay, eds. *How the World's Religions Are Responding to Climate Change: Social Scientific Investigations*. London: Routledge, 2013.

Whitehouse, Peter J. "The Rebirth of Bioethics: Extending the Original Formulations of Van Rensselaer Potter." *American Journal of Bioethics* 3, no. 4 (2003): W26–W31.

World Health Organization. "Climate Change and Human Health." Accessed November 27, 2017. http://www.who.int/globalchange/summary/en/index10.html.

PART III

Novel Approaches

14

Digital Medical Humanities and Design Thinking

Kirsten Ostherr

Introduction

This chapter describes a project that has developed out of ten years of pedagogical experimentation at the intersection of medicine and digital technologies. I will begin by describing the context for these experiments at the Medical Futures Lab, a collaborative creation space dedicated to bringing humanists, health professionals, artists, scientists, and pro-social hackers together under one roof to train the medical innovators of the future through creative, hands-on critical thinking and design. I co-founded the Medical Futures Lab in 2012 with Bryan Vartabedian, my colleague at Baylor College of Medicine, to develop research and teaching that would address what we saw (and continue to see) as a major gap in medical education.

In our respective experiences as a college professor and a practicing clinician, we observed that premed students lived in a fully digitally intermediated world, where social, educational, and extracurricular activities all took place through a complex blend of participation in online and offline spaces that, in their view, were seamlessly interconnected. For these students, the distinction between "online" and "offline" was irrelevant as their habits of social life moved frequently across these domains.[1] For example, when our students had a group assignment to complete, they would immediately establish their digital presence by creating a Facebook group, a shared Google document, a GroupMe chat, and other forms of connection as needed. They would interact through all of these platforms continuously, both synchronously and asynchronously, including when they were physically in the same location, sitting face-to-face around a table. Their use of information and communication technologies (ICTs) was unremarkable to the students themselves; the tools were ubiquitous parts of their lives that were familiar from years of use. Yet, we identified two major concerns that prompted us to form the Medical Futures Lab and, later, the Medical Media Arts Lab. First, we noted that despite our students' sophistication and seemingly intuitive ability to adopt new technologies as they emerged, they had little to no critical framework for assessing the broader cultural, political, economic, or ethical implications of their activities on the mobile, social Web. Second, we noted that our students' use of these tools enabled forms of social affiliation, creative expression, collaborative problem-solving, and sharing that were highly valued but completely absent from their training as medical professionals.[2]

The lack of a critical framework for reflecting on the implications of digital ICTs meant that our future health professionals had no training in how to assess their engagement with various forms of social media in their capacity as doctors, beyond the risk-containment-through-avoidance model promoted by many professional medical associations. The omission of critical reflection on the tools of the social Web from health professions training meant that educators were alienating their students, removing an important source of social support, diminishing their ability to perform at their highest level, and shutting down the potential for innovation through learner-centered pedagogy. Worse still, this meant lost opportunities to interact with patients using tools that both doctors and patients prefer in their nonclinical lives, potentially curtailing new forms of engagement that could lead to improved health outcomes, reduced cost, and better care.[3]

To address these gaps, we created the Medical Futures Lab as a multidisciplinary collaboration space that would engage in research and teaching on emerging technologies and social media, the quantified self, big data, mHealth, digital ethics, the doctor–patient relationship, health disparities, and patient engagement. Our goal was to cultivate a timely and necessary field of critical thought and creative practice that we might call "digital medical humanities." One of our core operating principles was that, in the age of user-generated content, there are no more passive consumers of information, if ever there were. For that reason, we argue that twenty-first-century learners need to cultivate new competencies, including content creation, curation, and sharing to facilitate transmedia storytelling that captures patients' full lived experiences of health, illness, ability, and disability beyond the limited context of the clinical encounter.

Our methods draw inspiration from Internet pioneer Howard Rheingold, who quotes new media anthropologist Mizuko Ito as stating, "When you start engaging in knowledge or media production, you tend to develop a much more sophisticated understanding of how knowledge and media is produced more generally."[4] To achieve this goal, we have crafted collaborative educational experiences that foster digital literacies across levels of training, from premed through continuing medical education. Our courses have been collaboratively taught by humanists and clinicians, with additional contributions from engineers, visual artists, designers, communication experts, health technology entrepreneurs, and media producers.

The Development Process: Connect, Pilot, Listen, Iterate

Our inspiration for developing the Medical Media Arts Lab came from numerous sources, including innovative humanist scholar-technologists,[5] media lab leaders and design thinkers,[6] as well as creative/critical practices in our local environments, such as architecture studio critiques and engineering design kitchens. I have described the theoretical framework for creating the Medical Futures Lab network of collaborators as part of an "applied media studies" practice elsewhere,[7] but it is worth emphasizing that the first, most important step in fostering digital medical humanities literacies through hands-on work is figuring out what kinds of partners you need, making connections, and building reciprocal, collaborative relationships.

In addition to my collaborative partnership with Vartabedian, the most significant formative relationships for the Medical Media Arts Lab were those we developed with colleagues in the School of Engineering at Rice University. Through conversations with Matthew Wettergreen, a bioengineer and artist at the Oshman Engineering Design Kitchen (OEDK), we learned how engineers approach "real-world," problem-based design projects in their "Freshman Design" class. Matthew, his co-instructor Ann Saterbak, and director of the OEDK Maria Oden generously shared their experiences of creating and refining a process for immersive, hands-on, client-based project work. With additional help from Tracy Volz, former director of the Rice Center for Engineering Leadership (and current director of the Program in Writing and Communication), we began the process of translating the engineering model of designing material artifacts that solve technical problems into the humanities model of designing visual and textual representations that solve human communication and information problems. I mention all of these collaborators and their formal roles at Rice because, in my experience, one does not always find the most helpful partners by looking in the most obvious places. On the surface, none of these colleagues does work that is related to my own, in terms of either topic or methodology. Perhaps that very distance allowed for a clarity in our conversations; we could not take anything for granted based on shared, field-specific knowledge because we had none.

In July 2013, we pilot-tested several of the design exercises we would later use in the "Medical Media Arts Lab" course. Embracing the experimental, rapid prototyping mentality that characterized the work at the OEDK, we ran a two-day "Transmedia Hackathon" within the Design Kitchen's summer internship program run by Wettergreen. Our goal was to explore how the visual and narrative representations of problems shape our ability to find solutions to those problems. With help from several Medical Futures Lab collaborators, including a visual artist (Allison Hunter), a clinician-informaticist (Peter Killoran), and a communications specialist (Volz) who provided expert feedback in mini-critiques, we engaged in hands-on practices that taught the engineers how to use images and words as tools.

Student teams were assigned specific complex problems in doctor–patient communication, such as addressing the risks and benefits of prenatal genetic testing and starting conversations on end-of-life preferences. We then engaged in a series of experiments using different communication and representational tools to develop the students' understanding of how the form of representation for a problem shapes the way we analyze and solve that problem. By exploring with metaphor, visual analogy, and storyboarding, students saw different dimensions of their problems. Based on this intensive two-day experiment, we refined some of the core processes we planned to employ in the Medical Media Arts Lab course and strengthened the existing ties between humanities and engineering faculty and students on campus.

Design Thinking: Medical Media Arts Lab

In January 2014, we launched the Medical Media Arts Lab, a collaborative, participatory design class that brings Rice undergraduate students together with physician mentors from the Texas Medical Center to solve real problems that clinicians face in their work. Following a process of human-centered design infused by readings on media theory, ICT research, digital health challenges and opportunities, and health policy, teams of students work with clinician "problem owners" for fifteen weeks to design solutions to complex but clearly defined health communication or visualization problems. The problems have specified parameters, and faculty provide guidance, feedback, technical skills, access to relevant environments for observation, and key people to interview. Students have worked on timely, pressing issues such as patient enrollment in clinical trials for personalized cancer drug therapies, goal-setting communication between doctors and patients with diabetes, and improving caregiver engagement on cardiovascular intensive care unit rounds. Projects have included production of short videos, graphic design, virtual three-dimensional models, infographics, game design, text-messaging campaigns, and app development.

Course planning begins long before the start of the semester, with recruitment of clinical "problem owners." We use the term *problem owner* to emphasize the status of the design projects as real, existing "problems" (not theoretical constructs) and to underscore that the team mentors claim "ownership" of these problems because they experience them in their daily, clinical lives.[8] Finding good "problem owners" is critical to the success of a design project, as is identifying an appropriately scoped and clearly defined design challenge. In my experience, the process of finding good problem owners is similar to the process of finding good collaborators: it takes a lot of lunches. Despite our emphasis on creative experimentation with digital technologies at the Medical Futures Lab, I still find that nothing is better than face-to-face conversation for cultivating a good working relationship with a problem owner.

We have worked primarily with medical doctors as problem owners in the past, in part because doctors make up the Medical Futures Lab's largest collaborative network and in part because doctors are often in a better position than many other health professionals to enact change in the clinical setting. An important aspect of the real problems that students work on is not only that their "owners" are committed to finding solutions to those problems but also that they can move forward with implementing a design solution if appropriate. In other words, the problem has to take place in a feasible test bed for piloting the design solution. Thus far, our projects have originated with doctors, though several have involved extensive consultations with other health professions stakeholders, such as nurses, nutritionists, and social workers. All of these professionals could be problem owners in their own right, and indeed, the engineering-based "MakerNurse" movement demonstrates the insights to be gained from diverse perspectives in healthcare teams.[9] Moreover, while our teams engage patients and caregivers as core stakeholders and critics in the design process, a truly patient-centered design practice would begin with patient-identified problems; and those patients would serve as the "problem owners" for the entire design process.[10]

Our primary methods for identifying problem owners have been networking and word of mouth, meeting colleagues of existing collaborators, connecting with audience members at public presentations about the Medical Futures Lab, occasional cold-calling based on publicity or publications by an intriguing Texas Medical Center clinician, and referrals from Medical Media Arts Lab alums—both students and problem owners. (Most of our students are premeds, and we have learned anecdotally that they often end up talking about their Medical Media Arts Lab projects during medical school interviews; on several occasions those conversations have led to introductions to future problem owners for the class, not to mention medical school admissions.)

When I meet with a problem owner, the first step is understanding both the broad and narrow contexts for the problem. The broad context might include incidence and prevalence data on a specific health condition, as well as demographics and cost, while the narrow context is a description of the problem as it occurs within the specific clinical context where the clinician works. For example, a recent broad problem was concerned with the incidence of sepsis in patients who were discharged from the hospital with an indwelling vascular catheter. This problem carries significant suffering, morbidity, mortality, and financial costs. The narrow setting for this problem was a pediatric ward of a hospital with a subpopulation of children with intestinal failure syndromes, where methods for training caregivers, patients, and home health aides on care of indwelling lines were not coordinated, standardized, or aligned with established best practices in the field. After extended conversation, we began to frame the problem in the form of a question: How might we ensure that we effectively educate parents, families, and other caretakers of children with intestinal failure syndromes on the appropriate use and care of indwelling vascular catheters to minimize the incidence of sepsis? Beyond this overarching goal, we focused more specifically: How might we effectively educate parents and families on the early signs of sepsis so that they can seek medical attention sooner and we can improve sepsis outcomes? In concrete terms, we wanted to know if there were tools we could develop and provide to caregivers and patients to help them meet these goals.

Good design problems are specific enough that a student team of non-experts can develop a viable solution that will truly benefit patients, caregivers, and/or health professionals. But the problems must also be challenging enough that the solution is not already known, they merit fifteen weeks of dedicated effort, and they provide the students with a rich opportunity for learning about the complexity of the healthcare system. I typically start cultivating problem owner relationships at least nine months before the semester begins. With a target size of four or five students per team, in a class capped at twenty to twenty-five students, this means finding at least five or six problem owners per semester. Given the unpredictability of clinical life, I encourage problem owners to pair up with a colleague who can step in if scheduling conflicts arise.

Process

The process for implementing the Medical Media Arts Lab draws inspiration from work that blends arts, humanities, and science, an emerging field of practice that I have described elsewhere as "applied media studies" work.[11] While we expect the process to be iterative as we encounter successes and failures, the basic format is a semester-long course that proceeds through the following steps (Figure 14.1).

The overall process of running the course consists of a mixture of discussion-based seminars focused on assigned readings in media theory, digital health technology, and other relevant topics, with in-class human-centered design exercises and in-class visits by problem owners. When the problem owners come to class, I provide structured exercises on identifying core stakeholders for the problem, understanding what they want or need relative to the problem, and exploring other dimensions of the problem through storyboarding and prototyping once the students have conducted sufficient end-user research. Outside of class, the student teams conduct deep end-user research, brainstorm with problem owners, engage in participant observation, conduct literature reviews, interview stakeholders, and pilot test solutions.[12]

At three points during the semester, we run critiques where the student teams give ten-minute presentations that are structured to address the current

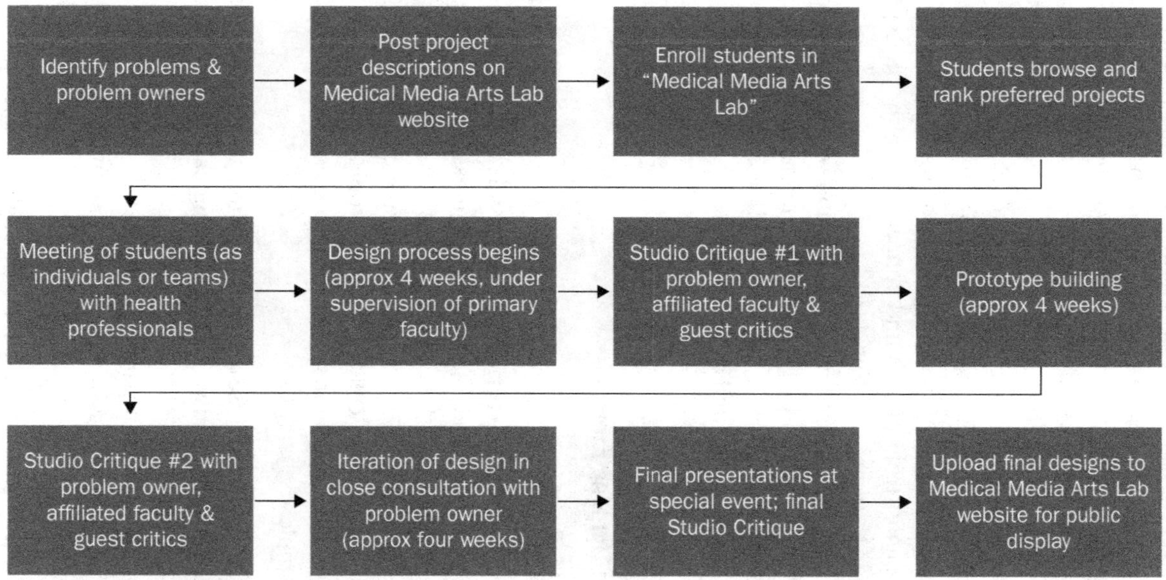

FIGURE 14.1 Medical Media Arts Lab logic model.

design phase, discoveries, unanswered questions, and next steps. Consistent with human-centered design practice, students spend a lot of time working to understand and empathize with their true end-users, primarily by listening to members of that group. The critiques are designed to ensure that students are reaching target design benchmarks and to help them frame their research insights in actionable forms. In addition to the problem owners, the varied contributors to the teaching team are present for the critiques, as are patients, caregivers, and other representatives of the "end-user" perspective.

The selection of assigned readings evolves throughout the semester to ensure that our students are up to date on current debates, policy decisions, new technologies, and research discoveries. Readings that I have found particularly valuable for setting out key concepts to anchor the design process focus on media theory, digital technologies and connected health, the e-patient movement, and design thinking in medicine.[13]

In addition to using class time for discussion of readings and design sessions with problem owners, I build in unstructured teamwork time to allow impromptu feedback, guaranteed availability of all team members, and dedicated time for teams to go off-site and conduct research.

Sample Design Thinking Exercises

Our design sessions build toward developing a multidimensional understanding of the core user's experience of the problem that the team is working to solve and then ensuring that their solution addresses all of the features of the problem that are most important to those users.

In our design sessions, we explore the power of metaphors, similes, and other kinds of analogies as creative thinking tools. We start by defining our terms with examples to demonstrate what we mean by "Doing things with words," for example,

> Metaphor: a word or phrase that uses one thing to mean another, to suggest likeness between the two things (fighting cancer, surfing the Internet, buried in email).
>
> Simile: a phrase that compares two things using "like" or "as" to suggest similarity (getting a mammogram is like making a panini with your breast).

Then we ask the teams to use these tools through exercises such as,

> Create ten metaphors or similes for your problem:
> My problem is ___________________________.
> My problem is like _________________________.

We introduce the broader concept of analogy,

> Analogy: extended comparison, often emphasizing similar structures between two things, using logical argument for the purpose of explanation or clarification.
> Example: machine or city analogy for human body

Some of the most illuminating results come from the absurdist-sounding exercise,

> Create five analogies.
> How is your problem like a . . .
> grocery store?
> airplane?
> puppy?
> cantaloupe?
> swimming pool?

We also use visual analogy exercises, instructing students to reflect on the physical characteristics of their problem by asking,

> What does this problem look like?
> What are its most salient features?
> What is its setting (mise-en-scène: costumes, props, backdrop, lighting, actors)?
> Sketch your problem, then sketch two other scenarios that visually resemble your problem.

Through these exercises, students develop the ability to explore affective, aesthetic, and narrative aspects of problems that typically escape a narrow biomedical frame for defining health and disease. For example, many of the barriers that patients face involve non-medical aspects of their lives, ranging from poverty and structural racism to feeling intimidated by medical jargon or feeling fatigued from being a caregiver of a chronically ill patient. What kinds of apps or other ICT interfaces do these patients use, and why? What do they find pleasurable about using some apps that keeps them coming back? What are the compelling stories that engage their interest? And how might a team's design solution be like those other experiences that effectively engage their users?

Many of the smaller design exercises become components of a storyboard, which we use extensively as a design tool for discovery, synthesis, and usability testing. I use examples from cinematic narrative to explain how stories take place in space and time and flow through a cause–effect chain that is often nonlinear and recursive. This framing provides the context for students to think through the constraints and conditions of possibility for their design solution. For example, if a team designs a mobile app that is meant to connect a surgical patient through the continuum of care, from pre-op to post-op to discharge, that means that the patient must not only have a device that can run the app but also gain access to the app, be motivated to install it, log in and use it, and then—most importantly—experience some incentive to return to the app to enter the status updates that the team expects will help solve their information or communication problem.

In thinking through and visualizing every single step in the process—before, during, and after—the design team members test their understanding of the target user population. I push them to identify the sources of their design decisions: Are they based on knowledge from direct observation or communication, from literature review, or from tacit assumptions? Might those tacit assumptions include implicit biases that could be unintentionally harmful to patients? I often encourage students to return to on-site research as often as their interlocutors allow, to ensure that they ground their design in genuine situated knowledges, a concept from feminist science and technology studies that informs much of the course design.[14] In addition to ensuring that a design is developed from the user's perspective, storyboarding helps address a common mistake in digital health design: the assumption that once a tool is available, users will automatically use it, exactly as intended. We address this fallacy by assigning a team member the role of devil's advocate. Along with this student, I question every step of the process through which the user encounters the design solution, and we add frames to the storyboard to map out spaces where the process could go awry so that the team can work on addressing those weak links (Figure 14.2).

Outcomes

We have found that long-lasting collaborative relationships are built on reciprocity, and for that reason, we work to ensure that the Medical Media Arts Lab generates benefits for all participants. Students develop their resumés or portfolios through an applied, relevant context, and they experience the gratification of helping to solve a real problem and thereby improve patients' lives. Health professionals gain tools and insights that help them improve their communication with patients, reverse mentoring by so-called digital natives, and work that forms the foundation for new research studies and publications. Patients develop greater understanding, confidence, and self-efficacy through collaborative engagement that empowers them to attain better health outcomes.

While it is difficult to precisely quantify the results of these efforts, the promise of our work thus far has attracted the attention of the Association of American Medical Colleges (AAMC), a national credentialing body for North American medical schools. Jennifer Salopek, editor of the AAMC blog *Wing of Zock*, conducted interviews with our faculty and students for a three-part

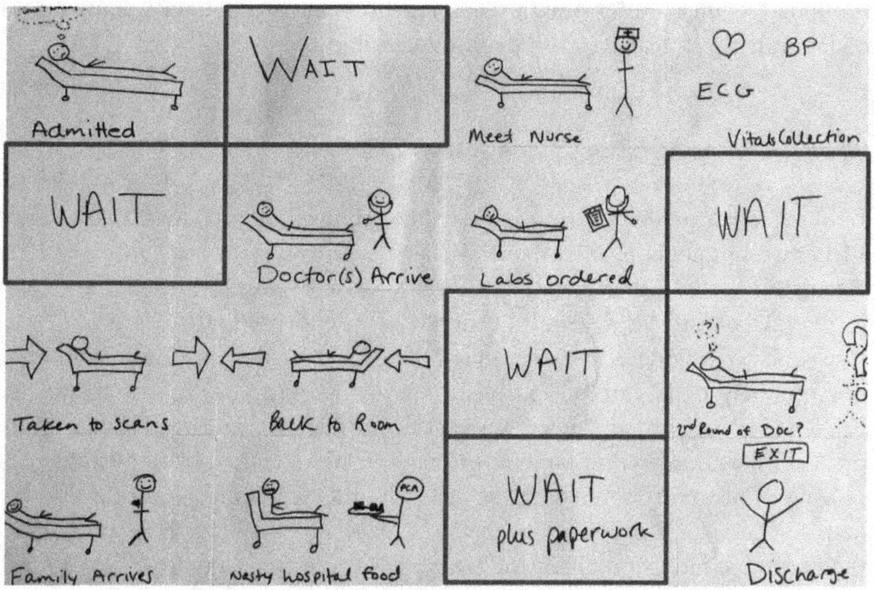
Admitted
WAIT
Meet Nurse
BP
ECG
Vitals Collection
WAIT
Doctor(s) Arrive
Labs ordered
WAIT
Taken to scans
Back to Room
WAIT
2nd Round of Doc?
EXIT
Family Arrives
Nasty hospital food
WAIT
plus paperwork
Discharge

FIGURE 14.2 Storyboard about inpatient communication identifies the recurring theme of waiting time (2017).
Credit students: Morgan Lewis, Catherine Dunaway, Winnie Wu, Chelsea Wu.

series on the course. Along with Dr. Ann Bonham, chief scientific officer of the AAMC, Salopek flew to Houston to attend our final critique for the class in spring 2014 and then invited us to present a panel on this innovative approach to premed pedagogy at the AAMC's annual meeting in Chicago in November 2014.

We are now in the process of seeking grant funding to develop several Medical Media Arts Lab projects into research studies that might validate the methods we have developed for specific challenges in doctor–patient/caregiver communication. Although at the beginning of every semester each group's problem seems very different from the others, once the teams develop sufficient confidence in their understanding of the biomedical particulars of their condition (for example, ventricular assist devices for pediatric patients with heart disease), they come to realize that most of the problems are at their core focused on communication of complex information to patients or caregivers in circumstances of emotional and cognitive exhaustion and vulnerability. The solutions, therefore, are often generalizable to other conditions and could prove beneficial to a much larger population. It is our hope that in the coming years we will streamline the process of moving from identifying problems to designing solutions to testing them in pilot studies and validating them through large-scale research. Apart from the scalability of the design solutions, however, it is clear that the benefit to the participants lies in the development of grounded techniques for building empathy, tolerating ambiguity, and working collaboratively in teams to solve complex problems.

Conclusion

Looking back at the logic model for the Medical Media Arts Lab (Figure 14.1), two initial goals and assumptions have proven inaccurate and are worth discussing here. Both issues relate to privacy and trust, two major concerns in digital health today. First, although we intended for the Medical Media Arts Lab to include a robust public-facing website, we have been unable to post publicly details of the problems we are working on. A second, related challenge is the subsequent limitation on posting our design solutions. In the process of working with potential problem owners, a critically important issue of establishing trust has become evident. In order for clinicians to identify and help solve existing problems in their clinical lives, they first have to describe the specific context in which the problem occurs. That context, also known as the site of employment, has a vested interest in presenting a positive and reassuring impression to the public and potential patients. While collaborating with a local university on an innovative design thinking project might seem to contribute to a positive public presence, acknowledging the existence of real problems in patient care might not. Our goal is to make healthcare better for patients, doctors, and other stakeholders, not to publicly criticize hospitals or other providers. Moreover, the open working relationships we enjoy are based on mutual respect and trust that extends beyond simply adhering to minimal ethical standards. Operating with the transparent, shared purpose of solving a health systems problem—that is, a problem that transcends any given site of care, even though we are working in one specific location—is therefore key to both identifying good design problems and ensuring a strong relationship of trust among collaborators.

The second assumption, that we would proudly display our design solutions on our website, hit a different kind of snag. We have found that each design team has a different stage of end product, dependent on variables such as the technological complexity of the solution, the ongoing availability of students to continue the project, and funding needs. Some of the projects have all of these elements lined up, and at the end of the semester, the team and its problem owner lay plans to scale up the work. This might include applying for grant funding, seeking internal seed development funds, working on a prospective research paper, and so on. In all of these cases, the possibility that the team has identified an innovative solution that might offer a competitive advantage for its hospital unit, for medical school admissions, for publication in a peer-reviewed journal, or for intellectual property and commercialization can end up pointing toward a proprietary posture toward the design, rather than an open-source approach to sharing. This limitation can be frustrating in that the concrete descriptions of our projects provide the most vivid depiction of our output and our students' achievements and could provide benefits for others in similar situations. I see the collaborative, participatory design process as pushing toward a more open model of healthcare, while nonetheless operating within the real constraints of the current system.

For now, I defer to the wishes of the problem owners and teams on how much detail to share and in what forms. In a very real sense, this stance is critical to the initiation of the projects and their continued ability to proceed without being hampered by legalistic procedural delays. This position also returns us to the importance of reciprocity. It must be noted that running the Medical Media Arts Lab is a lot of work. From finding problem owners to crafting well-defined problem statements, to coordinating logistics during the semester and lining up all of the necessary team members from different parts of the university and community, this approach to bringing design thinking into digital medical humanities is a significant undertaking. The expressions of appreciation at the end of the semester, along with my observation of the students' growth and learning throughout the course attest to the value of the process. Participating in Medical Media Arts Lab is also a substantial commitment for the problem owners. I work to lighten their load whenever possible through small gestures like providing parking passes and more meaningful efforts such as training my students to communicate succinctly, draft sections of journal articles or grant applications, and present their work to members of their problem owners' clinical departments. The most meaningful outcome for the problem owners is the development of the solutions themselves, from implementation of the design to collaboration on grant proposals.

Perhaps the most significant outcome for both the students and the problem owners is their newfound capacity to identify the human elements of medicine that are often at the heart of healthcare problems. Graduates of the Medical Media Arts Lab process know how to identify and describe problems, research and design potential solutions, and implement the results. In a healthcare system that is crying out for more humane treatment of both doctors and patients and more creative approaches to problem-solving, the ability and will to intervene and create change in local settings have enormous value that is well worth the effort.

Notes

1. For an insightful discussion of the new meanings of online and offline spaces for American youth, see danah boyd, *It's Complicated: The Social Lives of Networked Teens* (New Haven, CT: Yale University Press, 2014).

2. Henry Jenkins et al., *Confronting the Challenges of Participatory Culture: Media Education for the 21st Century* (Chicago: John D. and Catherine T. MacArthur Foundation, 2006); Jay Baruch, "Doctors as Makers," *Academic Medicine* 92, no. 1 (2017): 40–44.

3. Joseph Kvedar, Molly Joel Coye, and Wendy Everett, "Connected Health: A Review of Technologies and Strategies to Improve Patient Care with Telemedicine and Telehealth," *Health Affairs* 33, no. 2 (2014): 194–99.

4. Rheingold quotes Ito's comment in Howard Rheingold, *Net Smart: How to Thrive Online* (Cambridge, MA: MIT Press, 2012), 84.

5. Cathy Davidson, *Now You See It: How the Brain Science of Attention Will Transform the Way We Live, Work, and Learn* (New York: Viking, 2011); Jenkins et al., *Confronting the Challenges*; Anne Balsamo, *Designing Culture: The Technological Imagination at Work* (Durham, NC: Duke University Press, 2011).

6. John Maeda, "Artists and Scientists: More Alike Than Different," *Scientific American* (blog), July 11, 2013, https://blogs.scientificamerican.com/guest-blog/artists-and-scientists-more-alike-than-different; Frank Moss, *The Sorcerers and Their Apprentices: How the Digital Magicians of the MIT Media Lab Are Creating the Innovative Technologies That Will Transform Our Lives* (New York: Crown, 2011); IDEO, *The Field Guide to Human-Centered Design*, Ideo.org, 2015, http://www.designkit.org/resources/1.

7. Kirsten Ostherr, "The Medical Futures Lab: An Experiment in Applied Media Studies and Digital Medical Humanities," in *Applied Media Studies*, ed. Kirsten Ostherr (New York: Routledge, 2018), 60–78.

8. In engineering contexts, "real-world" design problems are often called "authentic" problems, but for our purposes, that term carries too many unwanted connotations.

9. For more on the MakerNurse movement, see http://makernurse.com/.

10. See Birnbaum et al., "Patient Engagement and the Design of Digital Health," *Academic Emergency Medicine* 22, no. 6 (2015): 754–56.

11. David Edwards, *ArtScience: Creativity in the Post-Google Generation* (Cambridge, MA: Harvard University Press, 2010); Kirsten Ostherr, ed., *Applied Media Studies* (New York: Routledge, 2018).

12. Many of these exercises are inspired by or adapted from the work of Dennis Boyle and his colleagues at IDEO; we have found their open-source *Field Guide to Human-Centered Design* (2015) to be particularly useful.

13. On media theory: Jonas Löwgren and Bo Reimer, *Collaborative Media: Production, Consumption, and Design Interventions* (Cambridge, MA: MIT Press, 2013); Mirca Madianou and Daniel Miller, "Polymedia: Towards a New Theory of Digital Media in Interpersonal Communication," *International Journal of Cultural Studies* 16, no. 2 (2012): 169–87. On digital technologies and connected health: Kristin L. Carman et al., "Patient and Family Engagement: A Framework for Understanding the Elements and Developing Interventions and Policies," *Health Affairs* 32, no. 2 (2013): 223–31; Susannah Fox and Maeve Duggan, *The Diagnosis Difference* (Washington, DC: Pew Research Center, 2013); Aaron Smith, *Older Adults and Technology Use* (Washington, DC: Pew Research Center, 2014); Kvedar, Coye, and Everett, "Connected Health." On the e-patient movement: Tom Ferguson and Giles Frydman, "The First Generation of e-Patients," *BMJ* 328 (2004): 1148; Fred Trotter, "Epatients: The Hackers of the Healthcare World," *O'Reilly Radar*, January 5, 2012, http://radar.oreilly.com/2012/01/epatients-empowered-patients.html; David deBronkart, "How the e-Patient Community Helped Save My Life," *BMJ* 346 (2013): f1990. On design

thinking in medicine: Arabella L. Simpkin and Richard M. Schwartzstein, "Tolerating Uncertainty—The Next Medical Revolution?" *New England Journal of Medicine* 375 (2016): 1713–15; Daniel Dohan et al., "The Importance of Integrating Narrative into Health Care Decision Making," *Health Affairs* 35, no. 4 (2016): 720–25; Joyce Lee, "The Role of Metaphor in Design: Impact on Health Outcomes," *Medium*, September 4, 2016, https://medium.com/@joyclee/the-role-of-metaphor-in-design-cd6d8f04daab; Baruch, "Doctors as Makers."

14. Donna Haraway, "Situated Knowledges: The Science Question in Feminism and the Privilege of Partial Perspective," *Feminist Studies* 14, no. 3 (1988): 575–99; Judy Wajcman, *TechnoFeminism* (Cambridge, UK; Malden, MA: Polity Press, 2004).

Works Cited

Balsamo, Anne. *Designing Culture: The Technological Imagination at Work*. Durham, NC: Duke University Press, 2011.

Baruch, Jay. "Doctors as Makers." *Academic Medicine* 92, no. 1 (2017): 40–44.

Birnbaum, Faith, Dana M. Lewis, Rochelle Rosen, and Megan L. Ranney. "Patient Engagement and the Design of Digital Health." *Academic Emergency Medicine* 22, no. 6 (2015): 754–56.

boyd, danah. *It's Complicated: The Social Lives of Networked Teens*. New Haven, CT: Yale University Press, 2014.

Carman, Kristin L., Pam Dardess, Maureen Maurer, Shoshanna Sofaer, Karen Adams, Christine Bechtel, and Jennifer Sweeney. "Patient and Family Engagement: A Framework for Understanding the Elements and Developing Interventions and Policies." *Health Affairs* 32, no. 2 (2013): 223–31.

Davidson, Cathy. *Now You See It: How the Brain Science of Attention Will Transform the Way We Live, Work, and Learn*. New York: Viking, 2011.

deBronkart, David. "How the e-Patient Community Helped Save My Life." *BMJ* 346 (2013): f1990.

Dohan, Daniel, Sarah B. Garrett, Katharine A. Rendle, Meghan Halley, and Corey Abramson. "The Importance of Integrating Narrative into Health Care Decision Making." *Health Affairs* 35, no. 4 (2016): 720–25.

Edwards, David. *ArtScience: Creativity in the Post-Google Generation*. Cambridge, MA: Harvard University Press, 2010.

Ferguson, Tom, and Gilles Frydman. "The First Generation of e-Patients." *BMJ* 328 (2004): 1148.

Fox, Susannah, and Maeve Duggan. *The Diagnosis Difference*. Washington, DC: Pew Research Center, 2013.

Haraway, Donna. "Situated Knowledges: The Science Question in Feminism and the Privilege of Partial Perspective." *Feminist Studies* 14, no. 3 (1988): 575–99.

IDEO. *The Field Guide to Human-Centered Design*. Ideo.org, 2015. http://www.designkit.org/resources/1.

Jenkins, Henry, Katie Clinton, Ravi Purushotma, Alice J. Robison, and Margaret Weigel. *Confronting the Challenges of Participatory Culture: Media Education for the 21st Century*. Chicago: John D. and Catherine T. MacArthur Foundation, 2006.

Kvedar, Joseph, Molly Joel Coye, and Wendy Everett. "Connected Health: A Review of Technologies and Strategies to Improve Patient Care with Telemedicine and Telehealth." *Health Affairs* 33, no. 2 (2014): 194–99.

Lee, Joyce. "The Role of Metaphor in Design: Impact on Health Outcomes." *Medium*, September 4, 2016. https://medium.com/@joycelee/the-role-of-metaphor-in-design-cd6d8f04daab.

Löwgren, Jonas, and Bo Reimer. *Collaborative Media: Production, Consumption, and Design Interventions*. Cambridge, MA: MIT Press, 2013.

Madianou, Mirca, and Daniel Miller. "Polymedia: Towards a New Theory of Digital Media in Interpersonal Communication." *International Journal of Cultural Studies* 16, no. 2 (2012): 169–87.

Maeda, John. "Artists and Scientists: More Alike Than Different." *Scientific American* (Guest Blog), July 11, 2013. https://blogs.scientificamerican.com/guest-blog/artists-and-scientists-more-alike-than-different/.

MakerNurse. MakerNurse website, powered by MakerHealth. http://makernurse.com/.

Moss, Frank. *The Sorcerers and Their Apprentices: How the Digital Magicians of the MIT Media Lab Are Creating the Innovative Technologies That Will Transform Our Lives*. New York: Crown, 2011.

Ostherr, Kirsten, ed. *Applied Media Studies*. New York: Routledge, 2018.

Ostherr, Kirsten. "The Medical Futures Lab: An Experiment in Applied Media Studies and Digital Medical Humanities." In *Applied Media Studies*, edited by Kirsten Ostherr, 60–78. New York: Routledge, 2018.

Rheingold, Howard. *Net Smart: How to Thrive Online*. Cambridge, MA: MIT Press, 2012.

Simpkin, Arabella L., and Richard M. Schwartzstein. "Tolerating Uncertainty—The Next Medical Revolution?" *New England Journal of Medicine* 375 (2016): 1713–15.

Smith, Aaron. *Older Adults and Technology Use*. Washington, DC: Pew Research Center, 2014.

Trotter, Fred. "Epatients: The Hackers of the Healthcare World." *O'Reilly Radar*, January 5, 2012. http://radar.oreilly.com/2012/01/epatients-empowered-patients.html.

Wajcman, Judy. *TechnoFeminism*. Cambridge, UK; Malden, MA: Polity Press, 2004.

15

Queer Bioethics for Everyday Medical Technologies

Jarah Moesch

Foundations

Electronic health records, digital health, diagnostic tools: "technologies" co-create meaning and knowledge throughout the medical–industrial complex. Bioethics is central to these ways of knowing. What does it mean to practice queer bioethical medicine in an age of technology? How do our knowledges shape and classify information to produce particular normativities? How might we use queer bioethics to change how knowledge is produced by the technologies of the medical–industrial complex? These designed technologies are part of larger sociopolitical assemblages with their own histories and complexities that are activated on, by, and through medical professionals and patients. This essay considers how queer theory can reformulate and extend bioethics to include the values imbricated in the design of technologies and systems within the medical–industrial complex.

To do so, this essay shows health humanities faculty how to incorporate critical bioethical approaches to "technologies" into course pedagogy, including a short syllabus. Students will take a hands-on theoretical approach, using multiple methodologies, from reading and discussion to editing Wikipedia, making games, and reconsidering the electronic health record.[1] Through a critical theoretical exploration of the values in the design and use of these tools and methods, we begin to understand that these methods and practices are structures that are themselves imbued with power and control and, as such, are foundational to creating and understanding a queer bioethics. By pairing hands-on learning/making with queer bioethics, we help those with little background in multimodal methods to activate these tools beyond the instrumental. This essay will focus on how a queer bioethical approach to understanding and activating these technologies can enable different forms of knowledge-making and therefore provide better care.

Understanding Queer Bioethics

Queer bioethics, as defined by Lance Wahlert and Autumn Fiester, is "a methodology of scholastic, bioethical, and critical scrutiny" that considers LGBT people's health needs as well as their collective histories and perspectives.[2] In their introductory article to this concept, their primary thinking is that the "mere inclusion of LGBT persons" does not remove stigma or marginalization.[3] To show how this occurs, they discuss two case studies where LGBT people were central to the question but were dealt with from a heteronormative, outsider view, leading to further stigma and marginalization. Stigma and marginalization become possible because within healthcare there is only one type of "normal," which prevents healthcare practitioners from recognizing how the US medical–industrial complex itself contributes to that marginalization.

Wahlert and Fiester's queer bioethics explores how to move beyond the "normative," by defining the word *queer* both as a noun and a verb—first as a noun, "that is, a lesbian, gay, bisexual, or transgender person" and, second, as a verb, "to employ a non-normative lens to what is taken to be standard and ordinary."[4] This first definition of LGBT people as queer (noun) is used as such in order to separate bodies from structures. Bias against individual bodies is personal: being attacked physically or emotionally is both dangerous and traumatic. Individual safety is crucial for a queer bioethics.

As both an embodied subject of healthcare and an educator, my fear is that people outside of queer theory may not understand the difference in calling someone queer versus LGBT. This possibility of conflation allows practitioners to make a common mistake: by using *queer* as an umbrella noun for LGBT people, they are speaking for and categorizing people without considering how they want to be named. Many LGBT people do not consider themselves queer, and many queer people do not consider themselves LGBT; these are not simply interchangeable terms. The word *queer* is fraught with historical meanings: odd or peculiar, a derogatory form of naming that ties suspicion of character to suspected bodies. It also means forged or fake, as well as living dishonestly.[5] *Queer* has also been used as a form of abuse, from being yelled at from a passing car to kids playing "smear the queer" on the playground. It is understandable, then, why some LGBT people might not want to be considered or called queer.

Naming is a process through which one becomes what other people think they should be. When one's body becomes someone else's discourse, trust is hard to build. How might a person who guards their sexuality or gender identity for physical and emotional safety feel about being asked to categorize themselves in medical settings, which have historically been dangerous places for LGBTQI people, LGBTQI/people of color, LGBTQI/women, and LGBTQI/people with disabilities? Naming also extends to include poor, noncompliant, and un- or underinsured as ways of naming within larger discourses, prejudices, and marginalization beyond the simplicity of the words themselves.

To not name oneself is to potentially become safer from bias and physical harm from the very practitioners who swore an oath to treat people according to ethical standards in care. LGBTQI people, LGBTQI/people of color, LGBTQI/women, and LGBTQI/people with disabilities have never been considered normative and therefore are not covered by the same set of ethics that white, heterosexual, able-bodied people are. Because ethical standards do not include non-normative people, not-naming is one way to protect oneself. This is what queer bioethics is trying to address when using *queer* as a noun.

At the same time, there are also many people who do wish to be called queer, for political and sociocultural reasons. Beginning in the late 1980s–early 1990s, being actively queer instead of gay or lesbian was an approach to fighting back against heteronormative laws, and policies, and anti-gay hate-mongering. It was also a way to differentiate from homonormative gay politics—a mostly white, Western, Christian, male, "we are the same as you only with different sexual preferences" kind of politics, which does not serve many queer people's needs or interests.[6]

Naming oneself as queer is to refuse to be statically assimilated into normative categories, even those such as gay, lesbian, bisexual, and trans that appear to be so open. To be queer is to break apart, or at the very least to blur the boundaries and categories that frame us. To be queer is to fight for justice and freedom and not only about being L, G, B, or T. To be queer is to be non-normative, perhaps in the interstices between genders and between sexualities, and to be intersectional with race, gender, dis/ability.

Wahlert and Fiester's second definition of queer as a verb, "to employ a non-normative lens to what is taken to be standard and ordinary," makes room for this kind of naming, or not-naming, of being outside, alongside, or in the interstices of categorizations and can be extended to include other boundaries, categories, and barriers to true healthcare.[7] But what is a non-normative lens, and how might we employ one for a queer bioethics?

My claim is that a queer bioethical, non-normative lens looks at and questions the histories and systems that create and produce the medical–industrial complex in the first place. This is separate from studying and making the individual person safe and instead focuses on the implicit, less recognizable issues within the structures of healthcare, the ones that make some people "normal" and others "deviant," causing unequal care, where access, diagnosis, and treatments vary considerably.

Within the US medical–industrial complex, there is only this one story, that of "normal" versus "deviant," defining who counts as human and who does not, who is healthy and who is sick and, therefore, needs to be "fixed."[8] Beginning with Chimamanda Adichie's "The Danger of a Single Story," we come to realize that stories make us understand other people in particular ways; and when we only know one story about a group of people, we come to know them as only that.[9] Currently, the "single story" of what it means to be healthy or sick within the US medical–industrial complex makes LGBTQI people, LGBTQI/people of color, LGBTQI/women, and LGBTQI/people with disabilities deviant, while heterosexual, white, able-bodied people are considered normal. It is a story of particular moralities, of "right" and "wrong," which prevents people from getting the care they need, while being forced to get care they do not want or need.

In her talk, Adichie references the Igbo word *nkali*, meaning "to be greater than another," explaining that stories "are defined by the principle of nkali: How they are told, who tells them, when they're told, how many stories are told, are really dependent on power. Power is the ability not just to tell the story of another person, but to make it the definitive story of that person."[10] The case studies that Wahlert and Fiester discuss are based on the definitive single story of LGBT people not being considered full adults, needing to be chided for not including their "family" and then not including the patient's same-sex partner in the decision-making. This, then, is the current status of non-normative people within the US healthcare system.

Queer bioethics deals first with LGBTQI people, LGBTQI/people of color, LGBTQI/women, and LGBTQI/people with disabilities as nouns and, second, with the systems in place that cause trauma to these bodies. Although they have been thus far discussed separately in order to clarify their differences, they cannot be separated in everyday life. Discourses of power and control have real, material consequences that affect individuals in various ways, from individual care and how machines and other technologies are designed and used to the overarching systems of policy, law, and bioethics itself, which are laden with historical and systemic racism, sexism, ableism, and homophobia.

A queer bioethics needs to first be able to work within the system. These structures, systems, policies, and codes all already exist; and it takes time to change them. Not only do practitioners need to be thinking and changing what is done and how it is done to ensure that people feel as safe and as comfortable as they can within the system, but they also must recognize that trust takes time. Understanding the patient's perspective (what is currently being called "patient-centered care") is therefore pertinent to queer bioethics. If patient-centered care does not recognize and understand the biased, hateful histories of "deviant" people and how they are still foundational to, and imbricated within, modern-day medical practice, the patient's experience cannot be truly centered.

Queer theorist José Esteban Muñoz's concept of disidentification is useful to understand how people manage being queerly embodied in the clinic. When faced with outsider status, disidentification, or the ability to exist in and against discourses of power, becomes a way of immediate survival.[11] To practice disidentification, a "deviant"/outsider patient may negotiate how their identity is perceived. This may fluctuate depending on their physical and emotional safety as well as their medical needs. They may not feel comfortable discussing their sexualities or genders, their preferred pronouns, or their mental health status as these are all potential pitfalls in gaining the care that is needed. Similarly, transmen might not disclose their need for cervical exams, regardless of medical necessity. Disidentificatory practices enable negotiation of a public sphere (or visit to the clinic) that "continuously elides or punishes the existence of such subjects who don't conform to . . . normative citizenship."[12]

Disidentificatory practices, then, are already being used by patients within the clinic, for protection from the moral and medical assumptions made about LGBTQI people, LGBTQI/people of color, LGBTQI/women, and LGBTQI/people with disabilities. Having to disidentify to protect oneself, to survive, is one of the dangers of the "single story" of normativity in medicine.

Becoming familiar with how disidentification is practiced enables medical practitioners and policymakers to gain nuanced understandings about the survival strategies marginalized people use to manage their healthcare experiences and interactions. Recognizing and acknowledging disidentificatory practices enables medical practitioners to work within the systems of knowledge that already exist, by reperforming, subverting, and questioning that which is "oppressive" (categories) in order to "displace," at least temporarily, the discourses of power inherent in the system.

The second responsibility for a queer bioethics is to change the system: from "norms" and "deviances" to how medicine is practiced. Wahlert and Fiester's Queer Bioethics Inventory is a good place to begin.[13] While their focus is on using their non-normative lens to question case studies in bioethics, their inventory of questions can be applied to other areas of medical practice: the space of the clinic, the emergency department, and even the physical exam. By asking these questions, medical practitioners can become more familiar with, and then change the way they and the rooms they work in are perceived by LGBTQI people, LGBTQI/people of color, LGBTQI/women, and LGBTQI/people with disabilities.

Queer bioethics begins with how to think away (or apart) from norms and deviance. How might we use a combination of Wahlert and Fiester's inventory and Muñoz's disidentificatory practices to conceptualize differently what is normal and what is queer? How might we assemble these queer analyses, theories, and bodies within medical practices? What are the ways that we might consider the multiple forms of interconnected violence(s), traumas, biases, and shame as central to queer bioethics? How can we rethink Western medicine's production, distribution, and acquisition of knowledge so that we can create alternate ways of centralizing queer analytics and methods within bioethics?

To begin this type of practice, medical practitioners must acknowledge the historical and structural role of medicine in the shaming, stigma, and continued bias against LGBTQI people, LGBTQI/people of color, LGBTQI/women, and LGBTQI/people with disabilities. In their clinics, they also must attend to the systemic everyday issues faced while interacting with the heteronormative medical–industrial complex, from the history of "homosexuality" to medicine and science as oppositional, pathologizing, and shaming. This is a must throughout medical education, but the health humanities can also begin to draw on science and technology studies and new media studies in order to apply queer bioethics to change how "norms" and "deviances" are constituted within the technologies, tools, practices, policies, and procedures used in everyday medical practice. To do so, it must necessarily include diagnostic categories and interface design, codes, and data collection, critically engaging with and changing the way knowledge is produced, controlled, and acquired. This is what this course, drawing from critical art, media, and cultural studies, seeks to teach undergraduates, regardless of their intended professions, as these knowledges will be beneficial whether one is a patient or practitioner.

Data, Normativity, and Its Discontents

Now that the students have been introduced to queer bioethics, we turn to how the medical–industrial complex furthers normative categories, marginalization, and stigma through the design of databases, policies, and rules in place to collect data and administer "care." Medical technologies have already changed how we treat illness and disease, the way we understand life and death, how we live, and how we die. It should be no surprise then that the ways patients are treated from before they walk into the clinic through the physical exam, blood draw, and diagnosis process are all affected by our databases, our digital policies and procedures, our interfaces, and our rules for collecting data.

The data we use in clinical practice are not neutral. Data are designed into information and knowledge through electronic medical and health records, *International Statistical Classification of Diseases and Related Health Problems* (ICD) diagnosis codes, insurance regulations, and even new patient registration forms (to name just a few). We frame particular information as "real" or "credible," and this forms the ways we use and understand our tools and the knowledge they give us. These tools used to obtain and distribute information are defined by their uses—collecting patient information, distributing test results, categorizing diagnosis codes, refilling prescriptions, sharing treatment plans. The decisions made about how and what these tools can do are responsible for how we organize our clinical practice, how we organize our patients' bodies, and what can and cannot happen in our clinic to individual bodies.

This is further impacted by the values of the people, policies, and economics of the companies that create and shape these databases and interfaces that medical professionals and patients use every day. The value-laden decisions of information technology design employees and health insurance "bean counters" plus ideas about morality go beyond the frustrating ways the screens freeze or the nonsensical drop-down menus to being central to how medical and health information is actually created, presented, distributed, and acquired in the first place. The design of the database itself determines the information we can even know in the first place. This information is how we come to understand difference.

LGBTQI people, LGBTQI/people of color, LGBTQI/women, and LGBTQI/people with disabilities have historically been entangled in the practice of diagnosis, treatment, norms, and stigma within and through medicine, from the creation of the "homosexual" as pathology or mental illness to surgical implantation of "normal" testes, genital mutilation, forced conversion therapy, and the (still) inclusion of "gender identity disorder" in the most current version of the *Diagnostic and Statistical Manual of Mental Disorders*. From the start (what we now "know" as) LGBTQI people, LGBTQI/people of color, LGBTQI/women, and LGBTQI/people with disabilities were in opposition to the medical establishment. The concept of "homosexuality" was co-constructed by medicine and law in order to produce discourses about sodomy for legal proof and conviction.[14] These medical discourses turned a "behavior" into a type of person, making heterosexual people "normal" and everyone else "deviant."

The word *homosexual* is still used in medicine today, but most LGBTQI people, LGBTQI/people of color, LGBTQI/women, and LGBTQI/people with disabilities have an aversion to its continued use. When broken into parts, *homo* is a slur, tossed out of car windows and yelled out in conjunction with the bat coming down on the heads, backs, and arms of LGBTQI people, LGBTQI/people of color, LGBTQI/women, and LGBTQI/people with disabilities; and *sexual* points to the act of sex in particular and not at a different way of being in the world, a different way of organizing one's life, such as queer temporalities, families of choice, how we live. Additionally, given its deployment by conservative politics as a weapon against so-called deviance, its lingering use within medicine reflects the systemic mistreatment found within the medical–industrial complex to this day.

The new patient registration form is a space to collect information about new patients, before they even meet the physician. This is, for most patients, the first contact they have had with the office. Many LGBTQI health organizations believe that this is a great place to ask people about their sexual orientation and gender identity, especially because this is the same space they already use to collect race and ethnicity data for population health purposes.[15] By collecting patient-level data, they feel that they will be better equipped to understand and correct disparities in care.

While one survey found that most LGBTQI people are open to having this question on their intake forms, there are a number of concerns as well.[16] According to the ACLU, only nineteen states and Washington, DC have protections from discrimination for sexual orientation and gender identity. A further three states have protections for sexual orientation only.[17] In 2016, there were over one hundred active bills in state legislatures that, if passed, would let businesses deny services to LGBTQI people, make it illegal for trans people to use bathrooms that match their gender identity, and, in Tennessee, even allow mental health professionals to refuse to treat LGBTQI patients.[18] Combine this with the historic mistreatment of LGBTQI people in medicine, and it is no wonder that people might be fearful of outing themselves on a patient intake form.

This is not to advocate against collecting such information; rather, this is a point for students to begin thinking about such collection through a queer bioethical lens. The biggest question when bringing new policies, procedures, forms, or systems into the clinic is, what is the actual purpose of collecting this information, and is this a valid reason for patients to comply? Why is this information collected in the first place? Many LGBTQI health organizations discuss the need to collect these data and give examples on how to do so properly. Yet, many of them are interested in aggregate data for population health issues, meaning that they want to have enough information on sexual orientation and gender identity in order to better understand long-term health issues and disparities in care and treatment as well as insurance coverage. While this may be beneficial (or detrimental) for the long haul, what is a specific clinic's purpose for collecting this information? What information could be included on the form that would help an individual decide—or consent—to offering up personal information? For example, if the purpose is to help with population health, perhaps the form itself could mention this.

Here, we can ask students to focus in on privacy concerns and consider in detail the context of filling out the patient form: patients either fill it out ahead of time at home, where they may not be "out," or fill it out in the waiting room, where other people are sitting nearby and can possibly see. The clinic receptionist and medical assistants will collect the paper and integrate the information into whatever electronic record system the clinic uses. What does the person at the front desk need to know? Is that person trained to understand what this information means and how to use it appropriately? Once it becomes electronic, is it secure? How is it being protected from potential hackers? From the staff? What about health insurance companies? Is this information being shared? What happens when insurance companies decide not to cover certain procedures because of sexual orientation or gender identity? Who protects patients?

Figure 15.1 shows an image of a "new patient registration form" that I received in the mail from my new primary care physician's office while writing this chapter. Bring a document like this into the classroom, and ask students to analyze the form as though it was any other text. Why is the word *queer* on this new patient form? Is it being wrongly conflated with LGBTI bodies as an umbrella term? If so, why then have other options? If not, what do they mean? Why do they want to know this? I find myself not sure whether to circle the word or not.

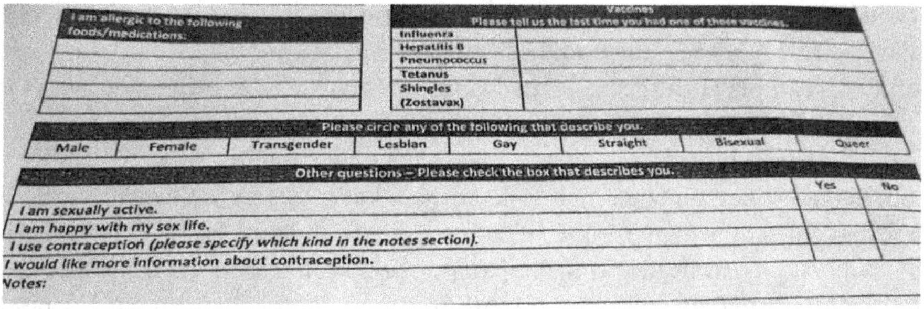

I am allergic to the following foods/medications:

Vaccines Please tell us the last time you had one of these vaccines.	
Influenza	
Hepatitis B	
Pneumococcus	
Tetanus	
Shingles (Zostavax)	

Please circle any of the following that describe you.							
Male	Female	Transgender	Lesbian	Gay	Straight	Bisexual	Queer

Other questions – Please check the box that describes you.	Yes	No
I am sexually active.		
I am happy with my sex life.		
I use contraception (please specify which kind in the notes section).		
I would like more information about contraception.		

Notes:

FIGURE 15.1 The image is of a new patient registration form asking people to circle any of the following that describes them. The list includes: Male, Female, Transgender, Lesbian, Gay, Straight, Bisexual, and Queer.

Photograph taken by the author.

I consider myself queer but not primarily or only due to my sexual orientation. What will circling it give me—or take from me—when I walk into that office? After a class discussion, ask students to create their own new patient registration form and to think intentionally about what kinds of data the form should ask for.

Shaping Information

In this next section, students look more deeply at how information is designed and shaped through the rules, policies, and procedures that produce the pathways to, and intrinsically are forms of medical knowledge. By understanding how population health management operates to design data, we begin to get other ways of knowing, allowing us to see the cracks, crevices, and interstices where patients reside.

Rules are a fundamental part of policies, procedures, health insurance claims, and diagnostic processes that organize systems and, in doing so, not only contribute to what we know but are foundational to how we know. They are our system. When a clinician follows a diagnostic algorithm, for example, they are looking for specific data and test results. The next step toward diagnosis depends on those results and the hierarchy of rule sets that make symptoms and results meaningful. These then integrate with the rules for the ICD-10 classification system, the rules for health insurance coverage, and the rules for how the body behaves for this potential diagnosis. Again drawing on new media studies methods, the course illuminates rules in health systems by looking at rule-making in game design. Using gaming, a genre most students are familiar with, we look at how rules formalize our interactions within the space of game play in order to understand the lived experience of the patient in a complicated system where the rules, values, and classifications enact and undermine each other and, at the least, render particular people invisible and, at the worst, can harm them. After reading and discussing how games are played through rules, students can play healthcare-related games and create their own game rules for queer bioethical healthcare.

Electronic health records not only shape how data are collected and used but define what counts enough to be included as a category. Electronic health records collect particular kinds of information in order to better care for individual patients, while also collecting population health data. Yet when it comes to gender, these data collection systems continuously fail due to a hardened set of categories that do not allow for the non-static reality of long-term gender transition, nor do they have space for those who are genderqueer or gender-questioning. How do you account for a person's legal name and gender used for insurance purposes, while at the same time provide a space for preferred name and current gender?[19] The process of transitioning from one gender to another can take years, making it imperative to make room in the electronic records for these realities. Transgender and genderqueer people also have routine gynecological needs to be attended to: transmen need pap smears, cervical exams, and mammograms, while transwomen who have a cervix created from the glans penis need routine cancer screenings.[20] These needs should be included within the electronic health record, regardless of what sex or gender they are legally required to use. During this section we again turn to a queer bioethics perspective, asking how the electronic health record can help to create a queer bioethics approach that keeps trans people safe.

The Production of Knowledge

The final part of the course considers the production of knowledge. We investigate how patients interact with their illness, disease, and health outside of traditional medical venues; how policy shapes knowledge; where patients get their information; and how that information is produced by the particular values of those who build our technologies. We enlist queer bioethics as an approach to understanding online health information research; we introduce concerns with collaborative information-building on Wikipedia; and we consider queer bioethical approaches to the five pillars of Wikipedia, from who can edit to how and what is allowed to remain on an edited page.

Wikipedia, a collaborative online encyclopedia, is currently ranked as the seventh most popular website in the world.[21] Two hundred million people read Wikipedia's twenty-five thousand health articles every month, making Wikipedia the most common site for accessing information about medical conditions.[22] This is a site that medical professionals should (and do) take seriously as patients are probably already using information from those pages to inform themselves before or after their clinical visit.

WikiProject Medicine, a volunteer community founded in 2004 to "manage and help in curation of Wikipedia's medical articles," has played a role in the amount and quality of medically related information on Wikipedia.[23] Currently, 671 editors are working to clarify, edit, and otherwise improve the one hundred most important medical topics, that "importance" determined by the combination of number of clicks on a page, the quality of the article, and the global health burden of disease.[24] Dr. Amin Azzam, associate professor at the University of California, San Francisco School of Medicine, takes this a step further by teaching fourth-year medical students how to "hone their information retrieval and assessment skills, practice communicating medical knowledge to an exceptionally broad global audience, and expand their sense of health care providers' roles" by editing Wikipedia, giving medical students the opportunity to contribute high-quality medical information to millions of people worldwide.[25] Together, these projects are changing the quality of medical information available on the Internet.

Some queer bioethical concerns are legibility and readability: WikiProject Medicine has a style guide that must be followed, which breaks down diseases into categories such as pathogenesis, pathophysiology, and epidemiology that are not necessarily understood by the layperson. All style guides on Wikipedia are recommended, not required; but in fact, content is continuously re-edited by interested parties until editors are forced to comply with those guidelines. Unfortunately, using this kind of jargon as section headers is off-putting at the least and impossible to comprehend for the average "reader" in the United States. According to the US Department of Health and Human Services, medical information should be written below a seventh-grade level for maximum understanding. This is due to the fact that "only 12 percent of adults have proficient health literacy. . . . In other words, nearly nine out of ten adults may lack the skills needed to manage their health and prevent disease."[26] This then is a foundational consideration for WikiProject Medicine and for queer bioethics.

There are three reasons why Wikipedia is significant to queer bioethics. First, according to the US Department of Health and Human Services, "Health literacy is lowest among the more vulnerable members of our communities—those with lower education levels, racial/ethnic minorities, the uninsured and publicly insured, and the elderly." LGBTQI people, LGBTQI/people of color, LGBTQI/women, and LGBTQI/people with disabilities fall into these categories, which therefore makes health literacy a significant concern within queer bioethics.[27] This is a structural problem within the medical–industrial complex that affects individual people's ability to understand medical information and to properly care for themselves and their loved ones. Importantly, readable and legible information on Wikipedia is central to queer bioethics.

Second, Wahlert and Fiester created a Queer Bioethics Inventory, where they present a series of questions for practitioners to use in order to center LGBTQI bodies and ways of knowing so that they can become caring partners in (the bioethics of) LGBTQI health. These questions help us "to better attend to the unique needs of LGBT parties in the clinic and in the biosciences by dwelling, not merely on the presence of queer people in bioethics cases, but (perhaps more importantly) on the need for decidedly non-normative and truly queer forms of analysis."[28] What happens when we expand these questions outward toward Wikipedia? How might these questions change the ways medical information is produced there? By focusing these questions on Wikipedia's medical content, we can begin to change how "normative" bodies, families, and timelines are inherently valued within its medical content. If the writers and editors of medical articles on Wikipedia were to consider various ways of living, of queer temporalities, of people who have medical needs but are very afraid, for good reasons, to make an appointment with a doctor, then perhaps it will help to assuage fears. If people find themselves within the stories, the data, they will feel more comfortable in assessing their own needs.

And finally, another way of extending queer bioethics is to consider the structures of Wikipedia itself from a queer analysis. What is Wikipedia but an encyclopedia? And what are the histories of the encyclopedia? Hint: encyclopedias make certain histories and knowledge legible while rendering others invisible. This means that Wikipedia itself is based on ways of knowing that already exclude certain bodies (LGBTQI people, LGBTQI/people of color, LGBTQI/women, and LGBTQI/people with disabilities) because they collect information from "reliable sources" that never included those people to begin with. By continuing to use only sources that are traditionally reliable for cisgendered, heterosexual, white, Western, Christian men, Wikipedia continues to reproduce the inequities and biases in our larger population. The encyclopedia produces both "normal" and "deviant" knowledges that are then taken up in collaborative form where editors continue to produce and maintain these ways of thinking and knowing by deleting content they feel is not up to these so-called standards. To help students think about these issues, we analyze Wikipedia content pages to see how and what kinds of knowledge are available. Then, we look to the "Talk" pages to consider how standards and practices that are ensconced within violent histories are foundational to the tools and knowledges in the medical–industrial complex. Finally, we analyze the WikiProject Medicine pages to understand how this set of policies contributes to the further obfuscation of basic health information.[29]

Conclusion

Bias is built into the standards, classifications, and design of information, creating acceptable norms and so-called morally corrupt deviances, affecting all areas of medical practice. This course investigated how multimodal tools and systems form medical knowledge: from the creation and use of "new patient" registration forms and the electronic health record to the rules and design of software and efficiency in data entry. In doing so, we were able to further the concepts originally deployed in Wahlert and Fiester's queer bioethics to enable a complex set of questions, interrogations, and reconsiderations of the systems, histories, and complexities of queer bodies within the medical–industrial practice. By questioning healthcare tools, systems, and structures, queer bioethics reconsiders the predetermined values in place, making room for various bodies and identities. A queer bioethical approach to understanding and activating medical technologies creates room for normativities and deviance to enable new ways of knowing, to allow people to be human and to be treated with the care and kindness they deserve.

PEDAGOGY EXERCISE SECTION

Syllabus

This shortened syllabus is split into three major themes over nine weeks: foundations in queer bioethics, shaping information, and the production of knowledge. Each theme focuses on tools or methods that further our understanding of that theme, and there is one workshop per theme, for a total of three workshops, allowing students to gain hands-on knowledge and apply critical analysis to the tools and systems themselves. Think of these as introductory workshops to the ideas, concepts, and process of creative inquiry. While no prior technical experience is necessary, students will be experimenting with and through various methodologies that incorporate fundamental themes in queer bioethics. Therefore, the key requirement for this course is curiosity and a willingness to explore new ideas in order to fully engage with the materials.

After completing this course, students should be able to do the following:

1. Describe queer bioethics in relation to the systems, structures, and tools in clinical practice
2. Critically investigate the predetermined values within digital systems in terms of the impact and consequences for everyday queer clinical interactions
3. Evaluate tools, systems, information sources, and arguments through a queer bioethical lens
4. Research, explore, and use design and creation tools to critically express theoretical arguments
5. Understand and critique their own role within the "medical–industrial practice"

Part I: Foundations

WEEK 1: UNDERSTANDING QUEER BIOETHICS

- Wahlert, Lance, and Autumn Fiester. "Repaving the Road of Good Intentions: LGBT Health Care and the Queer Bioethical Lens." *Hastings Center Report* 44, no. S4 (2014): S56–S65.
- Muñoz, José Esteban. "Introduction: Performing Disidentifications." In *Disidentifications: Queers of Color and the Performance of Politics*. Minneapolis: University of Minnesota Press, 1999.
- Adichie, Chimamanda Ngozi. "The Danger of a Single Story." TED (video). July 2009.

- Gert, Bernard, Charles M. Culver, and K. Danner Clouser, eds. *Bioethics: A Systematic Approach*. 2nd ed. New York: Oxford University Press, 2006.
- Choose one article from this special issue: Wahlert, Lance, ed. "Special Issue: Mapping Queer Bioethics: Space, Place, and Locality." *Journal of Homosexuality* 63 (2016).

WEEK 2: DATA, NORMATIVITY, AND ITS DISCONTENTS

- Winner, Langdon. "Do Artifacts Have Politics?" *Daedalus: Modern Technology: Problem or Opportunity?* 109, no. 1 (1980): 121–36.
- Bowker, Geoffrey C., and Susan Leigh Star. "Introduction: To Classify Is Human." In *Sorting Things Out: Classification and Its Consequences*, edited by Geoffrey C. Bowker and Susan Leigh Star, 1–32. Cambridge, MA: MIT Press, 2000.
- King, Katie, and Jarah Moesch. "Feminist Worlding: Media Ecologies Learning." In *Feminist Cyberspaces: Pedagogies in Transition*, edited by Sharon Collingwood, Alvina E. Quintana, and Smith J. Caroline, 14–31. Newcastle-upon-Tyne, UK: Cambridge Scholars Publishing, 2012.
- Enteen, Jillana. "Introduction: Life Skills." In *Virtual English: Queer Internets and Digital Creolization*. New York and London: Routledge, 2009.
- Crozier, Ivan Dalley. "The Medical Construction of Homosexuality and Its Relation to the Law in Nineteeth-Century England." *Medical History* 45 (2001): 61–82.
- Fenway Institute and Center for American Progress. *Asking Patients Questions about Sexual Orientation and Gender Identity in Clinical Settings: A Study in Four Health Centers*. Boston: Fenway Institute; Washington, DC: Center for American Progress, 2013.

WEEK 3: WORKSHOP

Create your own new patient registration form. Explain how you chose your data: what did you leave out, and why? What will you do differently in your clinical practice? Using Wahlert and Fiester's Queer Bioethics Inventory, decide what considerations should be built into clinical practice so that we are "queering" the ways we think about norms and deviance, the standards and practices we encounter every day. Remember that queer bioethics is not just about LGBTQI bodies but about rethinking the systems in place that make some bodies (LGBTQI, LGBTQI/people of color, LGBTQI/people with disabilities) deviant and others "normal."

Part II: Shaping Information

WEEK 4: CLASSIFICATION AND VALUES IN DESIGN

- Bowker, Geoffrey C. "The History of Information Infrastructures: The Case of the International Classification of Diseases." *Information Processing & Management* 32, no. 1 (1996): 49–61.
- Drabinski, Emily. "Queering the Catalog: Queer Theory and the Politics of Correction." *Library Quarterly* 83, no. 2 (2013): 94–111.

WEEK 5: RULES

- Flanagan, Mary. "Introduction to Critical Play." In *Critical Play: Radical Game Design*, 1–16. Cambridge, MA: MIT Press, 2009.
- Salen, Katie, and Eric Zimmerman. "The Rules of Digital Games." In *Rules of Play: Game Design Fundamentals*, 140–49. Cambridge, MA: MIT Press, 2004.
- Flanagan, Mary (producer). *Gut Check* (game). Tiltfactor.

WEEK 6: WORKSHOP

Using "Grow-A-Game" cards, game design cards that incorporate human values, have students design queer bioethical medical games. No experience is needed as there is a full curriculum for faculty to use.

- Tiltfactor. "Grow-A-Game." Accessed August 1, 2018. http://www.tiltfactor.org/grow-a-game/.

WEEK 7: ELECTRONIC HEALTH RECORDS

- HealthIT.gov. "Benefits of EHRs." Accessed August 20, 2016. https://www.healthit.gov/providers-professionals/benefits-electronic-health-records-ehrs.
- Callahan, Edward J., Nicole Sitkin, Hendry Ton, Suzanne W. Eidson-Ton, Julie Weckstein, and Darin Latimore. "Perspectives Introducing Sexual Orientation and Gender Identity into the Electronic Health Record: One Academic Health Center's Experience." *Academic Medicine* 90, no. 2 (2015): 154–60.
- Oram, Andy. "How Health IT Fails Transgender Patients." Last modified January 11, 2015. Accessed August 20, 2016. http://www.kevinmd.com/blog/2015/01/health-fails-transgender-patients.html.

Part III: The Production of Knowledge

WEEK 8: DR. GOOGLE AND WIKIPEDIA

- Silver, Curtis. "Google Will Offer Your Symptoms Better Medical Advice (But It's Probably Cancer)." *Forbes*, June 21, 2016. Accessed August 20, 2016. http://www.forbes.com/sites/curtissilver/2016/06/21/google-will-offer-your-symptoms-better-medical-advice-but-its-probably-cancer/#39ffdafe27ed.
- Heilman, James M. "Wikipedia and Medicine: Quantifying Readership, Editors and the Significance of Natural Language." *Journal of Medical Internet Research* 17, no. 3 (March 2015): 62.
- "Quick Guide to Health Literacy Fact Sheet." *Health.Gov*. Accessed August 24, 2016. https://health.gov/communication/literacy/quickguide/factsbasic.htm.
- Wikipedia. "WikiProject Medicine." Accessed August 20, 2016. https://en.wikipedia.org/wiki/Wikipedia:WikiProject_Medicine.
- Wikipedia. "Wikipedia: About." Accessed August 24, 2016. https://en.wikipedia.org/wiki/Wikipedia:About.
- Wikipedia. "Wikipedia: Five Pillars." Accessed August 24, 2016. https://en.wikipedia.org/wiki/Wikipedia:Five_Pillars.

WEEK 9: WORKSHOP

Find and read three Wikipedia medical pages for diseases that interest you. If you are not sure where to begin, look at the articles needing expert attention.[30] Take good notes: pay attention to what is simply explained yet well written. Note what might be confusing. Was it easy to read? Could the average seventh-grader (or someone who reads at a seventh-grade level) understand this? How might it be easier to understand? What might make it less confusing? What changes would you make? What would you need to know to make you comfortable editing the pages you viewed?

Bonus Weeks 10–12: Case Studies

- Singer, Ben. "The Human Simulation Lab—Dissecting Sex in the Simulator Lab: The Clinical Lacuna of Transsexed Embodiment." *Journal of Medical Humanities* 34, no. 2 (2013): 249–54.
- Guarrasi, Ivana. "Residual Categories in Medical Simulation: The Role of Affect in the Performance of Disease." *Mind, Culture, and Activity* 22, no. 2 (2015): 112–28.
- Roberts, Dorothy. *The Problem with Race-Based Medicine*. TEDMED (video). November 2015.

Notes

1. This proposed course is a mix of lesson plans, readings, and workshops I have taught to undergraduates from more than forty majors since 2006.

2. Lance Wahlert and Autumn Fiester, "Repaving the Road of Good Intentions: LGBT Health Care and the Queer Bioethical Lens," *Hastings Center Report* 44, no. S4 (2014): S56–S65. Wahlert and Fiester use *LGBT* in their work on queer bioethics, so I replicate it in this essay when I am specifically discussing their work. For my own work, I choose to use *LGBTQI people, LGBTQI/people of color, LGBTQI/women*, and *LGBTQI/people with disabilities* to show that LGBTQI people are not simply and only those identities, that they are intersectional with other identities. But I also use it because the disparities in healthcare I discuss here in regard to LGBTQI people also affect people of color, women, women of color, people with disabilities, and people of color with disabilities. All of these categories of identity overlap, are implicated and entangled with each other, and cannot be separated out. See Kimberlé Crenshaw's work on intersectionality for more information (Kimberlé Crenshaw, "Mapping the Margins: Intersectionality, Identity Politics, and Violence against Women of Color," *Stanford Law Review* 43, no. 6 [July 1991]: 1241–99). Here, I mean L = lesbian, G = gay, B = bi, T = transgender, Q = queer and questioning, I = intersex.

3. Wahlert and Fiester, "Repaving the Road," 57.

4. Ibid.

5. "Queer," adj.2 and n.1, OED Online, December 2007, accessed August 1, 2018, https://en.oxforddictionaries.com/definition/us/queer.

6. Lisa Duggan, "The New Homonormativity: The Sexual Politics of Neoliberalism," in *Materializing Democracy: Toward a Revitalized Cultural Politics*, ed. Dana D. Nelson and Russ Castronovo (Durham, NC: Duke University Press, 2002), 175–94. For me, it was also a way to describe myself as peculiar, not just in sexual preferences but in everything I was: given an unusual first name, Jewish, non-binary gendered. I never believed that any gender "covered" who I was, so I knew that if it didn't apply to me personally, it also didn't make sense in the world. I knew this early on because, as a Jew, I also understood that secular Christianity, what the United States practices in law, morals, and values, also didn't apply to me. What I thought, what I valued, came from different embodied ways of knowing, enabling me to see outside the systems of gender, sexuality, and politics and to know that there was something else. Once I became sick with a rare disease, I became even more sensitized to my own queerness.

7. Wahlert and Fiester, "Repaving the Road."

8. Look at Harriet A. Washington's *Medical Apartheid: The Dark History of Medical Experimentation on Black Americans from Colonial Times to the Present* (New York: Doubleday Books, 2007).

9. Chimamanda Ngozi Adichie, "The Danger of a Single Story," TED (video), July 2009, http://www.ted.com/talks/lang/eng/chimamanda_adichie_the_danger_of_a_single_story.html, 4:48.

10. Ibid., 10:11.

11. José Esteban Muñoz, "Introduction: Performing Disidentifications," in *Disidentifications: Queers of Color and the Performance of Politics* (Minneapolis: University of Minnesota Press, 1999): 1–34.

12. Ibid.

13. Wahlert and Fiester, "Repaving the Road."

14. Ivan Dalley Crozier, "The Medical Construction of Homosexuality and Its Relation to the Law in Nineteeth-Century England," *Medical History* 45 (2001): 61–82.

15. Look at Dorothy Roberts, "The Problem with Race-Based Medicine," TEDMED (video), November 2015, https://www.ted.com/talks/dorothy_roberts_the_problem_with_race_based_medicine, for the reasons why collecting data in this way can become problematic.

16. Fenway Institute and Center for American Progress, *Asking Patients Questions about Sexual Orientation and Gender Idenity in Clinical Settings: A Study in Four Health Centers* (Boston: Fenway Institute; Washington, DC: Center for American Progress), 2013, accessed August 15, 2016, http://thefenwayinstitute.org/wp-content/uploads/COM228_SOGI_CHARN_WhitePaper.pdf.

17. ACLU, "Non-Discrimination Laws: State by State Information—Map," accessed August 24, 2016, https://www.aclu.org/map/non-discrimination-laws-state-state-information-map.

18. Marina Fang, "Tennessee Passes Anti-LGBT Counseling Bill," *Huffington Post*, April 11, 2016, accessed August 24, 2016, http://www.huffingtonpost.com/entry/tennessee-lgbt-counseling_us_570c4c4de4b0836057a23d63; Jennifer Bendery, "Everything You Need to Know about the Wave of 100+ Anti-LGBT Bills Pending in States: Nine States Are Afraid to Let Transgender People Go to the Bathroom," *Huffington Post*, April 15, 2016, http://www.huffingtonpost.com/entry/lgbt-state-bills-discrimination_us_570ff4f2e4b0060ccda2a7a9.

19. Andy Oram, "How Health IT Fails Transgender Patients," KevinMD, January 11, 2015, accessed August 20, 2016, http://www.kevinmd.com/blog/2015/01/health-fails-transgender-patients.html.

20. Committee on Health Care for Underserved Women, "Health Care for Transgender Individuals," American College of Obstetricians and Gynecologists, December 2011, https://www.acog.org/Clinical-Guidance-and-Publications/Committee-Opinions/Committee-on-Health-Care-for-Underserved-Women/Health-Care-for-Transgender-Individuals.

21. Alexa.com, "Wikipedia.org Traffic Statistics: How Popular Is Wikipedia.org?" last modified August 29, 2016, accessed August 30, 2016, http://www.alexa.com/siteinfo/wikipedia.org. Google, YouTube, Facebook, Yahoo, and Baidu are the only sites that are consistently ranked higher.

22. Amin Azzam, "Medical Schools Making Wikipedia Better," Innovate with AMA, accessed August 24, 2016, https://www.innovatewithama.com/project/detail/327.

23. Ibid.

24. James M. Heilman, "Wikipedia and Medicine: Quantifying Readership, Editors and the Significance of Natural Language," *Journal of Medical Internet Research* 17, no. 3 (2015): e62.

25. Amin Azzam, David Bresler, Armando Leon, Lauren Maggio, Evans Whitaker, James Heilman, Jake Orlowitz, Valerie Swisher, Lane Rasberry, Kingsley Otoide, Fred Trotter, Will Ross, and Jack D. McCue, "Why Medical Schools Should Embrace Wikipedia: Final-Year Medical Student Contributions to Wikipedia Articles for Academic Credit at One School," *Academic Medicine* 92, no. 2 (2017): 194–200.

26. Health.Gov, "Quick Guide to Health Literacy Fact Sheet," accessed August 24, 2016, https://health.gov/communication/literacy/quickguide/factsbasic.htm. See also Office

of Disease Prevention and Health Promotion, "America's Health Literacy: Why We Need Accessible Health Information," accessed August 20, 2016, https://health.gov/communication/literacy/issuebrief/.

27. Health.gov, "Quick Guide."

28. Wahlert and Fiester, "Repaving the Road," 62.

29. Wikipedia, "Category: Medicine Articles Needing Expert Attention," last modified October 8, 2013, accessed August 24, 2016, https://en.wikipedia.org/wiki/Category:Medicine_articles_needing_expert_attention.

30. Ibid.

Works Cited

ACLU. "Past LGBT Nondiscrimination and Anti-LGBT Bills Across the Country." Accessed August 1, 2018. https://www.aclu.org/other/past-lgbt-nondiscrimination-and-anti-lgbt-bills-across-country.

Adichie, Chimamanda Ngozi. "The Danger of a Single Story." TED (video), July 2009. Accessed August 2016. http://www.ted.com/talks/lang/eng/chimamanda_adichie_the_danger_of_a_single_story.html.

Alexa.com. "Wikipedia.org Traffic Statistics: How Popular Is Wikipedia.org?" Last modified August 29, 2016. Accessed August 30, 2016. http://www.alexa.com/siteinfo/wikipedia.org.

Azzam, Amin. "Medical Schools Making Wikipedia Better." Innovate with AMA. Accessed August 24, 2016. https://www.innovatewithama.com/project/detail/327.

Azzam, Amin, David Bresler, Armando Leon, Lauren Maggio, Evans Whitaker, James Heilman, Jake Orlowitz, Valerie Swisher, Lane Rasberry, Kingsley Otoide, Fred Trotter, Will Ross, and Jack D. McCue. "Why Medical Schools Should Embrace Wikipedia: Final-Year Medical Student Contributions to Wikipedia Articles for Academic Credit at One School." *Academic Medicine* 92, no. 2 (2017): 194–200.

Bendery, Jennifer. "Everything You Need to Know about the Wave of 100+ Anti-LGBT Bills Pending in States: Nine States Are Afraid to Let Transgender People Go to the Bathroom." *Huffington Post*, April 15, 2016. http://www.huffingtonpost.com/entry/lgbt-state-bills-discrimination_us_570ff4f2e4b0060ccda2a7a9.

Bowker, Geoffrey C. "The History of Information Infrastructures: The Case of the International Classification of Diseases." *Information Processing & Management* 32, no. 1 (1996): 49–61.

Bowker, Geoffrey C., and Susan Leigh Star. "Introduction: To Classify Is Human." In *Sorting Things Out: Classification and Its Consequences*, edited by Geoffrey C. Bowker and Susan Leigh Star, 1–32. Cambridge, MA: MIT Press, 2000.

Callahan, Edward J., Nicole Sitkin, Hendry Ton, Suzanne W. Eidson-Ton, Julie Weckstein, and Darin Latimore. "Perspectives Introducing Sexual Orientation and Gender Identity into the Electronic Health Record: One Academic Health Center's Experience." *Academic Medicine* 90, no. 2 (2015): 154–60.

Committee on Health Care for Underserved Women. "Health Care for Transgender Individuals." American College of Obstetricians and Gynecologists, December 2011. https://www.acog.org/Clinical-Guidance-and-Publications/Committee-Opinions/

Committee-on-Health-Care-for-Underserved-Women/Health-Care-for-Transgender-Individuals.

Crenshaw, Kimberlé. "Mapping the Margins: Intersectionality, Identity Politics, and Violence against Women of Color." *Stanford Law Review* 43, no. 6 (1991): 1241–99.

Crozier, Ivan Dalley. "The Medical Construction of Homosexuality and Its Relation to the Law in Nineteeth-Century England." *Medical History* 45 (2001): 61–82.

Drabinski, Emily. "Queering the Catalog: Queer Theory and the Politics of Correction." *Library Quarterly* 83, no. 2 (2013): 94–111.

Duggan, Lisa. "The New Homonormativity: The Sexual Politics of Neoliberalism." In *Materializing Democracy: Toward a Revitalized Cultural Politics*, edited by Dana D. Nelson and Russ Castronovo, 175–94. Durham, NC: Duke University Press, 2002.

Enteen, Jillana. "Introduction: Life Skills." In *Virtual English: Queer Internets and Digital Creolization*, 1–20. New York and London: Routledge, 2009.

Fang, Marina. "Tennessee Passes Anti-LGBT Counseling Bill." *Huffington Post*, April 11, 2016. Accessed August 24, 2016. http://www.huffingtonpost.com/entry/tennessee-lgbt-counseling_us_570c4c4de4b0836057a23d63.

Fenway Institute and Center for American Progress. *Asking Patients Questions about Sexual Orientation and Gender Idenity in Clinical Settings: A Study in Four Health Centers*. Boston: Fenway Institute; Washington, DC: Center for American Progress, 2013. Accessed August 15, 2016. http://thefenwayinstitute.org/wp-content/uploads/COM228_SOGI_CHARN_WhitePaper.pdf.

Flanagan, Mary. "Introduction to Critical Play." In *Critical Play: Radical Game Design*, 1–16. Cambridge, MA: MIT Press, 2009.

Tiltfactor. *Grow-A-Game*. Accessed August 1, 2018. http://www.tiltfactor.org/grow-a-game/.

Gert, Bernard, Charles M. Culver, and K. Danner Clouser, eds. *Bioethics: A Systematic Approach*. 2nd ed. New York: Oxford University Press, 2006.

Guarrasi, Ivana. "Residual Categories in Medical Simulation: The Role of Affect in the Performance of Disease." *Mind, Culture, and Activity* 22, no. 2 (2015): 112–28.

Health.gov. "Quick Guide to Health Literacy: Fact Sheet." Accessed August 24, 2016. https://health.gov/communication/literacy/quickguide/factsbasic.htm.

HealthIT.gov. "Benefits of EHRs." Accessed August 20, 2016. https://www.healthit.gov/providers-professionals/benefits-electronic-health-records-ehrs.

Heilman, James M. "Wikipedia and Medicine: Quantifying Readership, Editors and the Significance of Natural Language." *Journal of Medical Internet Research* 17, no. 3 (2015): e62.

King, Katie, and Jarah Moesch. "Feminist Worlding: Media Ecologies Learning." In *Feminist Cyberspaces: Pedagogies in Transition*, edited by Sharon Collingwood, Alvina E. Quintana, and Smith J. Caroline, 14–31. Newcastle-upon-Tyne, UK: Cambridge Scholars Publishing, 2012.

Muñoz, José Esteban. "Introduction: Performing Disidentifications." In *Disidentifications: Queers of Color and the Performance of Politics*, 1–34. Minneapolis: University of Minnesota Press, 1999.

Office of Disease Prevention and Health Promotion. "America's Health Literacy: Why We Need Accessible Health Information." Accessed August 20, 2016. https://health.gov/communication/literacy/issuebrief/.

Oram, Andy. "How Health IT Fails Transgender Patients." KevinMD, January 11, 2015. Accessed August 20, 2016. http://www.kevinmd.com/blog/2015/01/health-fails-transgender-patients.html.

Roberts, Dorothy. *The Problem with Race-Based Medicine*. TEDMED (video). November 2015. Accessed August 1, 2018. https://www.ted.com/talks/dorothy_roberts_the_problem_with_race_based_medicine.

Salen, Katie, and Eric Zimmerman. "The Rules of Digital Games." In *Rules of Play Game Design Fundamentals*, 140–149. Cambridge, MA: MIT Press, 2004.

Silver, Curtis. "Google Will Offer Your Symptoms Better Medical Advice (But It's Probably Cancer)." *Forbes*, June 21, 2016. Accessed August 20, 2016. http://www.forbes.com/sites/curtissilver/2016/06/21/google-will-offer-your-symptoms-better-medical-advice-but-its-probably-cancer/#39ffdafe27ed.

Singer, Ben. "The Human Simulation Lab—Dissecting Sex in the Simulator Lab: The Clinical Lacuna of Transsexed Embodiment." *Journal of Medical Humanities* 34, no. 2 (2013): 249–54.

Wahlert, Lance, ed. "Special Issue: Mapping Queer Bioethics: Space, Place, and Locality." *Journal of Homosexuality* 63 (2016).

Wahlert, Lance, and Autumn Fiester. "Repaving the Road of Good Intentions: LGBT Health Care and the Queer Bioethical Lens." *Hastings Center Report* 44, no. S4 (2014): S56–S65.

Washington, Harriet A. *Medical Apartheid: The Dark History of Medical Experimentation on Black Americans from Colonial Times to the Present*. New York: Doubleday Books, 2007.

Wikipedia. "Category: Medicine Articles Needing Expert Attention." Last modified October 8, 2013. Accessed August 24, 2016. https://en.wikipedia.org/wiki/Category:Medicine_articles_needing_expert_attention.

Winner, Langdon. "Do Artifacts Have Politics?" *Daedalus: Modern Technology: Problem or Opportunity?* 109, no. 1 (1980): 121–36.

16

Moving Pictures

VISUAL CULTURE/VISUAL ACTIVISM IN THE HEALTH HUMANITIES CLASSROOM

Therese Jones

The whole world is watching.

—National Committee to End the War in Viet Nam, 1968

Occupy Wall Street, 2011

In *How to See the World*, Nicholas Mirzoeff opens with a snapshot of the visual world in which we and our students live.[1] It is a world where one hundred hours of video are uploaded every minute to YouTube and where six billion hours are watched every month (that is one hour of video for every person on earth), where Americans take more photographs in two minutes than were made in the entire nineteenth century, and where a worldwide total of 2.5 trillion were taken in 2016, 90 percent with smartphones.[2] All of these images, Mirzoeff writes, are our way of trying to see and make sense of a world actually too big to see but crucially vital to imagine—this is now the study of *visual culture*. Moreover, many of these images, such as the cellphone videos of police brutality in the United States or the student protests in Hong Kong, play a central and crucial role in rallying social and political response. Such *visual activism* confronts deep-seated hegemonies like racism, encourages silenced voices to emerge, and works as a catalyst for reform.

In health humanities classrooms, visual materials such as documentary films, photographs, and, yes, even YouTube videos often serve as accessible texts for the analysis and discussion of individual experiences of illness and disability or as evocative illustrations of issues such as access to care or end of life. Such works can foster empathic responses, sharpen critical thinking, and develop communication skills in health professions students. Moreover, visual materials can also serve as openings for students to critique the culture of healthcare itself and as opportunities for them to identify disparities, confront stigma and discrimination, and envision change. Thus, the visual arts not only encourage our students to see but also reveal to them how, what, and why they see what they see—sometimes prompting their action and provoking their transformation.

In this chapter, I will briefly describe and define visual culture and visual activism and illustrate them in the context of three health and human rights movements of the twentieth century—AIDS, breast cancer, and disability rights—which foreground the critical practice and political strategy of producing visibility and deploying testimony in forms such as documentary, video, photography, and poster art. I will then describe health humanities methodologies and materials in three content areas—mental illness, trauma of war, and disability—that I use in a variety of classroom settings to enable critical analysis and explore advocacy and intervention. For example, students consider the difference between looking and witnessing, how visual images influence attitudes toward patients and impact health policy, and the balance between inciting moral outrage from exposure to images and inducing compassion fatigue from overexposure to them.

From Visual Culture to Visual Activism

> Look art act.[3]

Visual culture came into academic view, so to speak, in the mid-1980s. It was more than an auspicious moment—it was a critical crucible. For example, William Gibson's term *cyberspace*, from his 1984 novel *Neuromancer*, was being appropriated to describe the new communication environment and social experience of computer networking. In 1985, the Guerrilla Girls began deploying outrageous visuals to expose gender and ethnic bias in art, film, and popular culture, while feminist academics and artists were critiquing high art and mixing it with pop culture and digital images. In 1986, W. J. T. Mitchell helped launch the field of visual studies with *Iconology*, which introduced ideas such as the pictorial turn, the image/picture distinction, the meta-picture, and the biopicture. In 1988, ACT UP activists and artists already committed to shining a light on the extreme levels of bias and stigma in the mainstream media and to creating alterative representations seized the opportunity of Nicholas Nixon's exhibit *Pictures of People with AIDS*, at the Museum of Modern Art, to mount their unforgettable condemnation of marginalization and exploitation: "STOP LOOKING AT US; START LISTENING TO US." In fact, AIDS as an "epidemic of signification"[4] would serve as a critical case study for what was becoming an epidemic of *theorizing* signification. By the end of the decade, the visual culture of performance also came into high relief, from Madonna's "strike a pose" to Judith Butler's groundbreaking book *Gender Trouble*, which revealed that gender itself is spectacle and speculative.

The myriad elements emerging and converging in the 1980s—the explosion and expansion of social media, the rejection and reappropriation of traditional Western iconography, and the eager and imaginative acceptance of identity as performance—helped shape and sharpen the new field of visual culture, which in the early 1990s centered on questions of visual and media representations in mass and popular culture,[5] namely, how we see others, how we see ourselves, and who has the power and the privilege to see or not be seen.

It should come as no surprise then that one of the most accessible "texts" for currently understanding what visual culture is and what it means is YouTube, where we can find a lecture series from the Royal College of Art as well as presentations by Mitchell himself on work in progress. Most appropriate and highly instructive is a lengthy and detailed description of the academic enterprise delivered by a cartoon fembot.[6] According to Mirzoeff, visual culture is both the name of an academic field and its object of study—a culture of the visual, "the relations between what is visible and the names that we give to what is seen as well as . . . what is invisible and kept out of sight."[7] Mirzoeff has been at the forefront of developing and chronicling the field. His *Visual Culture Reader* (1998) and *Introduction to Visual Culture* (1999) helped introduce the scope of inquiry as well as its prominent theorizers and practitioners to critics and educators around the world. As he noted then, the world-as-text was being effectively challenged by the world-as-picture, and images have only continued to disrupt and challenge any and all attempts to define culture in purely linguistic terms.[8]

However, visual culture practice cannot be and is not static. ACT UP's demand to be heard rather than simply seen exemplifies its turn toward social and political activism—not only questioning representations but using them to agitate for change. Indeed, since the early 1990s, visual culture has crystallized around visual activism[9]; and through organizations such as the International Association for Visual Culture, founded in 2009,[10] and conferences such as Visual Activism at San Francisco MOMA in 2014,[11] the areas of focus—analysis *and* engagement—are now coequal and intertwined. This is illustrated in descriptions of *visual activism* as cultural, critical, and political engagement with and responsibility for the *visual culture* in which we live (International Association for Visual Culture) and as a relationship between *visual culture* and *activist practices* (Visual Activism at San Francisco MOMA). For Mirzoeff, one of the defining moments of the evolution of visual culture to visual activism was the Arab Spring when social media outlets like Facebook allowed both for the dissemination of information and for the opportunity to see a crisis that a regime might, in the past, have kept unseen. His definition of *visual activism* is succinct: "the intersection of pixels and actions to make change," arguing that we can no longer simply study or simply see what is happening but must now actively engage in creating that change.[12]

Three health and human rights movements in the second half of the twentieth century—AIDS, breast cancer, and disability rights—can serve as compelling examples of the power and potential of visual activism for students in health humanities courses. For them, these issues (especially AIDS) may seem, at first glance, like historical artifacts; but students can quickly identify and appreciate the far-reaching effects of those activist agendas and strategies in their own political, cultural, and personal presents. In her book *Indirect Action: Schizophrenia, AIDS, and the Course of Health Activism,* Lisa Diedrich uses the phrase "multiple temporalities" to describe how illness and activism operate "chronically, persistently and randomly, directly and indirectly."[13] This perspective, activism as an expansive and multiplicitous experience rather than a singular and concrete event, fits especially well in a health humanities curriculum where the goals of introducing and analyzing visual materials may be as nebulous as a transformation in students' attitudes or opinions or as tangible as new visual works produced by them.

LET THE RECORD SHOW . . .

From the mid-1980s to the mid-1990s, we saw an expanded and deliberate use of cultural representations to effect political, institutional, and social change in response to HIV/AIDS. From the graphics of controversial artists such as David Wojnarowicz to less confrontational but highly emotional performances such as Tony Kushner's epic play *Angels in America* and Jonathan Demme's Academy Award–winning film *Philadelphia* to the collective mourning and memorial of the Names Quilt, visual materials served as instruments in the fight not only to modify healthcare policies and practices but also to educate people about the epidemic and transform their attitudes toward those infected with and affected by HIV/AIDS.

The single image most associated with AIDS activism in the United States is the pink triangle above the inscription SILENCE = DEATH—a simple graphic that originally served as the logo for ACT UP (AIDS Coalition to Unleash Power) and now figures as a singular icon for an organized and effective street response to issues of health and illness (Figure 16.1). In his contemporaneous examination of the dynamics and activities of the AIDS activism movement, Josh Gamson wrote about its mix of strategic action and material targets such as civil disobedience at the Food and Drug Administration (FDA) with expressive action and cultural targets such as guerrilla theater and die-ins.[14] Arguably, no cultural activity that ACT UP deployed was more impactful than its singular articulation of aesthetics and politics through visual images.

Let the Record Show . . . opened at the New Museum in late 1987 to provide current information regarding the epidemic, to depict the crisis in historical perspective, and to identify those national figures who were using AIDS "to promote their own political and religious agendas." The stated intention

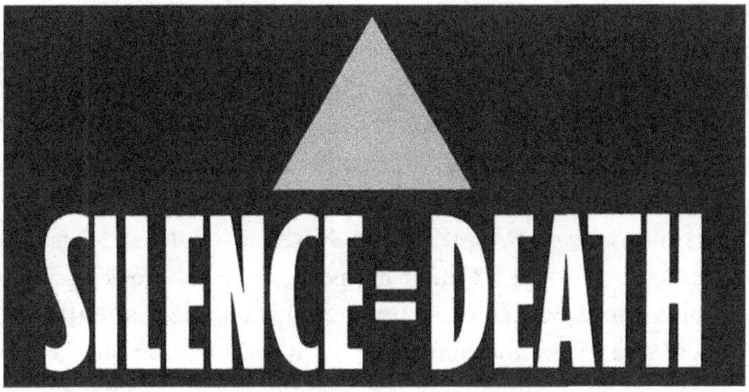

FIGURE 16.1 SILENCE = DEATH

of the project was "to make the viewer realize the depth of the problem and understand that history will judge our society by how we responded to this calamity, potentially the worst medical disaster of the century."[15] The exhibit included flyers and posters by Gran Fury, the activist artist collective, including the Silence = Death graphic; a photomural of the Nuremberg trials; images of AIDS criminals such as Jesse Helms, Ronald Reagan, and Jerry Falwell; and an LED display detailing the cost of government inaction.[16]

Andrew Weiner considers the lasting yet still immediate impact of *Let the Record Show . . .* in his discussion of the 2012 retrospective exhibition *ACT UP New York: Activism, Art, and the AIDS Crisis, 1987–1993* at Harvard University. He writes that the images and objects, despite having outlived their original purpose and context, "still retain considerable power, conjuring the life-and-death intensity of oppositional politics."[17] To situate and intensify that power, health humanities students can also view the 2012 documentary *How to Survive a Plague*, which chronicles the real and specific effects of AIDS activism including significant changes in FDA policies and practices as well as in the medical and media responses to HIV/AIDS. Students can recognize not only how the legacy of ACT UP shapes current healthcare including patient privacy and empowerment but also themselves and their own activist practices in that legacy. The medical student organization WhiteCoats4BlackLives, created to address racism especially enacted through police violence, began in 2014 with a demonstration taken right out of ACT UP's playbook: The National White Coat Die-In.[18]

"YOU CAN'T LOOK AWAY ANYMORE"

During most of the twentieth century, public testimonies and open discussions about breast cancer were simply unthinkable. What became known as the "breast cancer movement" was first solidified with the publication of *Our Bodies, Our Selves* by the Boston Women's Health Collective in the early 1970s and next transformed from relatively polite lobbying to an "in-your-face" militancy in the early 1980s, mirroring AIDS political activism. In 1993, the model Matuschka captured the next dynamic phase of the movement when she exposed her mastectomy scar on the cover of the *New York Times Magazine* in an aptly titled display of breast cancer exhibitionism: "You can't look away anymore"[19] (available for viewing at http://www.beautyoutofdamage.com/).

In her book *Staring: How We Look*, Rosemarie Garland-Thomson posits how staring actually makes things happen, and the shocking image of an amputated breast and scarred chest immediately captured attention, launching a new political awareness and activism.[20] Matuschka had made a career and a commodity of her body, showing it as a lingerie model, go-go dancer, and photographer of what we would now call nude "selfies." She well understood the dynamics of the male gaze: the ocular gesture of dominance that acts out the "gendered asymmetries of patriarchy and proliferates in institutionalized cultural forms such as films, beauty contests, advertising, striptease routines, and fashion shows"—many of the same forms in which she herself participated.[21] So when Matuschka showed up breast-less in the *New York Times Magazine*, sharply violating common expectations of women's breasts as visual fetish and sexual object, she immediately gave breast activism more than a face. According to Garland-Thomson, "It was a turning point for breast cancer advocacy, which has evolved an entire culture of visual symbolism, ranging from ubiquitous pink ribbons to intricate tattoos adorning mastectomy scars."[22]

Matuschka's pictorial revelation of breast cancer came ten years after the work of radical art photographer Jo Spence began her own documentation of diagnosis and treatment for breast cancer with exhibits such as *Cancer Shock* in 1982 and *The Picture of Health?* in 1982–1986. Spence's stated intention for a 1991 exhibit, *Narratives of Disease*, was to find a language that was counter to the biomedical discourse that speaks of "people as mechanical objects" and to a mainstream media "obsessed with the idealism of youth and beauty."[23] However, in contrast to Spence's confrontational and often grotesque images of her own body, Matuschka deliberately exploited the iconography of the conventional visual arena, displaying herself in the aesthetic tradition of the nude female figure and in the commercial attitude of the fashion model.

Matuschka's visual activism has inspired similar photographic displays and art projects, including the Breast Cancer Fund's 2000 public awareness campaign "Obsessed with Breasts," in which breast cancer removal scars were superimposed on professional models, mimicking the advertising imagery of Obsession perfume and Victoria's Secret catalogues. As Garland-Thomson notes, the public ads fuse two opposing visual genres—the medical photograph with its stark surgical imagery and the pinup model with its provocative posturing[24]—essentially merging the medical gaze and the male gaze. *The Scar Project* (2011) is a series of large-scale nude portraits of women in various states of treatment for and recovery from breast cancer created by photographer

David Jay. The project's immediate goal is to raise awareness about breast cancer, but what it articulates as its deeper message is an understanding of the human condition in which scars unite us all.[25]

For health humanities students, what Matuschka herself described as a "new vocabulary of images"[26] can serve as an explicit example of how visual activism works: from perception to action—from creating an opportunity to see differently (or for the first time) to prompting a responsibility to think and be differently. "You can't look away anymore" was just one dramatic strategy to make visible and present what had been unviewable and unmentionable in public.

VITAL SIGNS: CRIP CULTURE TALKS BACK

It was both an ironic and inspired move to employ the very visual medium—film—that had, for years, erased and exploited individuals with disabilities as a successful means of advancing the work of activists. For decades, viewers of American television and film have either not seen any representations of people with disabilities—accurately supporting the description of them as the invisible minority—or encountered them as one of six major stereotypes: "victim, hero, threat, unable to adjust, one to be cared for, one who should not have survived."[27]

David Mitchell and Sharon Snyder's 1995 edgy and raw documentary *Vital Signs: Crip Culture Talks Back* captured the political, social, and artistic revolution that had been emerging in disability culture. Filmed in the cinéma vérité mode with predominantly low camera angles, the filmmakers presented subjects who towered over "the viewer with their images punctuating their political positions and artistic caveats."[28] The participants, many in wheelchairs, shared their viewpoints and experiences about stigma, humiliation, public intolerance, and insensitivity in their own words and in their own way, contradicting the familiar visual images of isolation and powerlessness and controlling the terms of the body's portrayal in a visual medium. The film's intention was to foreground the ways that disability issues affect everyone: "visibility and invisibility, passing and coming out, accessibility and silence, mainstreaming and isolation, civil rights and public neglect, independence and institutionalization."[29] Its reach surprised even its creators, leading the front edge of a movement in film and video that narrated the experience of disability from the community itself. It is a distinct and powerful example of visual activism.

In health humanities classroom, films consistently serve as an effective pedagogical methodology to frame and reframe issues, provoke discussion and reflection, and encourage advocacy and activism. Schwartz et al. write of how films such as *Vital Signs* not only desensationalize and dispel stereotypes but also "signal a new paradigm in the way people with disabilities [are] represented."[30] In addition, Garland-Thomson writes about the impact of seeing disability in a culture that has hidden it or made it unusual: "we are stunned and alienated when it appears to us . . . we stare in fascinated disbelief and uneasy identification."[31] The defamiliarized and discomforting moment of recognizing how concealed disability has been creates an opportunity to challenge students, especially health professions students, who might not have, heretofore, critically interrogated the biomedical model of disability. Presenting the social model as an alternative in this context moves them forward as they recognize and apprehend a newness that can be transformative—one that disrupts both the visual and biomedical status quo.

From Looking to Acting/From Content to Creation

> Real art has the capacity to make us nervous.[32]

All health professions students are trained to observe—to look, to discern, to inventory discrete elements, to know the risks and benefits of pattern recognition—and many are motivated by a desire to serve, to advocate, and to care for people in need. This acquisition of scientific and technical expertise along with the inculcation of critical inquiry and caring behavior have been intrinsic to the predominant humanistic epistemological model in health professions education for over a half-century. In many health humanities programs, one common method of developing observational skills, enhancing critical thinking, and fostering empathy is through interaction with the visual arts—painting, photography, and sculpture—in classrooms, galleries, and museums. Much has been written about arts observation pedagogy and practice, most with a decided emphasis on its instrumental and restorative value.[33] However, more recently, scholars such as Caroline Wellberry and Rebecca McAteer have focused on art observation as an opportunity for disruption by "making visible the invisible or making strange what is ordinary" and as an opportunity for resistance by identifying and critiquing biomedical culture itself.[34] Their arts-based curriculum is designed to be a process, rather than an event, in which students move from the neutral position of looking to the implicated position of witnessing by realizing that seeing is more than description, that it is filtered through personal values and cultural norms which inhibit "nuanced, even contradictory, observations" to critically inform a final interpretation of the object in our sight line.[35] Their goal is to take their students from self-awareness to institutional self-criticism, which they describe as "the least exercised of all analysis": "Teaching observation in such a way . . . could go a long way in exploring the power of resistance as a pathway to a more humane approach to patient care."[36]

Such an approach invites and encourages the very act of observation to be scrutinized and critiqued, recognizing that looking itself can be "cruel, voyeuristic, traumatic and raw."[37] In essence, without such scrutiny and critique, health humanities educators run the risk of re-enacting and reifying the disciplinary, detached, and scripted "clinical gaze" despite our best intentions and stated curricular goals. The very structure and activity of observation are asymmetrical: by seeing and saying, we also dominate, objectify, and appropriate, as theorists such as Foucault (on the clinic), Sontag (on photography), Mulvey (on film), Haraway (on vision itself), and Garland-Thomson (on staring) have thoroughly examined and illustrated. Remaining aware of our own power and privilege is especially challenging in an academic environment in which the prerogative of looking inarguably belongs to an elite few who are educated and trained to do exactly that, while the exigency and vulnerability of the many make their ability to resist or deflect the clinical gaze nearly impossible.

Thus, how do we navigate between the contradictory positions of being inside and outside different systems at the same time in health humanities education? More specifically, how do we and our students apprehend that the intersections of privilege (gender, race, class, sexuality, age, ableness, etc.) can, simultaneously, reflect a commitment to change and a complicity with the status quo? And, finally, how do we negotiate the ethical and moral gray area of trying to do the right thing under the wrong conditions?[38]

One effective and accessible strategy is to confront directly the ambivalent position of spectator/critic and advocate/activist through visual materials that expose it with our selection of course content. Another more challenging and often less accessible method, because of limitations in time, materials, and opportunities, is an integrative art pedagogy that invites students not only to analyze critically their static and normative perspective of the other but also to explore the aesthetic qualities of visual materials and then use them as instruments of social activism.[39] Both critiquing and creating visual materials in health humanities courses demand that we and our students revisit and revise dichotomies such as the vernacular and the artistic, personal and private, representation and expression, isolation and engagement, and advocacy and exploitation.[40]

In the following section are selected visual materials—documentary films, an art exhibit, a personal video—that I have used with both health professions and undergraduate students in three content areas: mental health, trauma of war, and disability. Following the discussion of those materials, I will conclude with a description of one visual project by students, *What Worries You Most?* This exhibit vividly represents to all viewers the gap between the singular focus of emergency medicine to identify and address patients' presenting symptoms and the complicated responses from those same people to a simple question about their most important concerns.

Mental Health and Mental Illness

In an elective for senior medical students on cinematic representations of mental health and mental illness, we view and discuss two controversial documentaries: Frederick Wiseman's unflinching exposé of the Massachusetts Correctional Institution (MCI) for the "criminally insane" in *Titicut Follies* (1967) (Figure 16.2) and Eric Steel's visual record of people jumping to their deaths in *The Bridge* (2006). Because of the nature of filming inmates/patients warehoused in a state institution and of photographing the final, dark moments of a human being who steps over the edge of the Golden Gate Bridge, students must confront a number of moral contradictions and ethical conundrums raised by these films. For instance, they raise questions about the norms of privacy and the issue of public access, the rights of an individual and the responsibilities of a community, and the difference between bearing witness and being a voyeur. It is also crucial for students to understand and struggle with Wiseman's and Steel's explicit objective: making art to make change. Wiseman believed that public awareness of the terrible conditions at MCI would create an impetus for reform and a demand for improvement; at the time of filming, there were only two psychiatrists caring for over six hundred men in the hospital.[41] And after reading of the long history of suicides and concomitant arguments against the installation of preventive barriers at the

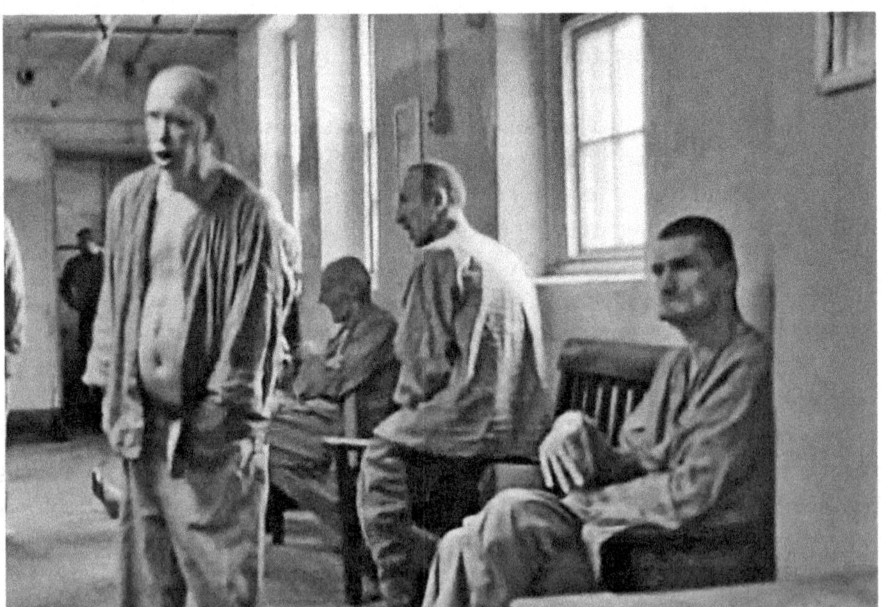

FIGURE 16.2 *Titicut Follies*

Golden Gate Bridge, Steel had clarity: "There are two choices: to do nothing or to pull someone back from the edge."[42]

But just how far should the artist-activist go? How does he or she cast light on human rights offenses and social justice concerns without inflicting further damage on those who are suffering and powerless? Both documentaries foreground this essential question about visual activism—do predominantly good intentions outweigh the potential of collateral violence to subjects *and* viewers? As noted by film scholar Bill Nichols, looking through the documentary keyhole can frequently exploit both subject and viewer; and students talk freely about feeling implicated and manipulated, about feeling a sense of responsibility[43]—what Meile calls the "unavoidable consequence of empathy"[44]—yet feeling a sense of revulsion. For health professions students, the discussion can be reframed for relevance in clinical settings—for example, advocating for a "difficult patient" after witnessing her or his mistreatment or disrespect by members of the healthcare team; identifying the cognitive dissonance between knowing the ethical obligations of informed consent and pragmatically performing it under time constraints, language challenges, and acute situations; and exploring the emotional cost of having to do harm to patients in order to care for them medically.

Seeing brutal violence or terrible suffering in a documentary engages us differently from that in other representations; its power to evoke a response is undeniable, and the visual evidence of *Titicut Follies* and *The Bridge* certainly provokes discomfort and indignation. However, there can be unintended consequences of such visual activist work that also resonate for medical students including a moral outrage that simply overwhelms the potential for bearing genuine ethical witness or a naive belief that exposure will induce compliance with human rights norms in institutions, states, and other systems of authority because of their shame and our reliance on the power of reason and knowledge.[45] Perhaps, related more directly to students' own experience, is the risk of overexposure or "compassion fatigue," the result of being overwhelmed by both the proliferation of visual evidence and the feeling of powerlessness when confronting it.

War and Trauma

It would seem counterintuitive that bringing visual representations of trauma suffered by American soldiers in the ongoing wars in Iraq and Afghanistan would qualify as making visible the invisible. Given that these are federally sanctioned and supported conflicts, which are being conducted as conventional military operations under continual review and with consistent reporting, there should not be that much unseen and unsaid. However, a documentary film, *Hell and Back Again* (2011), and an art exhibit, *The Joe Bonham Project*, provide visual evidence to the contrary—namely, the inescapable recognition of how invisible these wars have been and continue to be. By contrast, the Vietnam War was the first major military engagement of the television era; and once the military machine revved up its powerful engines through the beaches and jungles of Vietnam, the images of the war found prime space on the airwaves. Then, on any given day, viewers could turn on the nightly news and catch the Vietnam show, and artist-activists could deploy photographs that not only communicated the horrors of the war but also fueled protests against it. Now, on any given day, our students likely see nothing at all from Iraq or Afghanistan.

Afghan photojournalist and filmmaker Danfung Dennis was embedded with the US Marines Echo Company in 2009 during a major helicopter assault on a Taliban stronghold. The images of a devastated landscape, displaced villagers, constant miscommunications, and chaotic military actions are a vivid reminder of how little we have seen regarding how this war has been and is being waged. The narrative focus is Sergeant Nathan Harris, the twenty-five-year-old company commander, who is seriously wounded and returns home to North Carolina to his wife, Ashley, and a long, painful rehabilitation. A growing opioid dependence, marital conflicts, the emotional and psychological challenges as Nathan begins to question the reason for and cost of the war, an uncertain future, and the loss of identity as a career soldier provide a vivid contrast to the images of combat. The crosscutting technique of the film from soldiers moving through a war zone to Nathan negotiating the Wal-Mart parking lot, persuading a doctor to write another prescription, and struggling through the agony of physical therapy telegraph the film's argument—war is not hell; the consequences of war are hell.

For the pharmacy, medical, and physical therapy students who view and discuss this film in health humanities courses, it is both relevant and revelatory as they will very likely be encountering returning soldiers in multiple healthcare settings. I accompany it with an art exhibit, *The Joe Bonham Project: Drawing the Stories of America's Wounded Veterans*. After completing three tours in Iraq, Marine Corps artist Mike Fay organized a group of twelve colleagues—both military and civilian—to document with original drawings, paintings, and cartoons the grueling journeys of American soldiers who survived combat but did not survive "intact." The exhibit is named for the central character in Dalton Trumbo's 1938 novel *Johnny Got His Gun*, who is horribly wounded and lives out his days, alone and forgotten. The activist aim of this collective work is to ensure that a new generation of "Joe Bonhams" will not be forgotten (Figures 16.3 and 16.4).

These are the pictorial stories of the daunting challenges in trauma centers and rehabilitation facilities that soldiers and their caregivers—family members and health professionals—confront with dignity, courage, and compassion. Such images can be difficult for students, but they offer an opportunity to discuss the ethics of looking at images of suffering, pain, and death. Susan

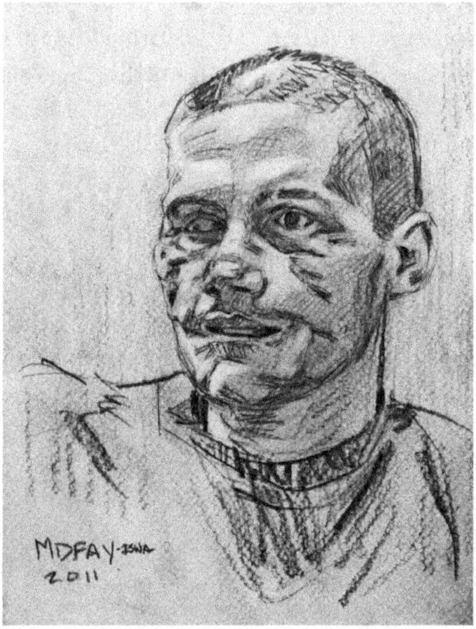

FIGURE 16.3 *The Joe Bonham Project.* Fay writes that Kyle was recognized with the Congressional Medal of Honor by President Barack Obama in June 2014 for throwing himself on a grenade to save his comrades.

Michael D. Fay, *Lance Corporal Kyle Carpenter USMC,* 2011. Graphite on paper (20 x 16). Reprinted with permission of the artist.

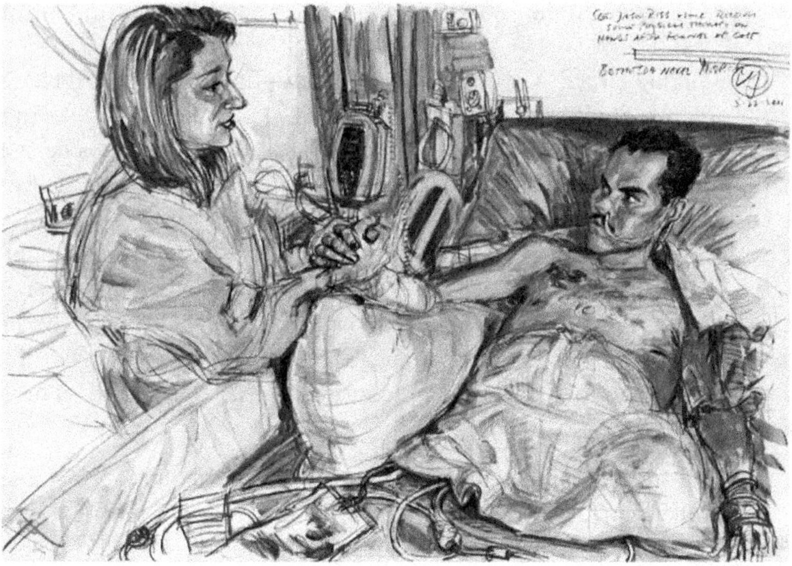

FIGURE 16.4 *The Joe Bonham Project.* Jason was an explosive ordnance disposal Marine who lost half his body and was given a 2% chance of survival by the medical staff at Walter Reed.

Victor Juhasz, *Sergeant Jason Ross USMC,* 2011. Acrylic on paper (31 x 38.5). Reprinted with permission of the artist.

Sontag's book *Regarding the Pain of Others* provides a helpful distinction for students between what she describes as an unethical gaze at mutilated bodies, which is prurient, passive, and indifferent, and an ethical gaze, which is empathic, engaged, and motivated toward political change.[46]

Disability

Since World War II, human rights activism has and continues to rely on testimony, and as Meg McLagan writes, it has been progressively refined in its production and circulation: "It has become a transnational cultural form, one that plays a crucial role in almost every human rights campaign."[47] The personal story of a survivor or the eyewitness account of a bystander can reach millions through social media, and the skillful deployment of visual images broadens the reach and intensifies the response. With an eight-and-a-half-minute YouTube post, "In My Language," Amanda Baggs found herself at the leading edge of an increasingly visible and highly networked community of people with autism.[48] I introduce this video to all learners in health humanities courses to explore how visual subversions of hegemonic body and social norms can destabilize our understanding of personhood, cognition, and communication and to demonstrate the power of visual activism (the approximate number of views is now 1.5 million). Baggs describes becoming mobilized after looking at gay pride websites, and the video was "a political statement, designed to call attention to people's tendency to underestimate autistics."[49]

It is a highly effective tool for teaching disability issues; students are immediately discomfited during the first half of the video as Baggs rocks in front of a window, tunelessly hums, strokes a keyboard repetitively, flaps her fingers under running water, and rubs her face against a book. The second half of the video—"A Translation" in the form of voiceover and subtitles—both reveals and confronts any assumptions we have made about her intellectual abilities or about others like her on the autism disorder spectrum who have experienced marginalization, exclusion, and even institutionalization because of difference. Artistic practices such as "In My Language" can effectively subvert the limiting and harming impact of normative practices on those constructed as other, as Baggs herself testifies:

> This has not been intended as a voyeuristic freak show where you get to look at the bizarre workings of the autistic mind, but it is meant as a strong statement on the existence and value of many different kinds of thinking and interacting.[50]

Mirzoeff writes that the implication of the identity politics protest, "they do not represent us," is that we must find ways to represent ourselves.[51] The visual activism of an Amanda Baggs is a compelling example of not only taking on that challenge but also using it to make change.

What Worries You Most?

In her book *Touching Photographs*, Margaret Olin explores photography's role in the world: it acts, it connects people, it creates communities. Olin presented the keynote lecture for the 2015 International Association for Visual Culture, whose theme was bearing witness. She titled her talk "Witnessing, Bystanding, Onlooking, Participating" in order to identify and understand the various ways we engage (or remain disengaged) in visual culture. The four words of her title offer an array of standpoints which presumably represent the most common reactions to the visual evidence of personal suffering, political oppression, and social violence. The first and fourth words signify a level of responsibility and involvement that bracket the more detached and less implicated positions of just standing by and looking on. Do our students make the leap over that relatively safe middle ground through the exposure to and exploration of visual materials like those I have described above? For the health humanities educator, it is often a leap of faith to believe that; but occasionally, there are students who respond creatively *and* concretely with visual work of their own in the hope that some witness, bystander, or onlooker will also make a leap toward change.

In February 2017, a group of senior medical students distributed cards to patients in the University of Colorado Hospital Emergency Department with a simple question printed at the top: "What Worries You Most?" Students encouraged people to be as honest as possible (the responses were anonymous), and when students returned to collect the cards, they discussed the content with the respondents. What emerged was a surprising disconnect or gap between the necessary and stark information supplied by the patient at the bottom of the card—chief complaint, age, sex, and acuity—and what was written on the card itself. A few patients were worried about their health, but most were concerned about family members, financial hardships, substance use, Medicaid status, and even the Trump administration. Wanting to be heard and understood and fearing isolation and loneliness were common responses (Figures 16.5 and 16.6).

The students next opened up the project with an exhibit of the cards, which they enlarged and curated for a public space. They effectively subverted the control and confinement of information in the healthcare setting, where what happens there usually stays there and is accessible to a privileged few, and the depersonalization and diminishment that patients experience in the medical encounter by revealing its inadequacy in getting crucial information—what really matters most to the person waiting in the Emergency Department. The visual evidence of each card literally subordinates clinical data to personal

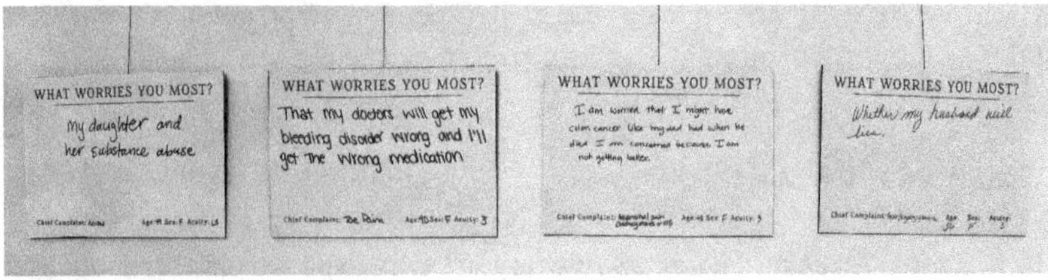

FIGURE 16.5 *What Worries You Most?*

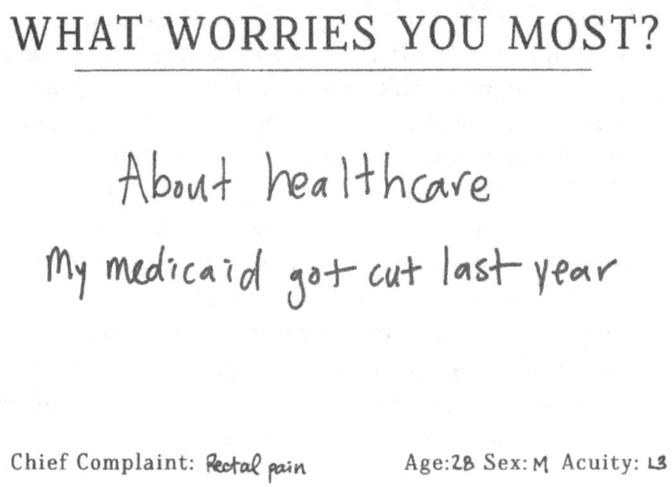

FIGURE 16.6 *What Worries You Most?*

response (medical and demographic facts are situated below the patient's handwriting), which may have been both restorative and empowering for the patients themselves.

Finally, the students installed an interactive element in which visitors to the exhibit could fill out their own cards. The results were even more startling and powerful as the cards became an opportunity for everyone to give voice to fears and concerns about being a patient *and* being a health professional, about encounters of bias and experiences of stigma, about access to care for our most vulnerable and marginalized citizens. With simplicity and directness, *What Worries You Most?* made the leap—engaging viewers, inviting their participation, and establishing a sense of community (Figure 16.7).

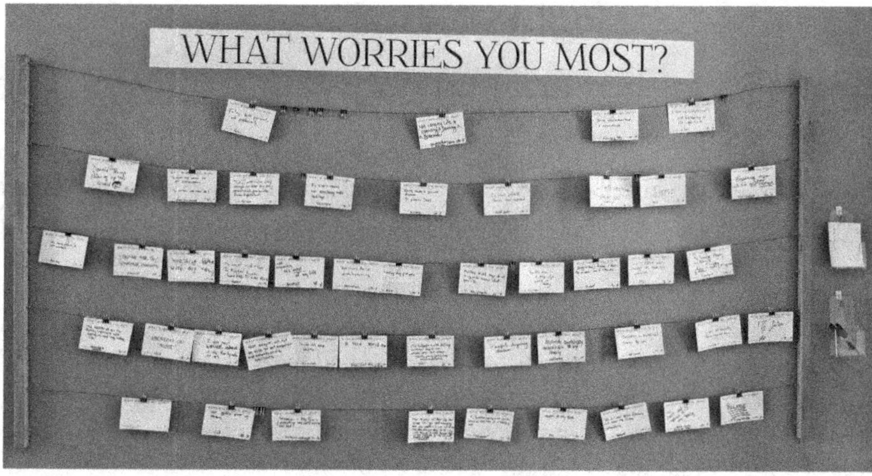

FIGURE 16.7 *What Worries You Most?*

In her work on staring and disability, Garland-Thomson outlines the process of seeing, thinking, and acting: "The impulse to look at novel sights and spectacular bodies . . . can be transformative. They disturb not just the visual status quo but the ethical status quo."[52] Critical to visual activism is empathy—how looking in and of itself can generate a sense of obligation to act differently, build the world differently, treat people differently. Health humanities educators and their students now have access to visual images that can expose injustice and incite rebellion, and they also have the opportunity to create visual images that can address problems and create communities—pictures that move us and move others.

PEDAGOGY EXERCISE SECTION

Exploring Health (Through a Personal Lens)

EXPLANATION OF EXERCISE

How can we recognize and understand the ways we see others *and* ourselves? How can we recognize and understand that we see illness not only through the lens of biology but also as a social, political, and narrative construct?

Using visual materials including a film clip and a comic, this ninety-minute session designed for first-year medical students provides an opportunity for them to explore how what we see is filtered through our own values and experiences. In this session, we use images to consider how stereotypes, biases, and preconceived notions impact how we see and how we react to individuals and situations that may be fraught with emotion or may have ambiguous or missing information. Learning goals are as follows:

- To analyze how personal perspectives and experiences impact our view of health and healthcare
- To employ self-reflection to acknowledge our own beliefs, biases, and practices
- To identify examples of personal bias that we have experienced or observed

STRUCTURE OF EXERCISE

The session begins with a large group presentation and discussion and then moves to small breakout groups, which are facilitated by individual faculty.

Part I: Large Group (25 Minutes)

1. Introduction of two-minute clip from 2004 American film *Crash*, including
   - Production details: Directed and written by Paul Haggis and set in Los Angeles with interlocking stories of whites, blacks, Latinos, Koreans, Muslims, cops, criminals, rich, poor, the powerful, and the powerless. Winner of three Academy Awards including Best Picture and Best Screenplay.
2. Screening of film clip, "Blind Fear" (scene 2, 7:48–9:42)
3. Open discussion, guided by the following questions:
   - Does the scene reinforce or undercut racial/gender stereotypes?
   - Did you see the woman do or say something to provoke the African American man's response?
   - Who do you most identify with in the scene and why?

Part II: Small Groups (60 Minutes)

1. More focused discussion of film clip, guided by the following questions:
   - What observations and responses do you have?
   - What is the general tone of the scene? Comic? Ironic? How does the tone work with the action?
   - How do the emotional states of the characters set up their reactions to one another?
   - How does the camera reinforce the question of what and how we see?
2. Introduction of "Fill in the Dialogue" exercise.
   - Distribute a selected comic with the original dialogue deleted.

     (We use a two-page chapter, "The Doctor Visit," from Paco Roca's 2016 graphic novel *Wrinkles*. There are many excellent health-related comics with situations that include children, adolescent, or elderly characters; disabled or chronically ill characters; transgender, gay, and minority characters.)
   - Read the following directions, and allow fifteen to twenty minutes for students to create their own narratives:

     The words to this short comic are missing. Taking your cue from the images, fill in the speech bubbles with your own imagined dialogue. As you look at the images, carefully consider the following:
     - What are the characters' demeanor and posture?
     - What is the setting?
     - What emotions might be in play?
     - What visual data are missing?
     - What is the story?
3. Sharing and discussing, guided by the following questions:
   - On plot:
     - What prompted your story?
     - How did you come up with that scenario?
     - Did the setting and situation remind you of something in your own experience?
   - On character:
     - Did you have a main character?
     - Did the characters seem familiar? Why? Who did they remind you of?
     - How did stereotypes influence your depiction of characters? Did you find yourself reinforcing stereotypes or working against them? Or did you even think about that?

- What was the most challenging element of this assignment for you?

4. Debriefing, guided by the following questions:
    - How do images tell us something about the ways in which we see?
    - What did you learn about your own perspective? About your colleagues?
    - Can we ever get beyond stereotypes? Aren't they often helpful in healthcare?

Notes

1. Nicholas Mirzoeff, *How to See the World* (London: Pelican Books, 2015), 6.

2. Deloitte, "Photo Sharing: Trillions and Rising," accessed May 17, 2017, https://www2.deloitte.com.

3. Antje Schuhmann, "How to Be Political? Art Activism, Queer Practices, and Temporary Autonomous Zones," *Agenda* 28, no. 4 (2014): 94–107.

4. Paula Treichler, *How to Have Theory in an Epidemic: Cultural Chronicles of AIDS* (Durham, NC: Duke University Press, 1999), 11.

5. Mirzoeff, *How to See the World*, 289.

6. "What Is Visual Culture?" YouTube video, 4:47, n.d., www.youtube.com/watch?v=qpDtbK6OiJQ.

7. Mirzoeff, *How to See the World*, 11.

8. Nicholas Mirzoeff, "What Is Visual Culture?" in *The Visual Culture Reader*, ed. Nicholas Mirzoeff (New York: Routledge, 1998), 5.

9. Mirzoeff, *How to See the World*, 289.

10. International Association for Visual Culture, accessed January 4, 2017, https://www.iavc.info/.

11. Visual Activism at San Francisco Museum of Modern Art, 2014, accessed January 4, 2017, https://www.sfmoma.org/event/visual-activism/.

12. Mirzoeff, *How to See the World*, 297.

13. Lisa Diedrich, *Indirect Action: Schizophrenia, Epilepsy, AIDS, and the Course of Health Activism* (Minneapolis: University of Minnesota Press, 2016), 1.

14. Josh Gamson, "Silence, Death, and the Invisible Enemy: AIDS Activism and Social Movement 'Newness,'" *Social Problems* 36, no. 4 (1989): 351.

15. William Olander (curator), *Let the Record Show . .*, New Museum Digital Archive, November 1987, accessed May 23, 2017, http://archive.newmuseum.org/index.php/Detail/Occurrence/Show/occurrence_id/158.

16. Andrew Weiner, "Disposable Media, Expendable Populations—ACT UP New York: Activism, Art, and the AIDS Crisis, 1987–1993," *Journal of Visual Culture* 11, no. 1 (2012): 104–105.

17. Ibid., 105.

18. White Coats For Black Lives, http://www.whitecoats4blacklives.org.

19. Susan Ferraro, "The Anguished Politics of Breast Cancer," *New York Times Magazine*, August 15, 1993, 24–27.

20. Rosemarie Garland-Thomson, *Staring: How We Look* (Oxford: Oxford University Press, 2009), 148–49.

21. Ibid., 41.

22. Ibid., 154.

23. Jo Spence, *Narratives of Disease*, 1989, accessed May 24, 2017, http://www.jospence.org/narratives_of_disease/narratives_of_disease_thumbs.html.

24. Garland-Thomson, *Staring*, 156.

25. David Jay, *The Scar Project*, David Jay Photography, 2011, accessed May 10, 2017, http://www.thescarproject.org/.

26. Matuschka, accessed May 1, 2017, http://www.matuschka.net/.

27. Diane Schwartz, et al., "Dispelling Stereotypes: Promoting Disability Equality through Film," *Disability and Society* 25, no. 7 (2010): 842.

28. David T. Mitchell and Sharon L. Snyder, "Talking about Talking Back: Afterthoughts on the Making of the Disability Documentary *Vital Signs: Crip Culture Talks Back*," *Disability, Art, and Culture* 37, no. 2 (Spring 1998), accessed May 16, 2017, http://hdl.handle.net/2027/spo.act2080.0037.206.

29. Ibid.

30. Schwartz et al., "Dispelling Stereotypes," 848.

31. Garland-Thomson, *Staring*, 20.

32. Susan Sontag, *Against Interpretation and Other Essays* (New York: Picador, 2001), 5.

33. See, for example, Charles L. Bardes, Debra Gillers, and Amy E. Herman, "Learning to Look: Developing Clinical Observation Skills at an Art Museum," *Medical Education* 35 (2001): 1157–61; Jacqueline C. Dolev, Linda Krohner Friedlander, and Irwin M. Braverman, "Use of Fine Art to Enhance Visual Diagnostic Skills," *Journal of American Medical Association* 2001, no. 286 (2001): 1020–21; Sona K. Jasani and Norma S. Saks, "Utilizing Visual Art to Enhance the Clinical Observation Skills of Medical Students," *Medical Teacher* 35 (2013): e1327–31; Craig Klugman, Jennifer Peel, and Diana Beckmann-Mendez, "Art Rounds: Teaching Interprofessional Students Visual Thinking Strategies at One School," *Academic Medicine* 86 (2011): 1266–71; Jo Marie Reilly, Jeffrey Ring, and Linda Duke, "Visual Thinking Strategies: A New Role for Art in Medical Education," *Family Medicine* 37 (2005): 250–52; Pamela B. Schaff, Suzanne Isken, and Robert M. Tager, "From Contemporary Art to Core Clinical Skills: Observation, Interpretation, and Meaning-Making in a Complex Environment," *Academic Medicine* 86 (2011): 1272–76; Johanna Shapiro, Lloyd Rucker, and Jill Beck, "Training Clinical Eye and Mind: Using the Arts to Develop Medical Students' Observational and Pattern Recognition Skills," *Medical Educator* 40 (2004): 263–68.

34. Carolyn Wellberry and Rebecca McAteer, "The Art of Observation: A Pedagogical Framework," *Academic Medicine* 90, no. 12 (2015), 1625.

35. Ibid., 1627.

36. Ibid., 1628.

37. Ibid.

38. See Antje Schuhmann, "How to Be Political? Art Activism, Queer Practices, and Temporary Autonomous Zones," *Agenda* 28, no. 4 (2014): 94–107.

39. See Sheng Kuan Chung and Michael S. Kirby, "Media Literacy Art Education: Logos, Culture Jamming, and Activism," *Art Education* 62, no. 1 (2015): 34–39.

40. See Connor Graham et al., "New Visual Technologies: Shifting Boundaries, Shared Moments," *Visual Studies* 26, no. 2 (2011): 87–91.

41. Therese Jones, "Another Kind of DNR (Do Not Record): *Titicut Follies*," in *The Picture of Health: Medical Ethics and the Movies,* ed. Henri Colt, Silvia Quadrelli, and Lester Friedman (Oxford: Oxford University Press, 2011), 91.

42. Therese Jones, "*The Bridge*," *American Journal of Bioethics* 9, no. 3 (2009): 52.

43. Bill Nichols, *Representing Reality: Issues and Concepts in Documentary* (Bloomington: University of Indiana Press, 1991).

44. Quoted in Garland-Thomson, *Staring*, 4.

45. Meg McLagan, "Introduction: Making Human Rights Claims Public," *American Anthropologist* 108, no. 1 (2006): 192.

46. Susan Sontag, *Regarding the Pain of Others* (New York: Farrar, Strauss, and Giroux, 2003).

47. McLagan, "Introduction," 193.

48. David Wolman, "The Truth about Autism: Scientists Reconsider What They Think They Know," *Wired*, February 25, 2008, accessed May 20, 2017, https://www.wired.com/2008/02/ff-autism/.

49. Ibid.

50. Amanda Baggs, "In My Language," YouTube Video, 8.36, January 14, 2007, accessed May 24, 2017, https://www.youtube.com/watch?v=JnylM1hI2jc.

51. Mirzoeff, *How to See the World*, 293.

52. Garland-Thomson, *Staring*, 188.

Works Cited

Baggs, Amanda. "In My Language." YouTube Video, 8.36, January 14, 2007. Accessed May 24, 2017. https://www.youtube.com/watch?v=JnylM1hI2jc.

Bardes, Charles L., Debra Gillers, and Amy E. Herman. "Learning to Look: Developing Clinical Observational Skills at an Art Museum." *Medical Education* 35 (2001): 1157–61.

Boston Women's Health Book Collective and Judy Norsigian. *Our Bodies, Ourselves,* Revised Edition. New York: Touchstone, 2011.

Butler, Judith. *Gender Trouble: Feminism and the Subversion of Identity*. New York: Routledge, 1990.

Chau, Mimi, and James Engeln (curators). *What Worries You Most?* Fulginiti Pavilion for Bioethics and Humanities, University of Colorado Anschutz Medical Campus, April 2017.

Chung, Sheng Kuan, and Michael S. Kirby. "Media Literacy Art Education: Logos, Culture Jamming, and Activism." *Art Education* 62, no. 1 (2015): 34–39.

Deloitte. "Photo Sharing: Trillions and Rising." Accessed May 1, 2017. https://www2.deloitte.com/content/dam/Deloitte/global/Documents/Technology-Media-Telecommunications/gx-tmt-prediction-online-photo-sharing.pdf.

Dennis, Danfung (director). *Hell and Back Again*. London: Roast Beef Productions, 2011.

Diedrich, Lisa. *Indirect Action: Schizophrenia, Epilepsy, AIDS, and the Course of Health Activism*. Minneapolis: University of Minnesota Press, 2016.

Dolev, Jacqueline C., Linda Krohner Friedlander, and Irwin M. Braverman. "Use of Fine Art to Enhance Visual Diagnostic Skills." *Journal of American Medical Association* 286 (2001): 1020–21.

Fay, Mike. *Joe Bonham Project* (blog). 2014. Accessed May 24, 2017. http://joebonhamproject.blogspot.com/.

Ferraro, Susan. "The Anguished Politics of Breast Cancer." *New York Times Magazine*, August 15, 1993, 24–27.

Foucault, Michel. *The Birth of the Clinic: An Archeology of Medical Perception*. Translated by Alan Sheridan Smith. New York: Vintage Books, 1994.

France, David (director). *How to Survive a Plague*. New York: Public Square Films, 2012.

Gamson, Josh. "Silence, Death, and the Invisible Enemy: AIDS Activism and Social Movement 'Newness.'" *Social Problems* 36, no. 4 (1989): 351–67.

Garland-Thomson, Rosemarie. *Staring: How We Look*. Oxford: Oxford University Press, 2009.

Gibson, William. *Neuromancer.* New York: Ace Publishing, 1984.

Graham, Connor, Eric Laurier, Vincent O'Brien, and Mark Rouncefield. "New Visual Technologies: Shifting Boundaries, Shared Moments." *Visual Studies* 26, no. 2 (2011): 87–91.

Haraway, Donna. "The Persistence of Vision." In *The Visual Culture Reader*, edited by N. Mirzoeff, 191–98. New York: Routledge, 1998.

International Association for Visual Culture. Accessed January 4, 2017. https://www.iavc.info/.

Jasani, Sona K., and Norma S. Saks. "Utilizing Visual Art to Enhance the Clinical Observation Skills of Medical Students." *Medical Teacher* 35 (2013): e1327–31.

Jay, David. *The Scar Project*. David Jay Photography, 2011. Accessed May 10, 2017. http://www.thescarproject.org/.

Jones, Therese. "Another Kind of DNR (Do Not Record): *Titicut Follies.*" In *The Picture of Health: Medical Ethics and the Movies*, edited by Henri Colt, Silvia Quadrelli, and Lester Friedman, 91–97. Oxford: Oxford University Press, 2011.

Jones, Therese. "*The Bridge.*" *American Journal of Bioethics* 9, no. 3 (2009): 51–53.

Klugman, Craig, Jennifer Peel, and Diana Beckmann-Mendez. "Art Rounds: Teaching Interprofessional Students Visual Thinking Strategies at One School." *Academic Medicine* 86 (2011): 1266–71.

Matuschka. Accessed May 1, 2017. http://www.matuschka.net.

McLagan, Meg. "Introduction: Making Human Rights Claims Public." *American Anthropologist* 108, no. 1 (2006): 191–200.

Mirzoeff, Nicholas. *An Introduction to Visual Culture,* 2nd edition. London: Routledge, 2009.

Mirzoeff, Nicholas. *How to See the World*. London: Pelican Books 2015.

Mirzoeff, Nicholas. "What Is Visual Culture?" In *The Visual Culture Reader*, edited by Nicholas Mirzoeff, 3–14. New York: Routledge, 1998.

Mitchell, David T., and Sharon L. Snyder. "Talking about Talking Back: Afterthoughts on the Making of the Disability Documentary *Vital Signs: Crip Culture Talks Back.*" *Disability, Art, and Culture* 37, no. 2 (Spring 1998). Accessed May 16, 2017. https://quod.lib.umich.edu/cgi/t/text/text-idx?cc=mqr;c=mqr;c=mqrarchive;idno=act2080.0037.216;g=mqrg;rgn=main;view=text;xc=1.

Mitchell, David, and Sharon Snyder (directors). *Vital Signs: Crip Culture Talks Back.* Brooklyn, NY: Fanlight Productions, 1995.

Mitchell, W. J. T. *Iconology: Image, Text, Ideology.* Chicago: University of Chicago Press, 1987.

Mulvey, Laura. "Visual Pleasure and Narrative Cinema." In *Film Theory and Criticism*, 7th ed., edited by Leo Braudy and Marshall Cohen, 711–23. Oxford: Oxford University Press, 2009.

Nichols, Bill. *Representing Reality: Issues and Concepts in Documentary*. Bloomington: University of Indiana Press, 1991.

Nixon, Nicholas. *Pictures of People with AIDS.* New York: David R. Godine, 1994.

Olander, William (curator). *Let the Record Show . . .* New Museum Digital Archive. November 1987. Accessed May 23, 2017. http://archive.newmuseum.org/index.php/Detail/Occurrence/Show/occurrence_id/158.

Olin, Margaret. *Touching Photographs.* Chicago: University of Chicago Press, 2011.

Reilly, Jo Marie, Jeffrey Ring, and Linda Duke. "Visual Thinking Strategies: A New Role for Art in Medical Education." *Family Medicine* 37 (2005): 250–52.

Roca, Paco. *Wrinkles*. Seattle, WA: Fantagraphics Books, 2016.

Schaff, Pamela B., Suzanne Isken, and Robert M. Tager. "From Contemporary Art to Core Clinical Skills: Observation, Interpretation, and Meaning-Making in a Complex Environment." *Academic Medicine* 86 (2011): 1272–76.

Schuhmann, Antje. "How to Be Political? Art Activism, Queer Practices, and Temporary Autonomous Zones." *Agenda* 28, no. 4 (2014): 94–107.

Schwartz, Diane, Elfreda Blue, Mary McDonald, George Giuliani, Genevieve Weber, Holly Seirup, Sage Rose, Deborah Elkis-Albuhoff, Jeffrey Rosenfeld, and Andrea Perkins. "Dispelling Stereotypes: Promoting Disability Equality through Film." *Disability and Society* 25, no. 7 (2010): 841–48.

Shapiro, Johanna, Lloyd Rucker, and Jill Beck. "Training Clinical Eye and Mind: Using the Arts to Develop Medical Students' Observational and Pattern Recognition Skills." *Medical Educator* 40 (2004): 263–68.

Sontag, Susan. *Against Interpretation and Other Essays*. New York: Picador, 2001.

Sontag, Susan. *On Photography.* New York: Picador, 2001.

Sontag, Susan. *Regarding the Pain of Others*. New York: Farrar, Strauss, and Giroux, 2003.

Spence, Jo. *Narratives of Dis-ease*. 1989. Accessed May 24, 2017. http://www.jospence.org/narratives_of_disease/narratives_of_disease_thumbs.html.

Steel, Eric (director). *The Bridge*. New York: Easy There Tiger Productions, 2006.

Treichler, Paula. *How to Have Theory in an Epidemic: Cultural Chronicles of AIDS*. Durham, NC: Duke University Press, 1999.

Trumbo, Dalton. *Johnny Got His Gun*. New York: Bantam, 1984.

Visual Activism Conference at San Francisco Museum of Modern Art. 2014. Accessed January 4, 2017. https://www.sfmoma.org/event/visual-activism/.

Weiner, Andrew. "Disposable Media, Expendable Populations—ACT UP New York: Activism, Art, and the AIDS Crisis, 1987–1993." *Journal of Visual Culture* 11, no. 1 (2012): 103–109.

Wellberry, Carolyn, and Rebecca A. McAteer. "The Art of Observation: A Pedagogical Framework." *Academic Medicine* 90, no. 12 (2015): 1624–30.

"What Is Visual Culture?" YouTube video, 4:47, n.d. www.youtube.com/watch?v=qpDtbK6OiJQ.

White Coats For Black Lives, http://www.whitecoats4blacklives.org.

Wiseman, Frederick (director). *Titicut Follies*. Cambridge, MA: Zipporah Films, 1967.

Wolman, David. "The Truth about Autism: Scientists Reconsider What They Think They Know." *Wired*, February 25, 2008. Accessed May 20, 2017. http://archive.wired.com/medtech/health/magazine/16-03/ff_autism.

17

The Baptism and the Butterfly

THE USE OF CREATIVE CLINICAL NARRATIVES IN TEACHING END-OF-LIFE SUBJECTS

Marcia Brennan

Pedagogical Reflections on "The Scale of Everything"

A typical day in my seminar "Life at the End of Life" may begin as follows: "Hello, everyone. As usual, last week I had an amazing day on the Acute Palliative Care Unit at M. D. Anderson. You just have to hear this story. I think you'll be intrigued. After you've listened to the narrative, we'll go around the table, and I want each of you to share your thoughts and insights on what is striking about the story you've just heard.

"My last visit of the day was with a youngish woman with advanced metastatic sarcoma. She only had limited mobility due to the multiple tumors pressing against her spinal cord. By the time our visit occurred, her pain issues were pretty well managed, and she was planning to leave for hospice care the next day. The occupational therapist helped the woman into a wheelchair, and I sat down beside her. As usual, I introduced myself, and I asked her where she was from. We chatted briefly about her family, and then we spoke about her work. I learned that the woman was a geologist. Until she became too ill, she had worked professionally, both in academia and in industry. Geology was her passion, and she was very proud of the fact that she had taught in this area for several years. I told her that I, too, am a teacher, and I briefly described our class. She was very interested in all of this. At the end of the visit I asked permission to share her narrative, so that others could hear her striking insights, and she generously agreed.

"When I asked the woman about the images that held special significance for her, she described a beautiful landscape that she had visited while working as a geologist. Yet it soon became clear that the meanings she associated with this landscape extended well beyond the scientific domain. The woman told a striking story about it.

The Scale of Everything

For my image,
I think of one of my favorite places in the world.
It's in the Canadian Rockies.
It's geological, of course.
It's a glacier valley, with one little meadow after another.

This place is out a ways,
And it's sort of the end of the road.
You can actually see the glacier retreating.
It's where geologists go.

You start at ground level and hike up.
There's a ridge line,
And there was a good group of us walking there.
That was a happy place to be.
It was very freeing.
When I was there I felt supported, and liberated,
In an absolutely spectacular natural place that I love.
It was beautiful.
That's why I'm a geologist, I guess.

It's also spiritual,
If you call transcendence by being in a happy place "spiritual."
At the Rockies, everything is so much bigger than you,
And that's very moving.

As geologists, we talk about the scale of something,
And we sometimes have difficulty conceptualizing that.
But this is one of the closest places to see it.
The scale of everything is quite stunning.

This opening vignette provides a glimpse within a glimpse of the way in which my practice as a literary Artist In Residence in the Department of Palliative Care and Rehabilitation Medicine at the University of Texas M. D. Anderson Cancer Center directly informs the seminars "Life at the End of Life" and "The Humanities of Care" that I teach at Rice University.[1] As this story exemplifies, as an Artist In Residence I serve not as a visual artist but as a creative writer. I assist patients and their caregivers in constructing poetic narratives to express their insights and experiences.[2] As people share their images, I gently encourage them to talk and make notes to help crystallize their thoughts. Once the literary artwork is complete, I read the person's words back to him or her, while making any additions or corrections that he or she indicates. The text is then inscribed into a handmade paper journal, which the person is able to keep and share with his or her family, either as a medium for further creative expression or as a legacy gift that performs a memorial function. The portable microenvironment of the text thus provides a durable yet tender memory of this transient moment in their lives.[3]

Narratives such as "The Scale of Everything" offer a suggestive framework for exploring some of the complex issues that emerge within our class discussions. While this story is based on an actual hiking trip that a woman took with fellow scientists, the artwork quickly progresses from the existential to the symbolic and the spiritual domains, as the woman described how her scientific work inspired a visionary perspective. Beginning in very concrete terms, the woman spoke of traveling a long distance, climbing through varied terrain, and ultimately encountering a breathtaking landscape "at the end of the road," a scene that presented a far more expansive perspective than is usually available. She also shared the ways in which the experience of being with good colleagues fostered a strong sense of support, friendship, and freedom. She then expressed an intriguing paradox as she described how her experience of the mountain glacier evoked a simultaneous sense of groundedness *and* of transcendence. In the woman's story, geological imagery thus referred to the natural landscape and to larger themes concerning the relations between size and scale, the microcosm and the macrocosm, and an individual's place in relation to something far greater than the self.

When reflecting on the immediacy and the immensity of this imagery, the woman observed that "the scale of everything is quite stunning." And with these words, she found a way to describe a state of being that lies well beyond the familiar boundaries of language. As the students heard her story and we discussed their individual and collective responses, so too did they find a vivid means to imagine otherwise unimaginable subjects. As the familiar world became invested with a heightened sense of intensity, themes that were otherwise too abstract, vast, and daunting suddenly became imaginable—and discussable—in ways that were deeply personal, relevant, and compelling.

Teaching "Life at the End of Life" and "The Humanities of Care"

Engaging such stories of presence and intimacy can create a sense of safety and relatability, which in turn can inform the overall tone and culture of the seminar in general. Much as in my creative clinical work, I approach my pedagogical practice in a spirit of open communication, a state that entails focused attention, careful listening, and the gentle affirmation of individual presences. On the first day of class, we go around the table and I ask everyone to introduce themselves, to explain briefly why they are drawn to a seminar on the end of life, and to share their feelings about the subject. I also ask them if they have ever personally attended a passing, and I ask who in the room plans to enter a healthcare profession.

After the introductions, I tell my students that, while we cover a great deal of material in this seminar—some of which may be difficult to engage—there is absolutely nothing that we cannot face together. I emphasize, "It's all right if these subjects make you feel uneasy, or sad, or scared. If you find this happening, just quietly catch my eye, take a deep breath, and you'll be okay in a minute. Everyone in this class is here for a very good reason, and together we have the great privilege of learning from one another. You will be amazed by the collective intelligence that emerges in the class. I always am."

We then go over the syllabus and review the course content. The common goal of my classes is to familiarize students with a methodologically diverse selection of texts and images associated with the end of life, from the classical through the contemporary periods. The materials provide a rigorous comparative framework to consider how death practices are visualized and enacted in a wide variety of historical, cultural, social, technological, spiritual, aesthetic, and disciplinary contexts. My classes engage the perspectives of medicine, bioethics, cultural studies, philosophy, anthropology, literature, art history, visual culture, media studies, and religious studies. Some of the specific topics we examine include the ethical choices and dilemmas associated with increased longevity and the use of life-sustaining technologies; the sometimes conflicting needs and perspectives of the dying and their caregivers; various cultural and anthropological conceptions of "the good death"; the philosophical paradox of "the gift of death"; the often fraught relations between bioethics, race, and healthcare disparities; historical, art historical, and technological representations of death and dying, monuments to the dead, and the personification of the figure of death itself; and finally, near-death experiences and representations of the afterlife.

In one of our sessions, we take a "field trip" to the center of the academic quad to view John Angel's bronze sculpture *William Marsh Rice* (1929), a life-size, seated statue of the university's founder. Notably, Rice's ashes are entombed in the base of the monument. The class stands around in a circle, and I tell everyone, "Please take a good, fresh look at this statue. I know that you've all probably seen this work hundreds of times. Yet now that we've spent this time together in class, I want to hear from each of you as to whether, in your opinion, we are standing in a sacred space. You cannot get the answer 'wrong,' but you must tell everyone: why or why not? And perhaps most importantly, *How do you know?* Then, I want you to consider how your answers to these questions will, or will not, change the way that you and your friends approach this sculpture in the future." Our conversations never fail to be intense, textured, humorous, and absolutely fascinating.

My classes at Rice are offered as advanced undergraduate seminars in religious studies and the medical humanities. Because the course enrollment demands exceed the capacity of the seminars, the classes typically fill up with seniors. Usually half or more of the students plan to enter healthcare professions. Yet the courses also attract a broad range of students from across the campus—from technically oriented STEM (science, technology, engineering, and mathematics) fields to humanistic disciplines to the applied creative fields of music and architecture. Just as end-of-life subjects are not the purview of any single group, the topics concern all of us and, thus, the courses are for *everyone*.

In turn, these themes emerge within the evaluations as students express their gratitude for the opportunity to broach difficult and meaningful subjects from a diverse range of personal and methodological perspectives. Regarding the seminars "Life at the End of Life" and "The Humanities of Care," students have remarked as follows:

> This course was unique and incredible. It challenged us to examine a somewhat difficult topic in order to understand the harsh realities and beauties found at the end of life and how that reflected on life itself. We covered such a wide array of topics that anyone can find an aspect that they are interested in. I would highly recommend this course to anyone and everyone!
>
> When people think about the "end of life," they think about a dismal and depressing outcome, but this course has opened my eyes to the importance of having such a conversation and such a class. We've learned about psychology, sociology, anthropology, bioethics, and so on. If you want to be challenged and are willing to open up, I highly recommend this class. It will hands down be the best class you will take at Rice.
>
> Amazing. A hidden gem. Wonderful course for all majors. I'm premed and it both challenged and engaged me. I feel as if I understand medicine differently—better because of it.
>
> Everyone is going to struggle with death, trauma, existentialism, and love at some point in their lives, and we need to learn how to do it with grace and care. Take this class!
>
> This course is unique and fun, despite the grim title. It's unlike any other course at Rice, and I appreciated the opportunity to have valuable discussions with my peers on a topic not often breached [*sic*] in other classes or in everyday life.
>
> The end of life seminar was amazing because it made me think about the part of life we all face but never talk about. This course combined different aspects of religion, philosophy, medicine, ethics, biomedical engineering, spirituality, and more through our discussions and readings.
>
> This course is a must-take for every student in any major. Guaranteed to develop critical thinking skills and [how to] think about a very natural part of life—not at all morbid or scary as people sometimes assume from the title.

> This class was absolutely incredible and greatly exceeded my expectations. I have learned so much about caregiving and the end of life. Topics were approached in a respectful and non-threatening way. At no point in the semester did I feel afraid or nervous about the topics being discussed, as Marcia was always there for us.[4]

In addition to my undergraduate seminars at Rice, I have engaged end-of-life narratives when teaching medical and dental students and when addressing practicing healthcare providers who undergo training as part of their continuing medical education (CME). In their evaluations, CME audiences have reported that learning about the arts and the humanities will impact their own healthcare practices by increasing their sense of humility, curiosity, perception, gratitude, and humanitarianism.[5]

Regarding medical school pedagogy, some especially striking insights were offered by a fourth-year medical student who shadowed me for several weeks on the Acute Palliative Care Inpatient Unit. In her final essay, the student emphasized the ways in which patients' voices can fill crucial gaps in medical school pedagogy. In particular, she noted that healthcare professionals who routinely deal with death rarely discuss it. Yet engaging in artistic work and hearing the actual voices of people facing the end of life can prepare medical students to think about death, which represents a vital step in preparing them to actually discuss the subject with vulnerable patients who may struggle with accepting a poor prognosis. She also observed that producing poetic narratives with a person at the end of life and with the caregivers who are present while a person is actively dying can demonstrate a sense of empathy and compassion that provides vital family support, a quality that can be especially valuable to meeting the needs of both patients and caregivers. She concluded that such responsiveness can be extremely empowering and play a valuable role in patient-centered care.[6]

Indeed, with the increasing emphases on medical technologies, the demographics of an aging population, and shifts in policies toward end-of-life planning at the national level, the need to cultivate such a humanistic perspective in medicine—and in the broader cultural sphere—remains both timely and pressing.[7] Moreover, people at the end of life represent a population that is often marginalized—if not altogether erased—within contemporary cultural discourses.[8] As the palliative care physician Michael Ashby has observed, within the medical literature "the patient's voice is not heard as loudly or often as it might be."[9] When commenting on these issues from a complementary perspective, the sociologist Allan Kellehear has noted that

> the problem-based concerns of both cancer medicine and palliative care have provided much useful information about symptom management, public health management and social management of illness-related

troubles but little in the way of description and understanding about positive aspects of dying.[10]

As both a teacher and a scholar, I have found that sharing end-of-life narratives can be beneficial for audiences in medicine and in the humanities. Just as the seminars "Life at the End of Life" and "The Humanities of Care" span multiple disciplines, the classes require a significant degree of openness, expansiveness, and self-overcoming. Throughout the discussions, the whole is always greater than the sum of the parts. This is particularly the case when we engage end-of-life narratives to enter spaces where "the scale of everything is quite stunning" and the subjects are even deeper and more significant than we can even imagine or than I can possibly tell you.

The Baptism and the Butterfly: A Study in Ultimate Things

I will conclude by taking you into the classroom—and into the clinic—one final time. As I tell my students, "This narrative is particularly complex and suggestive because it exemplifies the ways in which first and last things can become meaningfully conjoined through acts of personal, artistic, and spiritual creation. This story also aptly conveys one of the larger themes of the class, namely, that people have the capacity for self-creation, up to and including at the end of life. After you've heard the story, we'll go around the room and I want everyone to share what is striking and meaningful to them.

"One afternoon, I worked with a woman who had to use a white board to communicate. Due to the progression of her head and neck cancer, she had a trach (tracheostomy) tube, and she could no longer speak. Yet the woman was fully awake, alert, and oriented, and we had a great visit. I quickly learned that, while the woman had been raised in the Baptist faith, she had only been formally baptized two days before, in the interdenominational chapel at M. D. Anderson. After our staff chaplain performed a Christian baptism ceremony, the occupational therapist brought the woman and her family outside to the butterfly garden. The woman's adult children, and her brand new baby granddaughter, all attended the ceremony. While they sat together in the garden, several butterflies flew up to them.

"As we visited, I learned that this woman had experienced a very hard life. Yet she still had a quick sense of humor, a delicate presence, and a beautiful face. There were tears in her eyes as we created this narrative, especially as the woman expressed a sense of anticipatory grief as she faced what she saw as her own premature death, an event that only heightened her sadness and distress at not being able to see her new granddaughter grow up. Yet the woman loved hearing her story. Despite her limited range of motion, at the end of the visit she leaned forward so that I could kiss her cheek. Then I briefly told her about my teaching and scholarly work, and she kindly granted permission for the story to be shared. From the first sentences that appeared on the white board to the finished narrative, the words are all her own.

The Baptism and the Butterfly
I was baptized two days ago.
I wanted to be baptized because
I wanted to live on somehow.
I don't know how to express it.

Why baptism?
Maybe, and I'm not trying to sound too greedy,
But I'm too young to die.
I just had a grandbaby who I would love to see grow up.
Through baptism, it doesn't seem final for some reason.

The baptism felt like a deep breath.
I'm still feeling that now.

I would like to thank the chaplain.
She did a beautiful, elegant ceremony,
Which will live on.
She opened my eyes.

After the baptism, the therapist took us out into the garden,
And three butterflies followed through and landed as we sat around.
The therapist said these were monarch butterflies.

The butterflies reminded me of my mom.
She had lung cancer, and she passed away over twenty years ago.
The year she passed,
On my birthday,
My aunt gave me a present that my mom had bought earlier.
It was a butterfly necklace.
It hit me because, inside was a note that said,
"Butterflies are free."

I was going through a hard time at that time.
And two days ago,
Seeing those butterflies
Reminded me of her.

This woman passed away peacefully approximately three weeks after the ceremony. Thus, emerging at a critical juncture in her life, the woman's poetic narrative represents a study in ultimate things, one that unites images of the end of life with the promise of a new beginning.

All of this is to say that, at the very end of her life, this woman told a powerful story of creation.

PEDAGOGY EXERCISE SECTION

The Baptism and the Butterfly: The Use of Creative Clinical Narratives in Teaching End-of-Life Subjects

STEP I. PRELIMINARY REFLECTION

The end of life can represent an extremely challenging topic of discussion. As you begin the class, instruct the students to take out a blank sheet of paper and reflect on and complete the following sentence: "When I think about the end of life, the words that come to mind are _____."

STEP II. NARRATIVE INTERVENTIONS

Explain that you are now going to read aloud two literary artworks that were produced in a clinical setting and contain the actual words of people facing the end of life. After hearing the stories, you will ask the students to make some notes regarding what they find striking and meaningful in each of the narratives. Ask them to jot their thoughts down on the sheet of white paper, and tell them that you will then go around the room and ask each person to share her or his response and insights.

Read aloud "The Scale of Everything." Give the students a moment to note their reflections, and then invite them to share their thoughts.

Repeat this process with "The Baptism and the Butterfly."

STEP III. CONCLUDING REFLECTIONS

Tell the class, "Now that you have heard the stories and we have had an opportunity for discussion, I want everyone to take a moment to reflect on and complete the following sentence: 'When I think about the end of life, the words that now come to mind are _____.'"

Go around the room a final time, and invite everyone to compare their later responses with their initial answers. Invite the students to consider how their perspectives may have changed—and become more expansive—within the scope of this single class session.

Notes

1. My educational work unfolds primarily at the undergraduate level. For a discussion of the place of the humanities in the educational formation of medical professionals, see Nathan Carlin, Thomas R. Cole, and Henry Strobel, "Guidance from the Humanities for Professional Formation," in *Oxford Textbook of Spirituality and Healthcare*, ed. Mark Cobb, Christina M. Puchalski, and Bruce Rumbold (Oxford: Oxford University Press, 2012), 443–50.

2. For a discussion of the role of storytelling in end-of-life spiritual care, see Rachel Stanworth, *Recognizing Spiritual Needs in People Who Are Dying* (Oxford: Oxford University Press, 2004). For a related discussion of the power that narrative interventions can hold within a clinical context, particularly regarding their capacity to enhance the relations between communication and human dignity, see Rita Charon's influential study *Narrative Medicine: Honoring the Stories of Illness* (Oxford: Oxford University Press, 2006). In contrast to Charon's approach, the end-of-life narratives that I produce at M. D. Anderson are not "pathographies" or narratives of illness as there is no "symptom plot" or corresponding linkage between symptomology and selfhood, nor is there a therapeutic focus on the palliative value of "putting pain into words" by witnessing the suffering of others. Rather, the individuals with whom I work tend to characterize themselves primarily as human beings at the end of life and secondarily as patients, just as their stories often evoke themes not of disease, but of beauty, contingency, and transformation.

3. My hospital work is facilitated by COLLAGE: The Art for Cancer Network, a non-profit organization conceived and founded by Dr. Jennifer Wheler. For information on this organization, see http://www.collageartforcancer.org/index.htm. In addition to my teaching, this work represents the subject of my books *Life at the End of Life: Finding Words Beyond Words* (Bristol, UK: Intellect, 2017), and *The Heart of the Hereafter: Love Stories from the End of Life* (Winchester, UK: John Hunt Books, 2014).

4. These comments come from course evaluations collected by the university in December of 2015, December of 2016, and May of 2017.

5. These comments come from course evaluations collected at "The History and Culture of Disease and Healing Seminar Series" sponsored by the University of Texas School of Public Health on November 1, 2016.

6. I am grateful to Amberly Orr who shared her unpublished reflective essay, "Lessons on Dying: What Patients Taught Me That Was Missing from Medical School" (Spring 2017).

7. Regarding these themes, see Atul Gawande, *Being Mortal: Medicine and What Matters in the End* (New York: Henry Holt, 2014).

8. Regarding prominent cultural frameworks for approaching these issues, see Elisabeth Kübler-Ross's foundational work *On Death and Dying* (New York: Scribner's, 1969). For a qualification of Kübler-Ross's model and for detailed discussions of death from a medical perspective, see Sherwin Nuland, *How We Die: Reflections on Life's Final Chapter* (New York: Alfred A. Knopf, 1994).

9. See Michael Ashby, "The Dying Human: A Perspective from Palliative Medicine," in *The Study of Dying: From Autonomy to Transformation*, ed. Allan Kellehear (Cambridge: Cambridge University Press, 2009), 94. I use Kellehear's anthology as one of the textbooks in my seminar on "Life at the End of Life." For readers who are

contemplating teaching a course on death and dying at the college level, a valuable sourcebook is Christopher M. Moreman, ed., *Teaching Death and Dying* (Oxford: Oxford University Press, 2008). The various chapters address a range of practical, pedagogical, and philosophical issues that can arise for scholars working within the academic "death education movement."

10. Allan Kellehear, "What the Social and Behavioural Studies Say about Dying," in *The Study of Dying*, 19. Notably, Kellehear examines some of the key psychological aspects of dying in his text *The Inner Life of the Dying Person* (New York: Columbia University Press, 2014). Among the themes he explores are love, courage, hope, and transformation, as well as the challenges posed by fear, suffering, disconnection, resistance, and loneliness.

Works Cited

Ashby, Michael. "The Dying Human: A Perspective from Palliative Medicine." In *The Study of Dying: From Autonomy to Transformation*, edited by Allan Kellehear, 76–98. Cambridge: Cambridge University Press, 2009.

Brennan, Marcia. *Life at the End of Life: Finding Words Beyond Words*. Bristol, UK: Intellect, 2017.

Brennan, Marcia. *The Heart of the Hereafter: Love Stories from the End of Life*. Winchester, UK: John Hunt Books, 2014.

Carlin, Nathan, Thomas R. Cole, and Henry Strobel. "Guidance from the Humanities for Professional Formation." In *Oxford Textbook of Spirituality in Healthcare*, edited by Mark Cobb, Christina M. Puchalski, and Bruce Rumbold, 443–50. Oxford and New York: Oxford University Press, 2012.

Charon, Rita. *Narrative Medicine: Honoring the Stories of Illness*. Oxford: Oxford University Press, 2006.

Gawande, Atul. *Being Mortal: Medicine and What Matters in the End*. New York: Henry Holt, 2014.

Kellehear, Allan. *The Inner Life of the Dying Person*. New York: Columbia University Press, 2014.

Kellehear, Allan. "What the Social and Behavioural Studies Say about Dying." In *The Study of Dying: From Autonomy to Transformation*, edited by Allan Kellehear, 1–26. Cambridge: Cambridge University Press, 2009.

Kübler-Ross, Elisabeth. *On Death and Dying*. New York: Scribner's, 1969.

Moreman, Christopher M., ed. *Teaching Death and Dying*. Oxford: Oxford University Press, 2008.

Nuland, Sherwin. *How We Die: Reflections on Life's Final Chapter*. New York: Alfred A. Knopf, 1994.

Stanworth, Rachel. *Recognizing Spiritual Needs in People Who Are Dying*. Oxford: Oxford University Press, 2004.

18

Art as Disruption in Global Health Humanities

THE HUMUMENT TECHNIQUE, A SEXUAL AND REPRODUCTIVE HEALTH ARCHIVE, AND DEVELOPING FLEXIBLE STUDENT THINKING

Kearsley A. Stewart, Rachel Ingold, Maria de Bruyn, and Kelley K. Swain

Introduction

Narrative learning and reflective writing, two key pedagogies in medical and health humanities, have been shown to enhance physicians' empathy, improve clinical interview skills, and help practitioners better understand their patients' illness experiences.[1] These teaching techniques are well suited to the doctor–patient encounter, an intimate dyad that most often occurs in a highly controlled space and unfolds according to a mostly predictable, and regulated, script. In contrast, the aims of global health interventions are to improve health at a population level, identify the social determinants of health, and actively engage with reducing structural inequities that produce human suffering and inhibit human well-being. Yet, in practice, the spaces where global health initiatives and doctor–patient encounters unfold may be unpredictable, chaotic, fluid, and subject to multiple layers of regulation and intervention from local and global agents. Is there a role for the medical and health humanities in global health training and education? Could narrative learning and reflective writing enhance the practice of global health? Which pedagogies are best suited to developing a global health humanities education that prepares students to recognize and critique the structural features of health inequalities and barriers and, ultimately, to envision new perspectives and possible solutions?

This chapter describes a global health humanities undergraduate workshop that applies an art technique (*A Humument* by Tom Phillips)[2] to a reinterpretation of an archive of sexual and reproductive health literature including both published and gray literature (the Maria de Bruyn Papers at Duke University).[3] This assignment was developed over a yearlong, interdisciplinary collaboration among a global health educator (Stewart), the curator of the

History of Medicine Collections in the Rubenstein Rare Book & Manuscript Library at Duke University (Ingold), the donor of the archive (de Bruyn), and the poet who modified Phillips's Humument technique for the classroom (Swain).[4] In this chapter, we first describe the archival context in which the workshop took place. Next, we describe the pedagogical goals and how the workshop was structured to meet them. We then reflect on evidence of student learning and end with a discussion of lessons learned and future plans using this approach.

Our Archival Context

Global health archives exist in a variety of institutions, including, but by no means limited to, the US National Library of Medicine and Harvard University's Countway Library of Medicine. These collections may include gray literature,[5] such as organizational reports and newsletters, conference proceedings, policy statements, newspaper articles, journal notes, correspondence, audio and video clips, and much more. Such archival collections are rich repositories of materials created by public health and global health scholars, as well as clients and patients of health services, that are not always available in scholarly journals, in print, or online in a permanent manner.

Numerous special collection libraries and archives exist to preserve, and make available for research, primary source material. These primary sources range in date, format, and subject matter depending on the library, archive, institution, and collecting policies. At Duke University, the David M. Rubenstein Rare Book & Manuscript Library builds distinctive collections of original materials and preserves them for use on campus as well as with a global community of researchers. Within the context of the Rubenstein Library, the History of Medicine Collections seek to acquire, preserve, interpret, and make available for research and instruction materials documenting the history of medicine, biomedical science, and health and disease in the global context of the Western medical tradition. The collections seek to bring historical perspectives to bear on contemporary health issues and to facilitate an interdisciplinary understanding of the history of medicine. And the History of Medicine Collections in the Rubenstein Library, like other libraries and archives, seek to grow their collections of public health and global health materials.

In the summer of 2015, medical anthropologist Maria de Bruyn donated to the Rubenstein Library twenty-six boxes of materials collected from 1988 onward in the field of sexual and reproductive health and rights. The collection includes her own published and gray literature writings, as well as publications and artifacts (e.g., buttons, instructional health games, posters) produced by other authors, international agencies and non-governmental organizations (NGOs) in developing countries on topics such as HIV and AIDS,[6] sexual and reproductive health, human rights, condoms and contraception, stigma and discrimination, youth, sex work, and women's health. Materials of particular interest include first-person narratives and testimonies by adults and young people affected by HIV, violence, stigma, and discrimination. The value of the Maria de Bruyn collection lies in the opportunity to re-examine how various health issues have been addressed over time, particularly from the perspective of different geographical regions and ethnic groups.

The collection's arrival at the Rubenstein Library coincided with a discussion of how Stewart's global health seminar, Global Narratives of HIV and AIDS, could engage with archival material. At the time this collection was processed and made available to researchers (soon after its donation), Ingold and Stewart met to discuss the available collections at the library and the library services on offer. Their very first discussion initiated the project described in this chapter.

One of the most rewarding aspects of working in a special collection library is connecting researchers, particularly students, to archival collections. Many staff of special collections engage with students in bibliographic instruction sessions, giving students a chance to handle materials and experience archival research. Relationships with faculty have further provided opportunities for librarians and archivists to collaborate in developing assignments in which students utilize rare materials for coursework.[7]

Our Pedagogical Goals

Stewart had two goals in using the de Bruyn collection in her undergraduate seminar Global Narratives of HIV and AIDS: (1) to challenge global health students to conduct archival research in a new and innovative way and (2) to encourage global health students to explore how global health issues have been addressed by both the people affected and those working to mitigate and end these problems.

A NEW METHOD FOR ARCHIVAL RESEARCH

The workshop challenged students to consider using archival items in a new way. Many of these students hope to find work in the field of global health in the future; exposing them to such collections is a reminder that previous writing and literature can relate to current and future research. A traditional method for bringing students into contact with archival collections and primary sources is to assign them to write a historical analysis or analytical paper. The innovation of our new global health assignment is to require students to connect with archival material from a critical perspective and to develop their own reflections on these materials simultaneously in a creative and analytical way, specifically through a visual art technique. Assigning students to critically engage with NGO gray literature can reveal the political and sociocultural forces that shape global health.

When processing an archival collection, archivists often create a finding aid or collection guide to provide access to collection materials. After an introductory session on care and handling of archival materials, several workshop sessions were scheduled during class time so that students could spend significant time randomly browsing through the boxes and folders to identify potential items for their assignment. Students were advised to consult the collection guide for a more systematic introduction to the materials and encouraged to return to the reading room outside of class to spend even more time with the archival collection. In our increasingly digital world, there is something refreshing about seeing students pore over boxes of papers, pick them up, and point out sentences to their classmates. Archival research can take many forms, but a highlight for us was seeing students interact with physical materials, a skill, we reminded them, they are likely to need in their future work in resource-constrained environments where records are likely to still be on paper, not digitized.

LEARNING FROM THE PAST

In 2000, Emanuel et al. published a seminal paper observing that unnecessary duplication of previous research is perversely unethical in international clinical research.[8] In 2009, Chalmers and Glasziou published a provocative paper claiming that 85% of all biomedical research effort is wasted.[9] Most recently, a 2014 *Lancet* five-part series on research practices outlined ways to increase value and reduce waste in biomedical research.[10] Many of these recommendations are relevant to global health research, too. As educators, we wondered how to impart the message to increase value and reduce waste to our global health trainees. We know that too much global health research ends up as gray literature locked away in dusty filing cabinets.

If people working on sexual and reproductive health and rights can learn from archival materials recording what has been done in the past, they should be able to avoid, as it were, "reinventing the wheel," while applying lessons on what works and identifying gaps in coverage. The gray literature can help identify how issues such as HIV and AIDS, gender, sexual orientation, and reproductive rights have been tackled through behavior communication, education, training, activism, and, importantly, from the perspective of those who are directly affected and involved in the issues. Insights gained in this respect can lead to reuse and updating of successful approaches and further inform new approaches to ensure that health issues are tackled not only in a technically appropriate way but also with attention to the needs and desires of the human beings affected.

The Humument Technique Adapted to Global Health Humanities Learning

Swain's workshop takes as a starting point Tom Phillips's famous art book *A Humument*, a lifelong project now in its sixth and final edition.[11] Phillips collaged, painted, and deconstructed each page of a long-discarded Victorian novel to create a new text. He spent his creative life crafting something lively, poignant, political, and at times rude and funny, out of W. H. Mallock's dry, snobbish, anti-Semitic Victorian-era novel. This work, Phillips admits, "had its germ in idle play." He describes that he and a friend were "prowling a warehouse" in South London in 1966, looking for bargains: "Arriving at the racks of dusty books left over from house clearances, I boasted that the first one I found that cost threepence, I would make serve a serious long-term project." The next book he picked up happened to be one with a yellow cover, called *A Human Document*, by Victorian novelist W. H. Mallock. It cost threepence, so that book was to be Phillips's fated project. *A Human Document* became the go-to text for most of Phillips's multimedia art for fifty years, and its main creation has been *A Humument,* which Phillips calls "a treated Victorian novel."

"Treating" a text, in this case, means making artwork on every single page of the book, effacing most of the text, and, in a "word-search" style, leaving words, phrases, and letters on the page which flow together to create an entirely new story. Phillips usually treats the text by painting, but he has also used collage, cutting, folding, and even burning the pages in order to transform the text. He takes the technique from William Burroughs, who was inspired by the artist Brion Gysin. Burroughs began to experiment with the cut-up technique, where random lines of text were cut from a page and rearranged to form new sentences, with the intention of freeing readers' minds from conventional, linear modes of thought. The very title of Phillips's book emerged from folding the cover and turning *A Human Document* into *A Humument*, which Phillips says he liked for sounding "earthy" and "effortful." The artist acknowledges Mallock's book as his "resource of greatest use—and all thanks to a man who, from photographs and contemporary accounts of his personality, would seem to be someone I would not at all have enjoyed meeting." Mallock, writes Phillips, was an anti-socialist snob: "His snobbery pervades *A Human Document* and his attitude towards Jews (though not untypical at the time) supplies the crux of its love story. These negative aspects of his literary persona," writes Phillips, "assisted rather than impeded my scheme." What began as "idle play" became a half a century of work, creating something funny, and increasingly hopeful, out of an unpleasant text.

After students choose their original texts from their time browsing the archive, they scan the original documents and print copies to make facsimiles for their projects. Then, using the Humument technique, they each "treat" a page with color media, markers, crochet, glitter, stickers, ephemera, and other materials and methods. Upon completing their final pieces, they are assigned to write essays ("Final Reflections") in the form of a third-person review about the artwork. Students are prompted to reflect on why the artist (themselves) had chosen the original document and how the artwork, with its final word choices, transformed the meaning of the original document or helped them (and the viewers) gain fresh insights. These mock reviews were essential in requiring students to articulate how and why they had "translated" their selected archival document into artwork and the merits of the translation. It was important to require students to return to the original archival text and see it in a new way after giving it a hands-on transformation.

The completed student artworks were framed and displayed in a public, high-footfall exhibition space called the Student Wall, located within Perkins Library at Duke University, for a two-month period. In addition, three students presented their pieces during a World AIDS Day event at Duke University Library, which was open to the general public. One-minute video excerpts of the student oral presentations can be accessed on YouTube.[12] These were preceded by introductions by Ingold, de Bruyn, Stewart, and Swain, as well as reflections by a North Carolinian woman living with HIV, Alicia Diggs. Videos of these presentations are available on the Health Humanities Lab Facebook site. More information about the event can also be found online.[13]

Student Learning

Various aspects of the HIV and AIDS epidemic, as well as issues such as violence against women, were represented in the archival materials chosen by the students for this assignment. Materials included first-person narratives by persons living with HIV, policy position papers, project and program reports, and song texts. Students further selected items focused on different groups affected by the epidemic (children and youth, women, LGBTQ+ individuals, musicians), as well as various challenges faced by those groups (loss of innocence, rape, women's inequality, stigma, powerlessness and regaining power, taking medications). A common theme in the student artwork was transforming negative narratives focused on challenges associated with HIV, violence, and stigma into messages of hope and increased agency on the part of persons directly affected. The following two examples, taken from student essays and shown in Figures 18.1 and 18.2, illustrate this approach.[14]

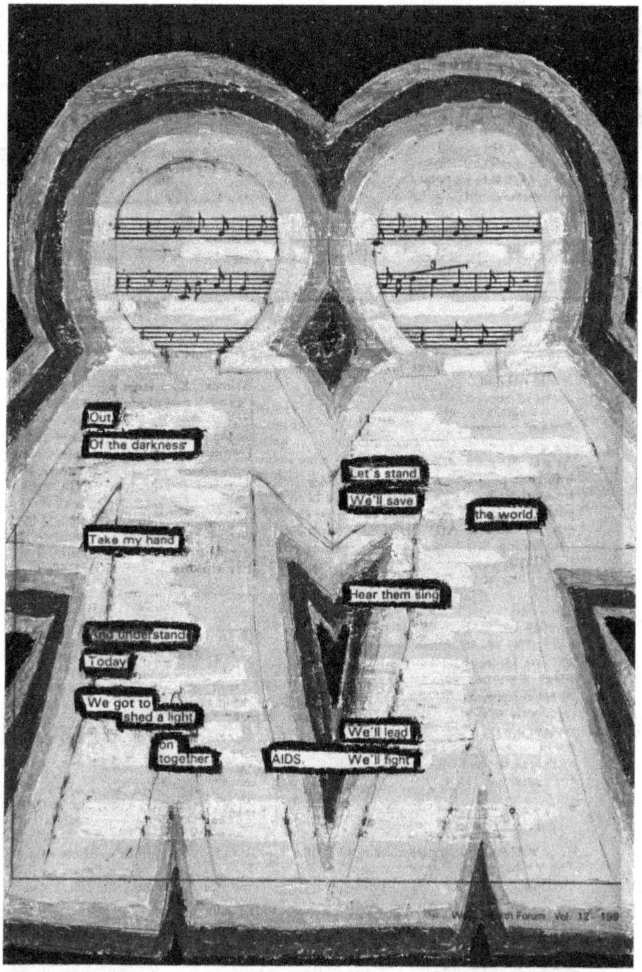

FIGURE 18.1 Brooke Whitfield, "Out of the Darkness, Into the Future." GLHTH 302 Global Narratives of HIV and AIDS. December 10, 2016. Used with permission.

"The original archival selection for this essay was a song written and composed by Ugandan artist Philly Lutaaya, upon learning that he was dying of AIDS. Brooke Whitfield,[15] *the artist of this Humument piece, said she was drawn to the original piece because of the "raw emotion" the song displayed and "the way in which it shows the pull of two apparent forces: one being the fear the singer is experiencing in his journey with AIDS and the other being the responsibility the singer feels towards the future generations to come." She continues in her essay by claiming that the piece "enabled her to mould a song that sang of despair, into one that reflected hope and strength. Not just the strength to face an HIV and AIDS diagnosis, but also the strength to fight it for the generations to come." Whitfield continues, "the words that [the] art piece chooses to highlight place the reader in*

an onward march towards HIV and AIDS solidarity, juxtaposing the original title Alone." To contrast some of the original work's lines, such as 'Out there somewhere/Alone and frightened' or 'No more loving arms/Thrown around my neck,' Whitfield transformed the lyrics to 'Out of the darkness let's stand/We'll save the world, take my hand' and 'We'll lead on together/AIDS we'll fight.' Whitfield explains this approach "not only places the original piece, Alone, at odds with her work through the transformation of lyrics, but also through the design of her art piece." Furthermore, she writes, "the title of her piece, Let's Stand, through this contraction, implies plurality, directly contrasting with the title Alone." The primary effect, Whitfield notes, "appears to counter the idea of being alone through choosing to depict two figures in the artwork."

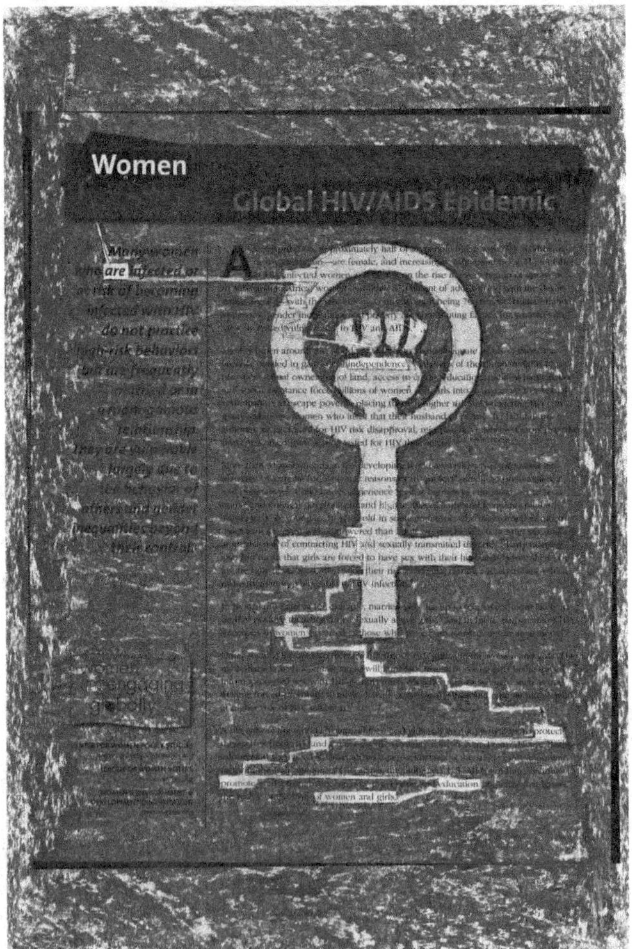

FIGURE 18.2 Simone Serat, "Recontextualizing Rights: Using Humumentism to Change the Rhetoric around Women's Reproductive Rights." GLHTH 302 Global Narratives of HIV and AIDS. December 12, 2016. Used with permission.

In another essay, Simone Serat[16] writes of her own Humument piece, "*The underlying text discusses facts women (especially women in the developing world) have come to know so well: females are more likely to be infected with HIV and AIDS because of biology, society, and culture. . . . The tone of the piece conveys that women have little say in protecting themselves from contracting HIV. Given this narrative, the sponsors for the factsheet are surprising: three organizations that focus on empowering women. . . . Serat's work seeks to alter this narrative, as a woman who has directly worked to empower women in protecting themselves from HIV, as well as the daughter of a midwife. 'Women . . . are . . . infected . . . with . . . independence,' the piece reads, the fist in the middle of the female symbol clenching the word 'independence' for dear life. 'we . . . women . . . will . . . protect . . . and . . . promote . . . education of women and girls.' Inspired by her time working with Kenyan women in an HIV clinic this summer, Serat uses bold, contrasting colours and a simple design to get her point across without mincing words.*"

Other students reflected on how the evolution of global health approaches can be seen through both successes and failures:

- One artist [name kept confidential at student's request] "*has chosen to focus her piece not on the fact of HIV and AIDS itself, but to indirectly comment on how the field of global health has grown with, and because of, the epidemic.*"[17]
- Using a booklet published by Amnesty International detailing human rights abuses faced by women in South Africa, *Joshua Grubbs, a "chemist by training," chooses to focus on antiretroviral drugs so that "out of the chronicles of suffering emerges a prophetic message of salvation through modern medicine"* (Figure 18.3).[18]
- "*Through a satirical presentation of censorship on the AIDS programme comic, Wei Xuan Lai invites viewers to take on a new lens when reading scientific journals. Are these journals truly illuminating key issues which the global community needs to focus on in combating the HIV and AIDS epidemic, or could they be unknowingly obscuring angles which have yet to be discovered?*"[19]
- "*Although HIV and AIDS stigma has deep roots today, Ellie Pasquale suggests there is a future, however distant, where it only exists as a forgotten past. . . . [I]t is the hope that through exposure, education, and narrative, tomorrow's Duke students will no longer shy away from someone who has HIV*" (Figure 18.4).[20]
- "*In examining a policy recommendation explaining how it can be useful for the media to 'give a face to HIV and AIDS' by encouraging HIV-positive individuals to share their stories for HIV and AIDS prevention and education campaigns, Sarah Beaverson transforms the meaning of the original and presents a poem that highlights the dangers*

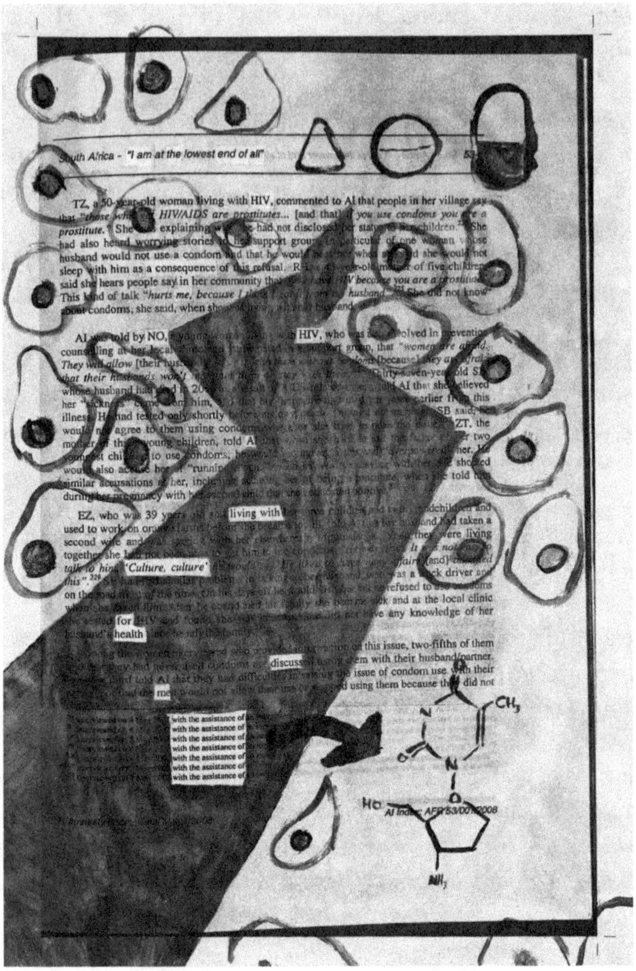

FIGURE 18.3 Joshua Grubbs, "Thus Spoke AZT." GLHTH 302 Global Narratives of HIV and AIDS. December 2016. Used with permission.

> *HIV-positive individuals face when society exploits their individual stories. . . . Their individuality is lost as they become a voice to speak on behalf of their community, country or race*" (Figure 18.5).[21]

Lessons Learned and Future Plans

The agencies funding global health-related research and interventions often want practitioners to develop entirely new and "innovative" materials for each new project and program. However, taking into consideration the critiques of "wasted research and resources" and an ever more evident need for us to learn from the past, we should avoid unnecessarily "reinventing the wheel" when a wealth of useful material can be updated to fit our current context.

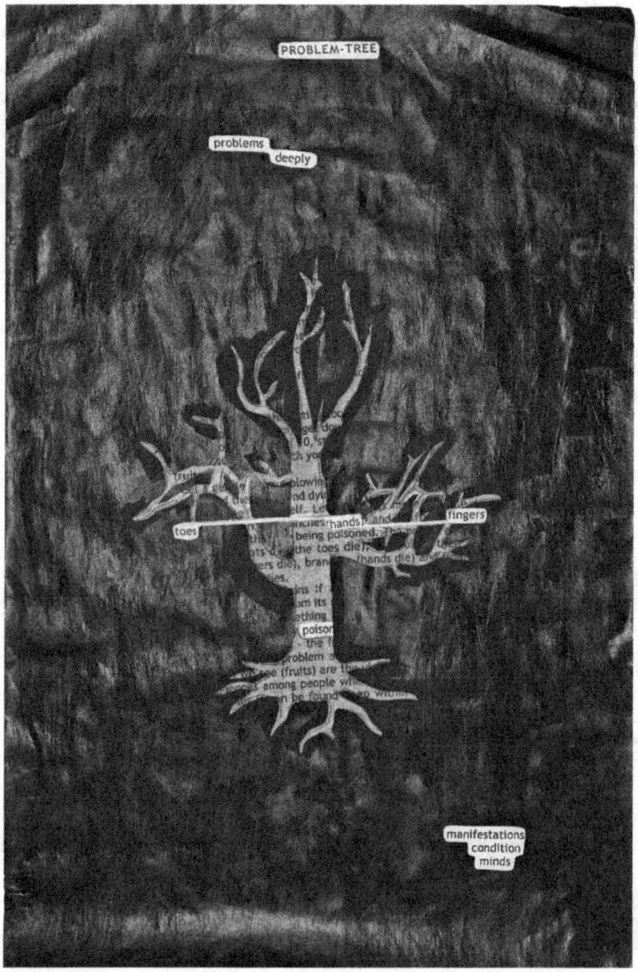

FIGURE 18.4 Ellie Pasquale, "The Problem with Stigma." GLHTH 302 Global Narratives of HIV/AIDS. December 2016. Used with permission.

As reflected in the student essays, the techniques used in the Humument workshop helped students become aware of the importance of archival material for the future of global health. They transformed relevant materials to explore the values that matter most to them by finding ways to express their analysis and thoughts visually and through the medium of concrete poetry. Rather than only "consume" text academically, the students investigated the language of the archival materials to find and reveal new logics and meanings. The artwork based on a pop song about AIDS in Uganda is evidence that different types of archival materials can be used in varied ways to help students engage with subject matter.

Other faculty have shown interest in the technique and the Maria de Bruyn papers as well. For example, Jules Odendahl-James, a member of the Duke

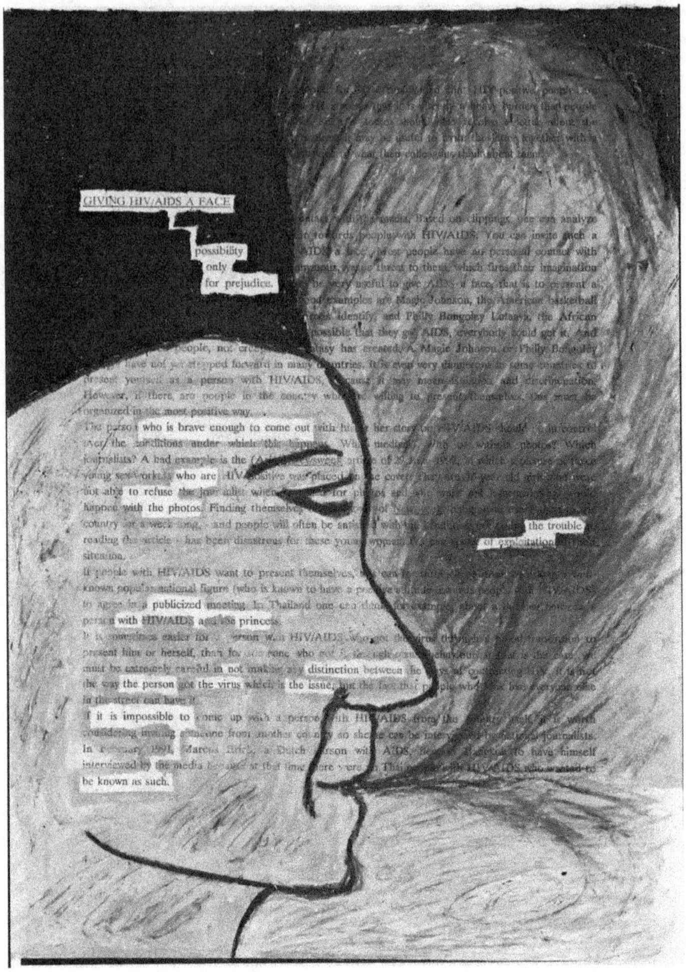

FIGURE 18.5 Sarah Beaverson, "Publicized with a Price." GLHTH 302 Global Narratives of HIV/AIDS. December 2016.

Theater Studies department, assigned students from her Medical Stories on Stage course to review materials with multimodal representations from the de Bruyn collection (activist ephemera, public health cartoons and booklets, educational reports and charts), as well as the Humument artworks displayed on the Duke Library Student Wall. She commented that it was particularly useful to show her students the transformation or adaptation of medical narratives from the educational, academic, and research context of the Maria de Bruyn papers (and their original creation/use prior to being archived) to this public, aesthetic, and activist engagement made possible by Kelley Swain's Humument workshop. She also commented that it enabled her students to know that other global health cross-listed courses use aesthetic, creative engagement with scientific and policy sources to highlight the human experience of health and illness. The visibility of the work made possible through humanistic lenses of analysis and creation gave them early license to see such an approach to analysis and research as rigorous and achievable even if they were newcomers to both subject matter and research method.

Since the Humument workshop will be offered for at least three years, student artwork and essays will be added successively to the Rubenstein Rare Book & Manuscript Library as a collection from Stewart's Global Narratives of HIV and AIDS seminar. Depositing student work from this course using the Maria de Bruyn collection is desirable for several reasons. The collaboration underlying the workshop has been one of many firsts:

- The first medical anthropological archive on sexual and reproductive health and rights with a special focus on HIV and AIDS in a global context for the History of Medicine Collections at Duke University
- The first use of the Humument technique in a US global health university setting
- The first event bringing together an archival curator, two medical anthropologists, a poet, an HIV activist a woman living with HIV (Alicia Diggs), and students to talk about their experiences and what is needed in addressing HIV and AIDS in the local and global contexts

Preserving the student work from this assignment and collaboration captures the essence of Duke University's mission of "knowledge in service to society." As noted, many of these students will continue to pursue careers in health professional fields. Giving them a broader context, a historical understanding, and a creative, nonlinear approach to experience using archival collections, all aid in their growth as scholars.

The Humument technique inspired us to develop this unique pedagogical exercise to immerse global health students in an archive of HIV and AIDS literature. We sought to increase student awareness of the ethical dimensions of value and waste in global health research by focusing on gray literature. Teaching global health trainees to use an archive of gray literature is an ethically and morally sound approach to improving the value of global health research in the future. We anticipate that these works will stimulate interest and debate and, ultimately, demonstrate the possibilities for fresh perspectives in global health to emerge from the creative animation of archival HIV and AIDS material.

As global health humanities at Duke University moves forward, we will engage additional critical issues, for example, the role of empathy in training global healthcare professionals (notably a recurring element in the student essays) and the urgency of establishing archival materials as a key resource for teaching and research in global health.

PEDAGOGY EXERCISE SECTION

The Humument and the Maria de Bruyn HIV and AIDS Archives

CLASS HANDOUT[22]

Resources: The Humument Technique

Tom Phillips, *A Humument: A Treated Victorian Novel*, 6th ed. (London: Thames & Hudson, 2016). http://www.tomphillips.co.uk

Resources: About *A Humument*

Steve Xerri, 1988,
http://www.tomphillips.co.uk/humument/essays/item/5860-trick-or-treatment-by-steve-xerri

Adam Smyth, 2012,
https://www.lrb.co.uk/v34/n19/adam-smyth/double-act

James Kidd, 2012,
http://www.tomphillips.co.uk/humument/essays/item/5858-every-day-of-my-life-is-like-a-page-by-james-kidd

Daniel Maidman, 2016,
https://www.huffingtonpost.com/daniel-maidman/rivers-in-the-sea-tom-phi_b_7941796.html

Resources: Influences on Tom Phillips's Humument Technique

Brion Gysin and William S. Burroughs, cut-up technique, 6:33 clip from a documentary on Burroughs,
https://www.youtube.com/watch?v=6NU3dIdqIBw

John Cage, 4:33,
https:// www.youtube.com/ watch?v=JTEFKFiXSx4

STEP 1

Identify an archive or a collection of materials that can provide the original, primary documents for the Humument exercise. If not already catalogued, develop a brief overview or guide of the items to help orient the students to the materials.

STEP 2

Prepare and deliver a lecture on Phillips's work, his influences (William S. Burroughs, John Cage, Samuel Beckett), and the techniques (cut-ups, concrete poetry, collage). Prepare and deliver a lecture on the archives and the basics of archival research and handling.

STEP 3

Select one item from the archive to use in a demonstration exercise. Scan and enlarge to 11 × 17. Supply crayons, colored pencils, markers, glitter, etc. Allow students to gain hands-on, in-class experience with the Humument technique using the instructor's preselected item. Ideally, have students "treat" the same text three or four times, encouraging them to make something different each time. This encourages nonlinear, creative thinking and motivates them to look at the text in a challenging and unfamiliar way.

STEP 4

Students then spend time on their own browsing in the archive. Encourage a random and exploratory approach. They choose one item from the archive for their Humument exercise. Students can use a cell phone or a scanner to make a reproduction of the item, subject to archival restrictions. Instruct them to make several 11 × 17 photocopies to have on hand for working on several drafts to achieve their final Humument piece.

STEP 5

Students bring in a first draft of their Humument project. This class session will include critique, editorial suggestions, and discussion of student first drafts. Their ability to articulate their choices in the artwork is as challenging and important as the artwork itself.

STEP 6

Students bring in the final version of their Humument project and discuss their intellectual and artistic process. As a class, they also discuss together how to organize their work for an actual, or in-class, show: for example, do they arrange these Humument pieces by themes, colors, content, etc.? Have students lay out their projects on the floor or on tables to see the overall effect. Hanging on the wall or organizing a show on campus is preferred.

STEP 7

In the third person, students write a review of their intellectual and artistic process, their global health goals, and assessment of the successes and shortcomings of the piece. Instruct them to follow a particular essay style, for example, review essays in *The Lancet Oncology* "CnS" (Cancer and Society) or *The Lancet* weekly's "Perspectives" section. The review style once again displaces students from the linear style of narrative and forces them into a different perspective.

For good examples, take a look at Swain's reviews, https://kelleyswain.wordpress.com/about/freelance/.

Criteria for writing a review-style essay:

1. No fewer than 700 words and no more than 800 words.
2. Written in the third person—you are critiquing your own piece of art as if you are reviewing it.
3. Include a quote/reference from Tom Phillips, *A Humument,* or a related review/interview such as those assigned in class or here: http://www.tomphillips.co.uk/humument/essays.
4. Include the proper citation. This will indicate the archives, box number, etc., from which you selected the original document you have "treated" and any citations of quotes.
5. Essay Prompt: Briefly describe the original document, then reflect on why the artist (you) has chosen it, and how "treating" the text transforms its meaning. Reconsider the original text. Does the artwork provide fresh insight into the original? How? Your essay should have a tight narrative arc.

STEP 8

Organize a public show. If not possible, organize a class showing: select a few students to read all or part of their essay while displaying their Humument piece enlarged on a projector screen.

Notes

1. The literature on this issue is extensive. For a recent evidence-based research paper, see Aileen Patterson et al., "Medical Humanities: A Closer Look at Learning," *BMJ Medical Humanities* 42, no. 2 (2016): 115–20.

2. Tom Phillips, *A Humument. A Treated Victorian Novel*, 6th ed. (London: Thames and Hudson, 2016).

3. Rubenstein Library, "Guide to the Maria de Bruyn Papers, 1988–2012 and Undated," Duke University Libraries, Durham, NC, 2015, https://library.duke.edu/rubenstein/findingaids/debruynmaria/.

4. Kearsley A. Stewart and Kelley S. Swain, "Global Health Humanities: Defining an Emerging Field," *Lancet* 388 (2016): 2586–87.

5. Gray literature is defined as "manifold document types produced on all levels of government, academics, business and industry in print and electronic formats that are protected by intellectual property rights, of sufficient quality to be collected and preserved by libraries and institutional repositories, but not controlled by commercial publishers; i.e. where publishing is not the primary activity of the producing body." Joachim Schöpfel, "Towards a Prague Definition of Grey Literature," paper presented at the Twelfth International Conference on Grey Literature: Transparency in Grey Literature. Grey Tech Approaches to High Tech Issues, Prague, Czech Republic, December 6–7, 2010, 11–26.

6. UNAIDS and organizations of people living with HIV and AIDS advise against the use of the term *HIV/AIDS*: "The expression HIV/AIDS should be avoided whenever possible because it can cause confusion. Most people with HIV do not have AIDS. The expression HIV/AIDS prevention is even more unacceptable because HIV prevention entails correct and consistent condom use, use of sterile injecting equipment, changes in social norms and so on, whereas AIDS prevention entails antiretroviral therapy, cotrimoxazole, good nutrition, isoniazid prophylaxis (INH), etc." UNAIDS, *UNAIDS Terminology Guidelines* (Geneva: UNAIDS, 2015).

7. Todd Samuelson and Cait Coker, "Mind the Gap: Integrating Special Collections Teaching," *Portal: Libraries and the Academy* 14, no. 1 (2014): 51–66. Melissa A. Hubbard and Megan Lotts, "Special Collections, Primary Resources, and Information Literacy Pedagogy," *Communications in Information Literacy* 7, no. 1 (2013): 24–38.

8. Ezekiel J. Emanuel, David Wendler, and Christine Grady, "What Makes Clinical Research Ethical?" *Journal of the American Medical Association* 283, no. 20 (2010): 2701–11.

9. Iain Chalmers and Paul Glasziou, "Avoidable Waste in the Production and Reporting of Research Evidence," *Obstetrics and Gynecology* 114, no. 6 (2009): 1341–45.

10. *Lancet*, "Research: Increasing Value, Reducing Waste," January 8, 2014, https://www.thelancet.com/series/research.

11. Marvin Sackner, "'Humumentism': The Works and Ideas of Tom Phillips," http://www.tomphillips.co.uk/humument/essays/item/5867-humumentism-the-works-and-ideas-of-tom-phillips-by-marvin-sackner.

12. Ryan Fitzgerald, https://www.youtube.com/watch?v=P9rLZ4KXFbo; Sarah Rapaport, https://www.youtube.com/watch?v=8zs-boBqh_c; Edom Tilahun, https://www.youtube.com/watch?v=QLx58OoKW7I&feature=youtu.be.

13. Susan Gallagher, "Combined with Art and Poetry, Historical HIV Papers Lend Fresh Perspective," *Duke Global Health Institute Newsletter*, November 22, 2016,

https://globalhealth.duke.edu/media/news/combined-art-and-poetry-historical-hiv-papers-lend-fresh-perspective.

14. Full-color reproductions of student Humument artwork cited here are available on: https://sites.duke.edu/glhlth302.

15. Brooke Whitfield, "Out of the Darkness, Into the Future," paper prepared for the course GLHTH 302 Global Narratives of HIV and AIDS, Duke University, Durham, NC, December 10, 2016. https://sites.duke.edu/glhlth302.

16. Simone Serat, "Recontextualizing Rights: Using Humumentism to Change the Rhetoric around Women's Reproductive Rights," paper prepared for the course GLHTH 302 Global Narratives of HIV and AIDS, Duke University, Durham, NC, December 12, 2016. https://sites.duke.edu/glhlth302.

17. Anonymous student, "The Development of Global Health," paper prepared for the course GLHTH 302 Global Narratives of HIV and AIDS, Duke University, Durham, NC, December 2016. https://sites.duke.edu/glhlth302.

18. Joshua Grubbs, "Thus Spoke AZT," paper prepared for the course GLHTH 302 Global Narratives of HIV and AIDS, Duke University, Durham, NC, December 2016. https://sites.duke.edu/glhlth302.

19. Wei Xuan Lai, "Silence Ill Address the Issue: Unnecessary Censorship in HIV/AIDS," paper prepared for the course GLHTH 302 Global Narratives of HIV and AIDS, Duke University, Durham, NC, December 12, 2016. https://sites.duke.edu/glhlth302.

20. Ellie Pasquale, "The Problem with Stigma," paper prepared for the course GLHTH 302 Global Narratives of HIV and AIDS, Duke University, Durham, NC, December 9, 2016. https://sites.duke.edu/glhlth302.

21. Sarah Beaverson, "Publicized with a Price," paper prepared for the course GLHTH 302 Global Narratives of HIV and AIDS, Duke University, Durham, NC, December 11, 2016. https://sites.duke.edu/glhlth302.

22. If you try this exercise, we are eager to hear from you. We are also happy to offer advice or guidance on the technique. Please contact Kearsley Stewart, k.stewart@duke.edu.

Works Cited

Anonymous student. "The Development of Global Health." Paper prepared for the course GLHTH 302 Global Narratives of HIV and AIDS. Duke University, Durham, NC, December 2016. https://sites.duke.edu/glhlth302.

Beaverson, Sarah. "Publicized with a Price." Paper prepared for the course GLHTH 302 Global Narratives of HIV and AIDS, Duke University, Durham, NC. December 11, 2016. https://sites.duke.edu/glhlth302.

Chalmers, Iain, and Paul Glasziou. "Avoidable Waste in the Production and Reporting of Research Evidence." *Obstetrics and Gynecology* 114, no. 6 (2009): 1341–45.

Emanuel, Ezekiel J., David Wendler, and Christine Grady. "What Makes Clinical Research Ethical?" *Journal of the American Medical Association* 283, no. 20 (2010): 2701–11.

Gallagher, Susan. "Combined with Art and Poetry, Historical HIV Papers Lend Fresh Perspective." *Duke Global Health Institute Newsletter*, November 22, 2016. https://globalhealth.duke.edu/media/news/combined-art-and-poetry-historical-hiv-papers-lend-fresh-perspective.

Grubbs, Joshua. "Thus Spoke AZT." Paper prepared for the course GLHTH 302 Global Narratives of HIV and AIDS. Duke University, Durham, NC. December 2016. https://sites.duke.edu/glhlth302.

Hubbard, Melissa A., and Megan Lotts. "Special Collections, Primary Resources, and Information Literacy Pedagogy." *Communications in Information Literacy* 7, no. 1 (2013): 24–38.

Lai, Wei Xuan. "Silence Ill Address the Issue: Unnecessary Censorship in HIV/AIDS." Paper prepared for the course GLHTH 302 Global Narratives of HIV and AIDS. Duke University, Durham, NC. December 12, 2016. https://sites.duke.edu/glhlth302.

Lancet. "Research: Increasing Value, Reducing Waste." January 8, 2014. http://www.thelancet.com/series/research.

Pasquale, Ellie. "The Problem with Stigma." Paper prepared for the course GLHTH 302 Global Narratives of HIV and AIDS. Duke University, Durham, NC. December 9, 2016. https://sites.duke.edu/glhlth302.

Patterson, Aileen, Danika Burke Sharek, Martina Hennessy, Matthew D. Phillips, and Susie Schofield. "Medical Humanities: A Closer Look at Learning." *BMJ Medical Humanities* 42, no. 2 (2016): 115–20.

Phillips, Tom. *A Humument. A Treated Victorian Novel*, 6th ed. London: Thames and Hudson, 2016.

Rubenstein Library. "Guide to the Maria de Bruyn Papers, 1988–2012 and Undated." Duke University Libraries, Durham, NC, 2015. http://library.duke.edu/rubenstein/findingaids/debruynmaria/.

Sackner, Marvin. "'Humumentism': The Works and Ideas of Tom Phillips." http://www.tomphillips.co.uk/humument/essays/item/5867-humumentism-the-works-and-ideas-of-tom-phillips-by-marvin-sackner.

Samuelson, Todd, and Cait Coker. "Mind the Gap: Integrating Special Collections Teaching." *Portal: Libraries and the Academy* 14, no. 1 (2014): 51–66.

Schöpfel, Joachim. "Towards a Prague Definition of Grey Literature." Paper presented at the Twelfth International Conference on Grey Literature: Transparency in Grey Literature. Grey Tech Approaches to High Tech Issues. Prague, Czech Republic, December 6–7, 2010, 11–26.

Serat, Simone. "Recontextualizing Rights: Using Humumentism to Change the Rhetoric around Women's Reproductive Rights." Paper prepared for the course GLHTH 302 Global Narratives of HIV and AIDS. Duke University, Durham, NC. December 12, 2016. https://sites.duke.edu/glhlth302.

Stewart, Kearsley A., and Kelley S. Swain. "Global Health Humanities: Defining an Emerging Field." *Lancet* 388 (2016): 2586–87.

UNAIDS. *UNAIDS Terminology Guidelines*. Geneva, Switzerland: UNAIDS, 2015.

Whitfield, Brooke. "Out of the Darkness, Into the Future." Paper prepared for the course GLHTH 302 Global Narratives of HIV and AIDS. Duke University, Durham, NC. December 10, 2016. https://sites.duke.edu/glhlth302.

19

Music, Music Therapy, Disability Studies, Bioethics, and Health Humanities

Alex Lubet

Introduction

I teach two courses offered jointly through the University of Minnesota's Center for Bioethics and School of Music, the latter my tenure home. Disability Ethics originated in bioethics and is cross-listed in music only because I am its instructor (although music occasionally appears in the course's media section). Music, Disability, and Society originated in my own department. It contemplates music from a variety of disability studies, health humanities, bioethics, medical, and engineering perspectives. That both course offerings can be justified within my teaching load within a music unit owes to their substantial enrollments, largely comprised of music therapy (MT) graduate students, for whom it is strongly recommended. While Disability Ethics attracts a diverse student body, mostly from health and science fields (including MT), Music, Disability, and Society is overwhelmingly taken by MT students and other music majors but few others, although the course carries no music prerequisites and requires no technical musical skills.

This essay begins with brief introductions to MT, to my professional and personal background, and to disability studies. It proceeds to descriptions of the abovementioned courses. Discussion of the intersection of MT in particular and music in general with health humanities and bioethics follows.

Music Therapy

Despite significant achievements, a sizeable research literature, and a record of continuous professional association since 1950, MT remains relatively unfamiliar to fellow health professionals and the general public. "What is Music Therapy?" from the American Music Therapy's Association's website thus bears quoting in toto:

> Music Therapy is the clinical and evidence-based use of music interventions to accomplish individualized goals within a therapeutic relationship by a credentialed professional who has completed an approved music therapy program.
>
> Music Therapy is an established health profession in which music is used within a therapeutic relationship to address physical, emotional, cognitive, and social needs of individuals. After assessing the strengths and needs of each client, the qualified music therapist provides the indicated treatment including creating, singing, moving to, and/or listening to music. Through musical involvement in the therapeutic context, clients' abilities are strengthened and transferred to other areas of their lives. Music therapy also provides avenues for communication that can be helpful to those who find it difficult to express themselves in words. Research in music therapy supports its effectiveness in many areas such as: overall physical rehabilitation and facilitating movement, increasing people's motivation to become engaged in their treatment, providing emotional support for clients and their families, and providing an outlet for expression of feelings.[1]

The University of Minnesota has had a highly regarded MT program for over forty years. My courses enroll mostly MT graduate students, most with bachelor's degrees in other music fields, seeking MT licensure and an M.A. degree. Students demonstrate their research competence with a thesis, always an experimental study.

The Instructor

My training is not in MT but music composition, a field without an overt relationship to health fields. I came to health humanities/bioethics through disability studies (DS). My interest in DS arose from my experience as a patient across numerous medical specialties, with conditions that have affected my ability to compose, perform, teach, and research, including performance-induced and -exacerbated injuries.

More than health challenges, though, it was return-to-work issues resulting from the first of two spinal neurosurgeries in 2000 that inspired my interest in DS. In particular, my engagement with health and disability law, policies, practices, and institutions, especially 3.5 years of workers' compensation litigation, convinced me that, at least for me, disability was a civil and human rights issue even more than a medical concern, a perspective enshrined in the "social model of disability," a theoretical foundation of DS. Since 2002, I have published in DS within and beyond my field, the first scholar of DS in music.[2]

Disability Studies

Mainstream DS posits an oppositional binary between the "social" and "medical models" of disability. The social model posits that "disability" is socially constructed, in contradistinction to embodied "impairment." DS defines as the social model's binary opposite the medical model of disability, characterized as defining disability as residing in pathologized individuals, whose challenges the medical and other service establishments (including, for example, education and social work) seek to address through individualized "cure." Notably, though, the late disability historian Paul Longmore saw the medical model—and thus the social versus medical binary—as an invention of DS itself.[3] Surely, the presence of quality-of-life concerns in bioethics demonstrates an acknowledgment that healthcare praxis concerns more than "cure." Still, much bioethics literature and praxis departs strongly from majority DS opinion.

I have never accepted the shunning of health science by DS scholars. From my earliest engagement with DS (and first publications), I have sought venues and collaborations within health fields and advocated for stronger relations. Among the greatest *pragmatic* potentials of DS is its role in professional training, including, but not limited to, health education. This has come to fruition in my own career, with an invitation to join the Faculty of the Center for Bioethics.

THE COURSES

Disability Ethics

This course was requested by the University of Minnesota Center for Bioethics, in response to a felt need for DS content. The course is offered semi-annually for three credits (the standard semester credit load) and meets once weekly for 2.5 hours. The enrollment was twelve, the highest among bioethics courses of its kind. In addition to six MT graduate students, six majors in bioethics, biology, health science communications, and genetic counseling enrolled.

Course Content

Disability Ethics includes three units: (1) Disability Studies, (2) Principles of Bioethics, and (3) Big Issues. In Disability Studies, students are introduced to that field's theoretical foundations, in particular the "social model" espoused by Simi Linton[4] (among others) and the newer "realist model" of the late Tobin Siebers,[5] which combines social and embodied concerns. Conversely, I assign readings by John Harris[6]that are critical of DS. In Disability Ethics, readings and media with sharply opposed opinions are presented, with as little of the instructor's viewpoint as possible, something I found challenging. Critiques of DS are, in my experience, rare in DS courses. This unit takes two weeks.

Principles of Bioethics employs the principlist approach of Beauchamp and Childress, whose textbook is required.[7] This unit requires five weeks, one per principle/chapter—(1) respect for autonomy, (2) beneficence, (3) non-maleficence, (4) justice, and (5) one week on the professional–patient relationship.

Beauchamp and Childress demonstrate that opposed conclusions can be reached when arguing cases on the basis of the four principles. Unlike DS's social and realist models of disability, principlism is less an ideology than a framework or method that permits, even encourages, ideological differences. The authors also describe an alternative to principlism in "casuistry," a method in which principles emerge from cases.

I am considering changing to a casuistical approach in this course. One attraction of having principles emerge from cases is an emphasis on the "bio" in bioethics, that is, proceeding to a significant degree from medical knowledge rather than philosophical concepts including, for example, religion, which are grounded in assumptions that are literally "leaps of faith."

Cases involving disability, including those at some remove from medicine, in, for example, education or housing, also benefit from casuistry. Similar to a process that proceeds from medical knowledge, a case-based approach to disability issues facilitates foregrounding specific impairments and accommodations, concerns that distinguish disability from other social justice issues and that might be shunted aside by social model arguments that emphasize disability as a unified minority group. It can also be difficult to distinguish between applicable principles, especially between beneficence and non-maleficence, and not always worth the trouble.

The final unit of Disability Ethics, presents three "Big Issues" in bioethics and DS: (1) physician-assisted death (suicide and euthanasia), (2) selective abortion, and (3) cochlear implants in children. The discussion of cochlear implants—and thus hearing—is particularly prescient for music therapists.[8] The readings for Big Issues (which are journal articles) present widely divergent perspectives, from DS scholars/disability rights advocates and often opposed, but arguably more mainstream, bioethical views of health professionals and policy advocates.

Class Session Structure

Disability Ethics is an ideal course for an active learning (as opposed to a lecture) approach. The course's most important learning outcome is the ability to apply principles of bioethics to healthcare and disability praxis, decisions which will, almost invariably, be made in discussions among colleagues, clients/patients, and other interested parties such as parents/guardians. Thus, the class functions as its own teaching team at nearly all times.

The class was divided into working groups of three students each. Each group was responsible for teaching part of the week's reading assignment. All students were expected to read the entire assignment, but since the reading was in a new and challenging field, one group's presentation of its particularly close reading of each portion was highly beneficial. Grounded in heretofore largely unfamiliar subjects and methods—DS and principlist bioethics—both more humanistic than students' own largely scientific majors, this approach proved quite effective.

Most class sessions also included cases for discussion and journal articles concerning the "big issues." Discussions were ultimately lively, though some students needed encouragement. The conversations of greatest intensity were, understandably, those concerning physician-assisted death, with emotions running highest—and almost universally against—the views of radical utilitarian bioethicist Peter Singer, a veritable anti-Christ in DS. By contrast, there was little sympathy for the deaf community's—and mainstream DS's—opposition to cochlear implants for children.

Each student also gave a brief weekly report, approximately three minutes, on a popular press or scholarly item of his or her own choosing concerning disability. (Popular press human interest items on disability are plentiful, especially in local news.) Media items were also posted on the (public) course Facebook page.

Finally, a portion of most class sessions was devoted to a (typically) longer, instructor-chosen media item and discussion thereof. Popular media play a significant role in framing public bioethical discussions. It is important for students to appreciate not only the subject positions of media makers but also strategies used to influence point of view, including filmic/visual effects and music, often despite a veneer of dispassion or objectivity. As a scholar of popular culture (music and beyond), this enabled me to instruct students in a particular area of expertise, mediated devices of persuasion. Not infrequently, the media I chose pertained to music, both my field of training and an activity whose intersection with disability is especially revealing.[9] Widely perceived as a talent—or "hyperability"—music-making is often juxtaposed with disability in popular media narratives as a recipe for potential tragedy that may or may not be "overcome."[10] I highly recommend using media in bioethics teaching. While I find music narratives very effective, instructors should foreground their own interests/expertise, not mine.

Among the longer films shown were (1) *The Blind Orchestra*,[11] about a blind women's symphony orchestra in Egypt, which raised issues about inclusive versus special education and cultural intersections of gender, religion, postcolonialism, modernism, and disability; (2) *Sound and Fury*,[12] about cochlear implants in children; and (3) *Dax's Case*,[13] about a burn victim's legal battle to obtain assistance in ending his life.

Each class session concluded with a brief preview of the next meeting, followed by office hours. Both the preview and office hours immediately after were well suited to course content that challenged students, regardless of their majors. Because students had such diverse majors—and thus came from across a huge campus—after-class office hours were a great convenience, even more for students with disability/mobility concerns.

Assignments

Disability Ethics included four types of assignments:

a) Presentations of weekly readings as described (pass–fail)
b) Weekly journals of 200–300 words, concerning any aspect of the students' prior week in disability: "readings, discussion, media, progress on your final project (see below), disability in your other studies/work/life, current events" (pass–fail)
c) Weekly media: an in-class report as described (pass–fail)
d) Final Project: completely open-ended, either individual or group (of any size). The only letter-graded activity (A–F). An informal proposal with at least a partial bibliography was due week eight, with presentations in the final three weeks of the semester. Two projects individual, with group projects including two to six students.

The preponderance of pass–fail activities, while initially appearing to heavily weight the final project as the only letter-graded assignment, was more balanced than at first seems, given the intense demands of completing three (pass–fail) assignments each week. Students also had the opportunity to have final projects reviewed at every phase of development, leaving no mystery regarding their final grade by the time of their end-of-term presentations. Letter grades have long struck me as an undesirable system of comparative human valuation, particularly inappropriate in a class on disabilities. Grades are unavoidable where I teach, but continuous engagement with students about their projects makes it possible for all who truly strive for excellence to achieve it in a relatively anxiety-free environment.

While the lack of a priori parameters for a final project should, I think, be exciting (it is typical that the student composers I teach have such wide latitude), at first such freedom is daunting for many students, whose other, largely science, courses are more fixed in their expectations. This anxiousness is eventually offset by the high level of readily available instructor assistance.

Music, Disability, and Society

While Music, Disability, and Society presents no skill barriers to enrollment by non-musicians, its enrollment has been overwhelmingly music majors, especially those in MT. The course is both largely tailored to MT's needs/interests and, by design, different from their MT coursework in its DS perspective and emphasis on qualitative methods. Like Disability Ethics, this is a three-credit course that meets once weekly for 2.5 hours, with office hours after.

Course Content

There are two units in this class. The first is Disability Studies, within and beyond music, based partly on my own research, in particular *Music, Disability, and Society*. Topics include social and realist models of disability, representations of disability and music in popular media, bioethics of music, adaptive music for people with mobility impairments, inclusive versus special education, and universal instructional design,[14] that is, inclusive pedagogy.

The second unit features guest presenters with a variety of viewpoints and expertise, in person and via Skype. Guests will surely vary from offering to the next of this course (which has heretofore been given twice), but to date they have included people with disabilities with expertise in disability accommodation and adaptation; engineers and other experts on adaptive technology, including new and modified musical instruments; scholars of sensory science, including speech and hearing (including cochlear implants and hearing aids), and vision (including Braille music notation); performing arts medicine physicians; music therapists with research agendas beyond the MT core curriculum; and medical librarians.

Class Session Structure

This is a more traditional course than Disability Ethics. While there is much discussion, my own teaching and that of guest presenters is largely lecture and demonstration. My presentations often include popular media, both fiction and documentary, principally concerning musicians with disabilities. (I have also taught a course just on this topic.) One session combines the film *Amadeus*[15] with speculative medical histories of Mozart's health, disability status, and cause of death.[16] Students have rarely thought of Mozart or Tom Hulce's film portrayal (or F. Murray Abraham's portrayal of the composer's rival Salieri) in terms of disability prior to this course. This session can thus be revelatory, particularly concerning the theory that Mozart had Tourette's syndrome.[17]

Assignments

This course utilizes project-based learning,[18] strongly compatible with the universal instructional design principles taught in the DS unit. There are three projects, which can be done (and turned in) in any order, but with set due dates for proposals and finished assignments (that is, on each due date, any proposal or project may be turned in):

a) Implementation Plan: a course the student has taken/taught/would like to teach is transformed according to the principles of universal instructional design.[19]
b) Field Journal: a narrative of the student's engagement with the disability community. MT students typically report on their practicums, a core element of the MT curriculum. The journal is

qualitative and personal and thus does not duplicate the (mostly) quantitative data kept for practicum assignments in the MT major. Non-MTs typically conduct fieldwork at a 7–12 charter school in St. Paul with a high (25%–33%) enrollment of students with "invisible" disabilities,[20] where I volunteer.

c) Research Project: as in Disability Ethics, this is open-ended but must be done individually. Typically, MT students create literature reviews on topics of interest that will serve as preparation for their theses. Non-MTs tend toward musicological projects, focusing on well-known musicians with disabilities. Students are typically more relaxed about the open-endedness of this project than in Disability Ethics because of greater familiarity with the subject matter and, in the case of MTs, extensive prior exposure to research in their specialty.

Music and Music Therapy as/in Bioethics and Health Humanities

Music and MT can make unique contributions to bioethics and health humanities. Although there are now degrees and certificates in bioethics, bioethics faculty themselves come from nearly thirty disciplines,[21] rather than typically from bioethics programs. Music is a recent addition that will benefit both musicians and others exposed to music from this new perspective.

As a visiting scholar of medical humanities at the University of Texas–Medical Branch in 2003, I was struck by the diverse backgrounds of scholars with roles in life-and-death medical decisions and in shaping law and policy with life-and-death (and otherwise serious) ramifications. Despite a higher education almost entirely in music, I felt utterly capable of holding my own in any bioethical/health humanities discussion with colleagues, at times even able to offer fresh and needed insights, owing to my experiences as both patient and plaintiff and my DS expertise.

But the training of musicians in general and composers in particular also offers an interesting potential for health education. Unlike verbal text, aesthetic or expository, music is polyphonic (many simultaneous melodies and rhythms can be perceived as coherent) and polydimensional (each individual musical sound must be understood as having dimensions of frequency, duration, amplitude, timbre ["tone color"], and spatial location, often in addition to bearing linguistic information in the form of lyrics). My specialty, composition, especially, is taught Socratically. Students must be able to account for every one of the aforementioned musical dimensions in every note/combination of notes, often in extended works for many performers. Composition instruction is typically in private lessons, where the questions posed by an instructor can be many, rapid-fire, and challenging, technical, and aesthetic. Simply put, what I have described here is the same kind of rich, nuanced complexity required in every biomedical consideration, decisions that are simultaneously scientific and humanistic, sociocultural and philosophical, engaging extracorporeal questions of quality of life and just allocation of limited human and material resources. The need to balance science and quality-of-life concerns is strongly analogous to the technical versus aesthetic choices that challenge composers. Were it possible to export the sensibilities of musicians to health practitioners, it would be invaluable. Physician Paul Haidet offers useful suggestions for how health practitioners can benefit from understanding the work of great jazz improvisers.[22]

When I was in residence at the University of Texas–Medical Branch, the Institute for Medical Humanities had a small theater program (it has since closed). Since then, though, the field of "medical improvisation"[23] has emerged, utilizing the techniques of improvisational theater in medical education through workshops. Little, though, has been published about the potentials of musical improvisation and even less attempted. (A notable exception is ongoing work using the Adaptive Use Musical Instrument (AUMI).)[24] There is potential in medical education for sharing improvisational experiences that facilitate active and reactive listening. A leading role is played by the mostly Canadian International Institute for Critical Studies in Improvisation, whose ideas emanate from music and among whose "formal partnerships with over 30 community-based organizations [are] health centres."[25]

Majoring in music can be good preparation for health professionals, something I have observed in music students who become physicians, including two of my own doctors. There are also more direct benefits to including music topics in health education, as in the media unit in Disability Ethics. The aforementioned juxtaposition of "hyperability" and disability in the service of potential tragedy appears in many films about music, including *Amadeus*.[26] It has great value in enlightening health communities about perceptions of disability in the public consciousness. Documentaries,[27] memoirs,[28] and essays[29] are all highly informative, sometimes even in their lack of emphasis on an artist's disability.

Bioethics across Health and Music Curriculums

MTs benefit from health humanities/bioethics curricula, not only for course content but for their interaction with colleagues in allied fields. In its premiere offering, Disability Ethics enrolled students with backgrounds in genetic counseling, biology, technical communication, bioethics, law, and medicine. Of course, students in all of these allied professions benefit from interacting.

The implications of the inclusion of students (and faculty) of health/clinical practices such as MT—non-invasive, non-prescribing, typically low-risk—in bioethics are significant. For example, Beauchamp and Childress's *Principles of Biomedical Ethics* references physicians and nurses by and large (though they do discuss research scientists as well as perspectives from public health professionals). In any case, other health professionals, including dentists; psychotherapists; physical, occupational, speech, and arts therapists; dieticians; audiologists; optometrists and opticians; genetic counselors; and cosmetic surgery aestheticians, also face ethical choices and would benefit from bioethics and DS.

Recent studies show that the majority of health facilities in the United States are not compliant with the Americans with Disabilities Act.[30] And an ethical issue common among MTs, according to my students, is that parents of young clients often offer to purchase additional MT services beyond those specified in their treatment regimen. Though potentially beneficial to clients and practitioners alike, these are in violation of the regulations and ethics of the field. Health and disability ethics questions extend beyond such "big" issues as life and death, grave illness, unbearable pain, significant impairment, and major surgery and are needed in the training of all health practitioners.

Further, among musicians, MTs are only the most obviously in need of bioethics training. Any music teacher or musician who assigns repertoire and/or directs rehearsals and performances is prescribing mind/body work intended to build facility and technique in a manner analogous to physical, occupational, and other therapies. Once, a major symphony orchestra was at odds with its new music director for his having programmed several works of a prominent "minimalist" composer throughout their performance season, music that included extended passages of injury-provoking pattern repetition. The following season, after protests by the musicians, the orchestra's programming was less unreasonably taxing, a bioethical lesson that would better have been learned during the maestro's training.

Conclusions

MTs in particular, but also musicians in general, can benefit from curricula in health humanities, bioethics, and DS. Music studies can also enrich the education of health professionals and students of DS. My teaching of two very different health humanities/bioethics/DS courses—one musical, the other ethical—demonstrate both of these benefits. Music, Disability, and Society offers an immersion in DS as well as disability applications in technology and medicine from a uniquely valuable musical outlook. Disability Ethics offers a perspective that is rare in health/medical education programs, one that benefits students in health-related professional programs across the curriculum, of which MT is an exemplar but hardly unique. While there are a handful of disability ethics taught from a variety of perspectives in universities worldwide, my own inspiration was musical, derived from a work-related injury and subsequent battles with law and policy as related to the idiosyncrasies of my profession.

Anyone contemplating developing either course should adopt a mixed perspective that combines the standpoints of DS and the health professions. Students need every opportunity to form and share their own opinions. In both courses, but especially Disability Ethics, time was allotted for informal discussion, with special encouragement for students to engage with those in other majors.

PEDAGOGY EXERCISE SECTION

Disability Ethics: A Weekly Session

A TYPICAL WEEK'S ACTIVITIES

Disability Ethics meets once weekly for 2.5 hours (including a mid-class break of five to ten minutes). While the first week is, of necessity, instructor-led and the closing weeks (the number determined by enrollment) are devoted to presentations of the students' final research projects, the interim weeks all follow a similar sequence of highly varied activities, with an emphasis on "active," that is, student-led, work:

1. **Unrestricted discussion (fifteen minutes):** The class begins with students and the instructor mingling and conversing freely on any topic. Even without preordained structure, conversations revolve around topics pertinent to the course, typically as they relate to the students' majors. The course meets in the evening, and easing into the material of the course semi-socially is an effective preparation for more focused activities. One of the attractions of the course is the wide variety of student majors, and free discussion is a good forum for interdisciplinary sharing.
2. **Student media presentations (five minutes per student):** Every student is expected to give a short presentation on a reading or otherwise mediated publication. These may come either from the previous week's mass culture—typically news items—or scholarly articles from any time. The purpose of including mass culture items is to illustrate the ubiquity of disability in popular culture, essential to the patient–client interface that looms large in the professions to which most of the class aspires. Alternatively (and somewhat less frequently), students share articles from their research.
3. **Presentation of assigned readings (forty-five minutes–one hour):** The week's readings are explicated to the class by a team of two or three students. While all students will have been expected to have prepared the readings, taking turns teaching the selections will enrich their understanding and enhance the teamwork and communication skills essential to their future careers.
4. **Teacher-selected media (time remaining):** The typical class ends with a film, typically a documentary (such as *Sound and Fury*) or news clip but also at times a fiction feature or even an artistic performance. Students require something relatively less intense at the end of class. More important, given the ubiquity (not always obvious) of disability in popular culture, students need to learn to critique what they see and hear. Always open to a variety of interpretations, these films function as the course's principal case studies. Because the instructor's field is the performing arts, this is also an opportunity to model the application of the course material to one's own field.

Notes

1. American Music Therapy Association, "What Is Music Therapy?" http://www.musictherapy.org/about/musictherapy/.

2. Joseph Straus, *Extraordinary Measures: Disability in Music* (New York and Oxford: Oxford University Press, 2011); Alex Lubet, "Disability Studies and Performing Arts Medicine," *Medical Problems of Performing Artists* 17, no. 2 (2002): 59–62.

3. Paul Longmore, "The State of Disability Studies: Observations and Suggestions" (plenary address given at the Society for Disability Studies Annual Meeting, San Francisco State University, 2005).

4. Simi Linton, *Claiming Disability: Knowledge and Identity* (New York: New York University Press, 1998).

5. Tobin Siebers, *Disability Theory*, Corporealities: Discourses of Disability (Ann Arbor: University of Michigan Press, 2008).

6. John Harris, "One Principle and Three Fallacies of Disability Studies," *Journal of Medical Ethics* 27, no. 6 (2001): 383–87; John Harris, "One Principle and a Fourth Fallacy of Disability Studies," *Journal of Medical Ethics* 28, no. 3 (2002): 204.

7. Tom Beauchamp and James Childress, *Principles of Biomedical Ethics*, 7th ed. (New York and Oxford: Oxford University Press, 2013).

8. See, for example, Kate Gfeller et al., "Music Perception with Cochlear Implants and Residual Hearing," *Audiology and Neurotology* 11, no. S1 (2006): 12–15.

9. Alex Lubet, *Music, Disability, and Society* (Philadelphia: Temple University Press, 2011).

10. Alex Lubet and Ingrid Hofmann, "Classical Music, Disability, and Film: A Pedagogical Script," *Disability Studies Quarterly* 26, no. 1 (2006): doi:10.18061/dsq.v26i1.657.

11. Sabine König (director), *The Blind Orchestra* (Amsterdam, The Netherlands: Cobos Films and IKON, 2002).

12. Josh Aronson (director), *Sound and Fury* (New York: Aronson Film Associates, 2000).

13. Donald Pasquella (director), *Dax's Case* (Somerset, NJ: Video Corporation of America, 1984).

14. Jeanne Higbee and Emily Goff, eds., *Pedagogy and Student Services for Institutional Transformation: Implementing Universal Design in Higher Education* (Minneapolis, MN: Center for Research on Developmental Education and Urban Literacy, 2008).

15. Milos Forman (director), *Amadeus* (Berkeley, CA: Saul Zaentz Company, 1984).

16. For example, Benjamin Simkin, "Was PANDAS Associated with Mozart's Personality Idiosyncrasies?" *Medical Problems of Performing Artists* 14 (1999): 113–16.

17. Ibid.

18. Joseph Krajcik and Phyllis Blumenfeld, "Project-Based Learning," in *The Cambridge Handbook of the Learning Sciences*, ed. R. Keith Sawyer (New York: Cambridge University Press, 2006), 317–34.

19. Higbee and Goff, *Pedagogy and Student Services*.

20. Ann Davis, "Invisible Disability," *Ethics* 116, no. 1 (2005): 153–213.

21. Alex Lubet, "The Bioethics of Music, the Music of Bioethics," *Medical Problems of Performing Artists* 30, no. 4 (2015): 255.

22. Paul Haidet, "Jazz and the 'Art' of Medicine: Improvisation in the Medical Encounter," *Annals of Family Medicine* 5, no. 2 (2007): 164–69.

23. Katie Watson and Belinda Fu, "Medical Improv," accessed June 22, 2016, http://www.medicalimprov.org.

24. Oliveros, Pauline, Leaf Miller, Jaclyn Heyen, Gillian Siddall, and Sergio Hazard, "A Musical Improvisation Interface for People with Severe Disabilities," *Music and Medicine* 3, no. 3 (2011): 172–81; Tucker Sherrie, Jaclyn Heyen, Christine Sun Kim, Leaf Miller, Pauline Oliveros, Neil Rolnick, Clara Tomaz, and David Whalen, "Stretched Boundaries: Improvising across Abilities," in *Negotiated Moments: Improvisation, Sound, and Subjectivity*, ed. Ellen Waterman and Gillian Siddall (Durham: Duke University Press, 2016), 181–98.

25. "International Institute for Critical Studies in Improvisation," accessed June 22, 2016, http://improvisationinstitute.ca.

26. Some such films are discussed in Lubet and Hofmann, "Classical Music."

27. For example, Michèle Hozer and Peter Raymont (directors), *Genius Within: The Inner Life of Glenn Gould* (Toronto: White Pine Pictures, 2009).

28. Including Thomas Quasthoff, *The Voice: A Memoir* (New York: Pantheon, 2008).

29. Most notably Oliver Sacks, *Musicophilia: Tales of Music and the Brain* (Toronto: Vintage Canada, 2010).

30. Among many such studies is Nancy Mudrick and Michael Schwartz, "Health Care under the ADA: A Vision or a Mirage?" *Disability and Health Journal* 3, no. 4 (2010): 233–39.

Works Cited

American Music Therapy Association. "What Is Music Therapy?" http://www.musictherapy.org/about/musictherapy/.

Aronson, Josh (director). *Sound and Fury*. New York: Aronson Film Associates, 2000.

Beauchamp, Tom, and James Childress. *Principles of Biomedical Ethics*. 7th ed. New York and Oxford: Oxford University Press, 2013.

Davis, Ann. "Invisible Disability." *Ethics* 116, no. 1 (2005): 153–213.

Forman, Milos (director). *Amadeus*. Berkeley, CA: Saul Zaentz Company, 1984.

Gfeller, Kate, Carol Olszewski, Christopher Turner, Bruce Gantz, and Jacob Oleson. "Music Perception with Cochlear Implants and Residual Hearing." *Audiology and Neurotology* 11, Suppl. 1 (2006): 12–15.

Haidet, Paul. "Jazz and the 'Art' of Medicine: Improvisation in the Medical Encounter." *Annals of Family Medicine* 5, no. 2 (2007): 164–69.

Harris, John. "One Principle and a Fourth Fallacy of Disability Studies." *Journal of Medical Ethics* 28, no. 3 (2002): 204.

Harris, John. "One Principle and Three Fallacies of Disability Studies." *Journal of Medical Ethics* 27, no. 6 (2001): 383–87.

Higbee, Jeanne, and Emily Goff, eds. *Pedagogy and Student Services for Institutional Transformation: Implementing Universal Design in Higher Education*. Minneapolis, MN: Center for Research on Developmental Education and Urban Literacy, 2008.

Hozer, Michèle, and Peter Raymont (directors). *Genius Within: The Inner Life of Glenn Gould*. Toronto: White Pine Pictures, 2009.

International Institute for Critical Studies in Improvisation. Accessed June 22, 2016. http://improvisationinstitute.ca.

König, Sabine (director). *The Blind Orchestra*. Amsterdam, The Netherlands: Cobos Films and IKON, 2002.

Krajcik, Joseph, and Phyllis Blumenfeld. "Project-Based Learning." In *The Cambridge Handbook of the Learning Sciences*, edited by R. Keith Sawyer, 317–34. New York: Cambridge University Press, 2006.

Linton, Simi. *Claiming Disability: Knowledge and Identity*. New York: New York University Press, 1998.

Longmore, Paul. "The State of Disability Studies: Observations and Suggestions." Plenary address given at the Society for Disability Studies Annual Meeting, San Francisco State University, 2005.

Lubet, Alex. "Disability Studies and Performing Arts Medicine." *Medical Problems of Performing Artists* 17, no. 2 (2002): 59–62.

Lubet, Alex. *Music, Disability, and Society*. Philadelphia: Temple University Press, 2011.

Lubet, Alex. "The Bioethics of Music, the Music of Bioethics." *Medical Problems of Performing Artists* 30, no. 4 (2015): 255–59.

Lubet, Alex, and Ingrid Hofmann. "Classical Music, Disability, and Film: A Pedagogical Script." *Disability Studies Quarterly* 26, no. 1 (2006): doi:10.18061/dsq.v26i1.657.

Mudrick, Nancy, and Michael Schwartz. "Health Care under the ADA: A Vision or a Mirage?" *Disability and Health Journal* 3, no. 4 (2010): 233–39.

Oliveros, Pauline, Leaf Miller, Jaclyn Heyen, Gillian Siddall, and Sergio Hazard. "A Musical Improvisation Interface for People with Severe Disabilities." *Music and Medicine* 3, no. 3 (2011): 172–81.

Pasquella, Donald (director). *Dax's Case*. Somerset, NJ: Video Corporation of America, 1984.

Quasthoff, Thomas. *The Voice: A Memoir*. New York: Pantheon, 2008.

Sacks, Oliver. *Musicophilia: Tales of Music and the Brain*. Toronto: Vintage Canada, 2010.

Siebers, Tobin. *Disability Theory*. Corporealities: Discourses of Disability. Ann Arbor: University of Michigan Press, 2008.

Simkin, Benjamin. "Was PANDAS Associated with Mozart's Personality Idiosyncrasies?" *Medical Problems of Performing Artists* 14 (1999): 113–16.

Straus, Joseph. *Extraordinary Measures: Disability in Music*. New York and Oxford: Oxford University Press, 2011.

Tucker, Sherrie, Jaclyn Heyen, Christine Sun Kim, Leaf Miller, Pauline Oliveros, Neil Rolnick, Clara Tomaz, and David Whalen. "Stretched Boundaries: Improvising across Abilities." In *Negotiated Moments: Improvisation, Sound, and Subjectivity*, edited by Ellen Waterman and Gillian Siddall, 181–98. Durham: Duke University Press, 2016.

Watson, Katie, and Belinda Fu. "Medical Improv." Accessed June 22, 2016. http://www.medicalimprov.org.

20

Using Podcasts in Health Humanities Education

Nathan Carlin

Introduction

Health humanities has emerged out of certain criticisms of medical humanities as well as bioethics. Also, bioethics has enjoyed considerably more success than either medical humanities or health humanities. As a consequence, pedagogical methods in bioethics education are considerably more developed.[1]

The discussion of cases in bioethics education—especially clinical ethics education in medical schools—has been the leading pedagogical strategy for several decades.[2] There are good reasons for this. One is that because time spent on bioethics education in health professional schools is limited, students need to be introduced to key issues quickly. Cases accomplish this, with the added benefit that this pedagogical approach is structurally similar to the teaching of other clinical topics (e.g., morbidity and mortality rounds, team-based learning classes, and standardized patient encounters). Another is that the dominant theoretical approach to teaching bioethics is principlism, which involves the application of principles (especially the principles of autonomy, nonmaleficence, beneficence, and justice[3]) to scenarios in clinical ethics, research ethics, public health ethics, etc. Sometimes the discussion of cases centers on "classic cases," such as that of Karen Ann Quinlan or of Terri Schiavo.[4] Other times the discussion of cases entails focusing on short, fabricated, and specialty-related vignettes in, for example, psychiatric ethics.[5] But a problem with case-based approaches is that the presentation of these cases often seems too "thin," and therefore the discussion of the issues raised by a given case may be superficial—thus, other pedagogical approaches in health professional education have emerged in recent years, narrative medicine being one of the most prominent.[6] In this chapter, a new approach will be introduced: using podcasts in health humanities education. This approach retains the advantages of using cases but adds the advantages of narrative approaches.

The Need for Something New

Several years ago I began using podcasts in medical education. I did this for three reasons. The first was that in my third-year clinical clerkship teaching I found that many—but not all—students were not willing to do the reading that I assigned, despite the fact that I would ask students to read a very small amount (such as an article or a chapter). Because my sessions with students are not graded—though they are required—students felt no pressure to do the reading. Moreover, they had more important matters to attend to, such as studying for various exams. So I decided to stop asking students to read. "You have to pick your battles," I thought to myself.

Still, I needed something to focus our discussion, if not a reading. A lecture could do just this. In academic medicine, a common approach to teaching is to introduce some topic by means of a case discussion (in grand rounds, for example, a lecture is often given, followed by a discussion of a case). I've used this approach during clerkship teaching, but I felt that the dynamics of these discussions, perhaps because we were talking about matters of ethics, seemed to be leading or chiding or pedantic. It was hard for students to trust that the discussion was to be genuinely open.

So I abandoned the lecture method. This leads to the second reason I began using podcasts—namely, the use of podcasts changes the dynamics of the conversation in that students do not know if I, as a teacher, support what is being said in the podcast or if I disagree with it. Thus, it opens the discussion up for genuine debate.

A third reason I began using podcasts is that no one else, to my knowledge, was using podcasts at my medical school; thus, this presentation of material makes students curious about the session, especially because my time with students was scheduled for the end of the day, after students had lectures for six hours. At the end of the day, students were bored and anxious to get home before rush hour. I needed something to hold their attention, and while students commonly see videos during their education (they also have the opportunity of not attending many classes in person, "streaming" lectures at home instead), the idea of an audio-only experience is different for them. While it is true that young people today do listen to podcasts—especially since production of *Serial*, which many people "binge," like various shows on Netflix such as *House of Cards*—it is less common to listen to podcasts in educational environments and as a group activity. My choice of podcasts is strategic. I use selections of episodes from *This American Life*, an extremely popular podcast (*Serial* is an offshoot of *This American Life*), and it often has segments on health-related matters.

I teach in three rotations. In internal medicine, I teach a session on breaking bad news to patients. In psychiatry, I teach a general session on psychiatric ethics. And in family medicine I teach a session on disability benefits. I use podcasts in the family medicine session and the psychiatry session; this chapter will focus on these sessions.

Trends with Benefits

In the family medicine clerkship the podcast that I use, "Trends with Benefits,"[7] focuses on the recent rise of persons in the United States filing for disability benefits. I play twelve minutes from this episode.

According to the episode, which aired on March 22, 2013, fourteen million Americans receive disability benefits; and there are pockets in the country where one in four adults receive them—a curious percentage of the population. Hale County, Alabama, is one such place. Chana Joffe-Walt, the journalist covering this story, went there to find out why.

Joffe-Walt noted that possible explanations for the high percentage of persons receiving disability benefits in Hale County could include the following:

- People in Hale County take poor care of themselves because they eat bad food and/or "party too hard" (i.e., drink and smoke too much)
- People are living longer, so a larger number of people need disability benefits as they age
- They are cheating (i.e., they can work but are choosing not to do so)
- Some other reason

When she began interviewing people, Joffe-Walt discovered that one doctor in particular seemed to be responsible for signing off on all of the disability claims in Hale County: Dr. Perry Timberlake. So she wondered if Dr. Timberlake was running some kind of disability scam. When she interviewed him, Joffe-Walt found that, while Dr. Timberlake was not personally profiting in any significant way from seeing disability patients, he did have a liberal or expansive understanding of what disability is, in that he asked about a patient's educational level when considering supporting his or her application for social security benefits. Dr. Timberlake reasoned as follows: because there are few desk jobs in Hale County, if a patient who had, say, back pain (and therefore cannot stand for long periods of time) and also if this patient did not have a high school diploma, he (Dr. Timberlake) should fill out the paperwork because he felt that it was unlikely that this patient would be able to find meaningful work. Thus, what Dr. Timberlake defined as "disability" was contingent upon whether one could procure a job in Hale County; his decision was not purely medical or bodily.

A poignant moment in the podcast is when Joffe-Walt asks a woman on disability what kind of work she would be willing to do in order to accommodate her back pain. The woman says that "she hadn't really thought about it," which leads the listener to believe that this woman does not want to work, that she is, in all likelihood, cheating the system. And this suspicion seems to be confirmed when the woman suggests that she would like to be the person sitting at the desk at the social security office so that she "could weed out the ones who don't need it" (i.e., social security benefits). In class there is sometimes a lot of laughter at this point because the class, or some in the class, assume that the speaker is being disingenuous.

But then the podcast takes a twist. Joffe-Walt discovers the primary reason that this woman wants to work for the social security office: because she gets to sit at a desk. In other words, the nature of the work did not matter to her at all. This woman simply never saw a desk job that could be attainable for her, until she applied for disability benefits. Joffe-Walt, in disbelief, later went to the jobs listings for the area and found that there were, in fact, no sit-down jobs, only jobs at places like fast-food restaurants, plants, and loading docks, as well as in health professional fields, such as nursing. All of these jobs require a lot of standing. There were literally no sit-down jobs in the area.

The issue of deciding who/what condition qualifies as disabled is especially relevant to the students whom I teach because most, if not all, will encounter at least one patient requesting disability benefits. Students observe their clinical professors navigate when to sign off on disability paperwork and when to say no, but this teaching, as is so often inherent in clinical teaching, is indirect and not uniform. So in my session with students, one of the learning objectives includes articulating a rationale for approving or disapproving an application for disability benefits so as to address this issue directly.

For a couple of years I played this podcast and then opened up the floor for discussion. Co-led with a family medicine physician, sometimes the discussion went well, but other times it did not. The quality of the sessions seemed to depend on whether there was a critical mass of students willing to talk (usually three or four). This variation displeased me because I felt deflated after a session went poorly.

Later, I became acquainted with another podcast: *Intelligence*^{2}. I learned of this podcast from an upper-level resident. Since the podcast was appealing to this young physician, I guessed it might be appealing to medical students. *Intelligence*^{2} is a podcast that hosts Oxford-style debates where two teams, each comprised of two experts, consider a simple yes/no motion that is addressed in three rounds. The winner of the debate is determined by a live audience (the audience takes a pre-/posttest with regard to the motion being debated, and the team that induces the greater change wins). During the 2015–2016 academic year, I incorporated *Intelligence*^{2} into the exercise. I did not change the audio portion of the class (so students do not listen to any segments of *Intelligence*^{2}), but I did explain to them what *Intelligence*^{2} is and informed them that we would be having a mock debate, very similar to *Intelligence*^{2}.

The advantage of this approach is that it requires students to be active. My previous strategy of playing the podcast and then facilitating an open discussion, as noted, would work well sometimes but not others. Using the mock-debate format has worked well every single session.

Here is how it works. I divide the class into two groups, one that argues that Dr. Timberlake is doing a good thing and one that argues that Dr. Timberlake is doing a bad thing. After listening to the podcast, we have the debate in three rounds. But first each team is given ten minutes to come up with their arguments, both for their assigned assessment of Dr. Timberlake and for their critiques of the other team's expected arguments. To begin the debate, a representative from each team presents to the front of the class, and each team offers opening arguments. In round two, questions and critiques are offered by each team toward the other team, with the purpose of exposing weaknesses in arguments. In round three, each team has the opportunity to offer a closing argument, in light of critiques made in round two.

Key issues typically raised by the debate include the following:

- What is disability?
- To what extent should psychosocial issues, such as education level, be considered when making a medical diagnosis?
- What is the role of a family medicine doctor in a community with limited resources?
- What is the difference between helping and enabling?
- Would it be a better use of resources to create more job and educational opportunities in such counties, rather than giving money to individuals?

The result of this format is that ethics arguments are made—far beyond a mere opinion about an issue—which is another learning objective for the session. In other words, the purpose of this session is not to convey particular substantive knowledge regarding consensus opinion among clinical ethics experts. Rather, the purpose of this session is to help students apply ethics principles they have learned previously so as to make an ethics argument, to demonstrate critical thinking skills.

Guided by Voices

In the psychiatry clerkship where I teach, I also use, as noted, another podcast from *This American Life*, from the episode "Edge of Sanity," specifically the segment titled "Guided by Voices."[8] Since this segment is ten minutes long, I play all of it.

The segment consists of a brief interview conducted by Ira Glass with Dr. Patricia Deegan, a clinical psychologist and disability rights activist, who also hears voices. Dr. Deegan finds much of the language about mental illness to be stigmatizing and prefers the term *voice hearer* (in contrast to the diagnosis of schizophrenia). As a girl, Dr. Deegan heard voices that were mostly positive; but as a teenager, the voices became critical, so she was diagnosed with schizophrenia.

Dr. Deegan thinks that the only way healthcare professionals who care for persons who hear voices can understand their patients is if they themselves hear voices. Dr. Deegan and others produced a recording of voices, created by voice hearers, to be worn by healthcare professionals while they do their job, as well as other tasks. Here is an excerpt from the tape:

> That's right. That's right. Look at them. Their eyes are filled with disgust. They know how disgusting you are. Stop it now. Stop, stop, stop, stop. I see you. I see you. They see you. Everyone sees you. They hear you. They know you. They know how foul you are. Ugh. You are foul. Don't touch it. Don't touch it. Don't touch it. Don't touch it. Don't touch it.

Glass asks Dr. Deegan if voices are usually negative, and Dr. Deegan responds that this a common characteristic for those who are showing up for help, meaning that others, who do not hear negative voices, often do not present in psychiatric settings.

An issue that Glass talks with Dr. Deegan about at length is the idea of a continuum between mental health and mental illness. Specifically, Glass notes that he has wondered if he hears voices, though in a low-level way, because he often hears songs in his head. But Dr. Deegan, while indicating that the idea of a continuum is a nice one—in that a continuum, if true, could possibly destigmatize the experience—she points out that it is not accurate because, for voice hearers, the experience is fundamentally auditory. In other words, for voice hearers it is as though one really hears the sound—it is not experienced differently from other sounds that one actually does hear—so they are not intrusive thoughts but actual auditory voices (or other sounds) that one experiences. This is why the recording that Dr. Deegan produced is so effective.

They also discuss some of Dr. Deegan's self-help suggestions for voice hearers. One involves putting an earplug in one ear when one is hearing voices. Putting an ear plug in both ears does not tend to work, Dr. Deegan has found, both in her own experience and in the experience of others. Glass asks Dr. Deegan why this might be, wondering if simply a change—any change—can disrupt the voices for some voice hearers. Dr. Deegan thinks that anything that promotes a sense of power can contribute to well-being, and using an earplug, for some, does provide this sense of agency.

Dr. Deegan here also criticizes American psychiatry for being too pharmacological. American psychiatry, she argues, too often assumes that individuals who hear voices and have other such experiences have "broken brains" and that the only thing that they can do is take medication in order to take a stand against their mental illness. Dr. Deegan thinks that persons diagnosed with various forms of mental illness can take control of their well-being in ways beyond or other than medication.

Dr. Deegan still hears voices, and Glass asks her about this. He asks about voices and selfhood, about whether she considers the voices to be a part of herself or whether she thinks that the voices are foreign, coming from outside, as it were. Dr. Deegan thinks that the voices are indeed a part of herself, and she finds it helpful to think of them as such. She thinks that the voices represent her feelings, and it is her goal to think of the voices as a part of herself. The podcast ends on this insight.

After playing the podcast, I open the class up for discussion, asking for general reactions. These discussions have tended to go well, though (as with the family medicine clerkship) some groups are more talkative than others. I think these open-ended discussions go well because the podcast so directly relates to their clinical experience about an issue that is usually neglected, even in psychiatry—namely, the *experience* of psychosis. There are, of course, ethical issues brought up by the podcast (e.g., what language should we use to destigmatize mental illness?); but the podcast, because of its focus on subjectivity, makes it ideal for health humanities education, in distinction to from clinical ethics education.[9]

Often, what students comment on first is the point that the experience of hearing voices is profoundly auditory. Many students, like Glass, do not appreciate this at first; and learning this reframes their previous clinical experience of working with psychiatric patients, many of whom do suffer from hearing distressing voices. This insight enables students, they say, to be more empathetic, in that they feel as though they do understand their patients better. Strikingly, however, when I ask students if we should simulate the experience (i.e., create our own recordings and have students perform tasks while listening to distressing voices, just like Dr. Deegan did), students almost always respond by saying that this is unnecessary, that hearing excerpts from Dr. Deegan's recording on *This American Life* is enough.

Another theme that students often raise is Dr. Deegan's comments about ear plugs. Because the teaching of psychiatry at our medical school is, for the most part, neurobiological and psychopharmacological, this excerpt from the podcast comes across to them as humorous and perhaps somewhat gimmicky. But, after the laughter, I probe further. I ask students to reflect on why this method does appear to work for some, including Dr. Deegan. This steers the conversation in a way that invites others in class to speak about psychiatry from a different angle, usually from the angle of psychotherapy. The (usually unspoken) logic that connects this transition in the conversation is this: *if ear plugs can help patients, why not talking, and vice versa?* And once the conversation is steered toward the direction of psychotherapy, often some student will point out that patients do the best with both medication and therapy—that it is a false dichotomy to force choosing one over the other.[10] Part of the role of health humanities education is to move, or at least expose, health science students beyond biomedically reductive ways of thinking.

An issue that I bring up is why the voices are negative. Students are intrigued by the question but do not know how to respond. I lead them further, with a seemingly unrelated question about religious ideation. I ask, "How many of you have 'met' Jesus during this rotation, or how many of you have talked with patients with religious delusions or hallucinations?" Every hand always goes up. Students now want some explanation for this. I tell them about Sigmund Freud's theory that delusions are an attempt at recovery,[11] that psychotic experiences are protective, defensive in some way, however inefficient they may be; and I point out that this is congruent with Dr. Deegan's suggestion that voices are an expression of feelings. In other words, psychiatric patients in the county hospital where students rotate really do feel badly about their lives (many, for instance, are addicted to drugs and/or alcohol, and many are homeless), so their experience of distressing voices is what they are feeling about themselves. But these negative feelings are too strong. So, in a defensive manner, these same patients also hear voices that they are God, that the CIA has a special mission for them, etc. They are not failures in life but rather leaders of the world, important to such a degree to even have God's ear and, in some cases, to be God's own son.

Student feedback is usually positive for this session. Here are some typical comments for the course evaluations:

- I loved it. Maybe one of my favorite sessions during our [didactic sessions]. That piece on schizophrenia impressed my understanding of what my patients experience.
- I liked the format in that it was an open discussion rather than a lecture.
- It was too open-ended. I felt that we have too much "discuss your experience."
- Interesting lecture, although I would've liked a little more structure.[12]

As indicated by the latter two comments, a consistent critique that I have received for this session, unlike the session in family medicine, is that students sometimes perceive this session to be "off the cuff" or disorganized, likely because of my inductive approach. I know how I want the session to go, and, as indicated, I guide the discussion in certain directions. Every session goes pretty much the same way. But to some students this appears to be meandering, leaving them wondering if they have covered the learning objectives for the day. Some of these students have suggested that I add a ten-minute PowerPoint presentation to the class to give it more structure. I may do so in the future.

Conclusion

Using podcasts as a vehicle for health humanities education retains the advantages of using cases in clinical teaching but adds the advantages of narrative approaches by "thickening" the discussion because podcasts can attend to human experience in a substantive way. Podcasts such as *This American Life* provide hundreds of hours of professional labor that offer polished and interesting material for discussion, in contrast to the detached and decontextualized clinical case vignettes that are so common in medical education.

At the end of this chapter is the actual handout that I distribute to students in the family medicine clerkship. If you would like to do a mock debate, this handout can serve as a guide. In the psychiatry clerkship, I do not distribute a handout but rather, as described, guide the discussion. In either case, or if you can think of another model for class discussion, in what remains of this chapter I conclude with some practical suggestions about using podcasts in your own teaching.

First, do not use Google or some other search engine to find a podcast that you can use in class. Instead, find two or three podcasts that you really enjoy, such as *This American Life, Being Human*, or *Philosophy Bites*, and listen to them on a regular basis. When the podcast happens to address an issue that intersects with your teaching, begin thinking about how to employ it in class. Let your own interest and curiosity be your guide. Do not attempt to use a podcast simply "to make your teaching more 'relevant' or 'up-to-date'" because students will likely see through these attempts. *Second, once you find a topic on a podcast that you find interesting, select a short segment to be played, something between ten and fifteen minutes.* This is enough time for the podcast to develop some issue in considerable detail but short enough so that it will not bore students. *Third, the segment selected should focus on an open-ended issue—that is, it should invite discussion.* It can be an unsettled, contemporary debate in bioethics (as in the podcast I use in the family medicine clerkship), or it can be material that encourages personal reflection (as in the podcast I use in the psychiatry clerkship). It should not, in other words, be a selection that attempts to convey a normative lesson in professionalism, such as "tell the truth to patients" or "don't cheat on exams." *Fourth, pick out at least three questions you would like the class to consider.* If the segment you have selected does not yield at least three questions, then it is unlikely that it will be able to sustain a discussion. *Finally, decide how you will raise these issues for the class to consider.* Mock debates work well for large groups (thirty students or more), while small group discussion would be more appropriate for a humanities seminar (twelve students or fewer).

PEDAGOGY EXERCISE SECTION

Mock Debate

CLASS HANDOUT

Explanation of Exercise

In most of your clerkships you have at least an hour dedicated to some topic in humanities and/or ethics and clinical practice. During this session we will be talking about ethical issues related to disability benefits. In order to get a handle on the discussion, we will be listening to twelve minutes of a podcast from *This American Life*. The episode is "Trends with Benefits."

After we listen to the podcast, we will have a debate, modeled after another podcast (*Intelligence²*), a podcast that hosts debates on various topics in which there is a single motion that is debated in a yes/no fashion. There are three rounds. Round 1 is for opening statements. Round 2 is for questioning. And Round 3 is for closing statements.

For us, the motion to be debated is this:

> Dr. Perry Timberlake is doing a good thing by signing paperwork to extend disability benefits to persons who, from a strictly medical perspective, may not be eligible for them.

Structure of Hour

1. The class will be divided into two equal teams, and each team will be assigned a position to argue (one side will argue that Dr. Perry Timberlake is doing a good thing and the other will argue that Dr. Perry Timberlake is doing a bad thing).
2. A fact sheet on disability benefits will be distributed.
3. The podcast will be played.
4. Teams will have ten minutes to do the following things:
    a. Pick a debater to represent your team.
    b. As a group, make the strongest arguments possible for your position (using ethics principles where viable), also identifying potential weaknesses in the other team's position.
    c. Look up or brainstorm material beyond the fact sheet and the podcast for the purposes of the debate.
5. The debate will happen in this way:
    a. Round 1: Each team will make an opening statement (only debaters may talk).
    b. Round 2: Each side can question the other side, trying to poke holes in arguments (anyone may speak).
    c. Round 3: Each team will make a closing statement (only debaters may talk).
6. Voting will take place, and we will discuss what we really think about the issue.

Notes

1. Ellen Fox, Robert Arnold, and Baruch Brody, "Medical Ethics Education: Past, Present, and Future," *Academic Medicine* 70, no. 9 (1995): 761–69.

2. Ronald Carson, "Case Method," *Journal of Medical Ethics* 12, no. 1 (1986): 36–38.

3. Tom Beauchamp and James Childress, *Principles of Biomedical Ethics*, 7th ed. (New York and Oxford: Oxford University Press, 2013).

4. See, for example, Gregory Pence, *Classic Cases in Medical Ethics: Accounts of Cases that Have Shaped Medical Ethics, with Philosophical, Legal, and Historical Backgrounds*, 3rd ed. (Boston: McGraw-Hill, 2000).

5. Brief clinical vignettes are commonly used in all specialties.

6. See, for example, Rita Charon, *Narrative Medicine: Honoring the Stories of Illness* (Oxford: Oxford University Press, 2006).

7. Chana Joffe-Walt, "Trends with Benefits," *This American Life*, March 22, 2013, http://www.thisamericanlife.org/radio-archives/episode/490/trends-with-benefits.

8. Ira Glass, "Edge of Sanity," *This American Life*, January 31, 1997, http://www.thisamericanlife.org/radio-archives/episode/52/edge-of-sanity.

9. In point of fact, because in the past my class session in the psychiatry clerkship was labeled "ethics" (this was not my decision), a common criticism I have received from students is that the session, while interesting, did not cover ethics. Medical students, then, intuitively pick up on the difference between ethics and health humanities, even if they do not have the vocabulary to articulate this distinction.

10. See, for example, T. M. Luhrmann, *Of Two Minds: An Anthropologist Looks at American Psychiatry* (New York: Vintage Books, 2001), 284.

11. Sigmund Freud, "Psychoanalytic Notes on an Autobiographical Account of a Case of Paranoia (Dementia Paranoides)," in *The Standard Edition of the Complete Psychological Works of Sigmund Freud*, ed. and trans. James Strachey, vol. 12 (London: Vintage, 2001), 1–82 (first published 1911).

12. These comments come from course evaluations collected by the Department of Psychiatry on July 16, 2014; August 27, 2014; and October 22, 2014.

Works Cited

Beauchamp, Tom, and James Childress. *Principles of Biomedical Ethics*. 7th ed. New York and Oxford: Oxford University Press, 2013.

Carson, Ronald. "Case Method." *Journal of Medical Ethics* 12, no. 1 (1986): 36–38.

Charon, Rita. *Narrative Medicine: Honoring the Stories of Illness*. Oxford: Oxford University Press, 2006.

Fox, Ellen, Robert Arnold, and Baruch Brody. "Medical Ethics Education: Past, Present, and Future." *Academic Medicine* 70, no. 9 (1995): 761–69.

Freud, Sigmund. "Psychoanalytic Notes on an Autobiographical Account of a Case of Paranoia (Dementia Paranoides)." In *The Standard Edition of the Complete Psychological Works of Sigmund Freud*, edited and translated by James Strachey. Vol. 12, 1–82. London: Vintage, 2001. First published 1911.

Glass, Ira. "Edge of Sanity." *This American Life*, January 31, 1997. http://www.thisamericanlife.org/radio-archives/episode/52/edge-of-sanity.

Joffe-Walt, Chana. "Trends with Benefits." *This American Life*, March 22, 2013. http://www.thisamericanlife.org/radio-archives/episode/490/trends-with-benefits.

Luhrmann, T. M. *Of Two Minds: An Anthropologist Looks at American Psychiatry*. New York: Vintage Books, 2001.

Pence, Gregory. *Classic Cases in Medical Ethics: Accounts of Cases That Have Shaped Medical Ethics, with Philosophical, Legal, and Historical Backgrounds*. 3rd ed. Boston: McGraw-Hill, 2000.

APPENDIX

Resources on Health Humanities Teaching

General Sources on Health Humanities and Medical Humanities

Atkinson, Sarah, Bethan Evans, Angela Woods, and Robin Kearns. "'The Medical' and 'Health' in a Critical Medical Humanities." *Journal of Medical Humanities* 36, no. 1 (March 2015): 71–81.

Berry, Sarah, Therese Jones, and Erin Lamb. "Editors' Introduction: Health Humanities: The Future of Pre-Health Education Is Here." *Journal of Medical Humanities* 38, no. 4 (December 2017): 353–60.

Bishop, Jeffrey P. "Rejecting Medical Humanism: Medical Humanities and the Metaphysics of Medicine." *Journal of Medical Humanities* 29, no. 1 (March 2008): 15–25.

Bleakley, Alan. "The Health Humanities: A Democratizing Force for Medicine." In *InSight: Visualizing Health Humanities*, edited by Bonnie Sadler Takach, Pamela Brett-Maclean, Aidan Rowe, and George F. Takach, 1–23. Edmonton, AB, Canada: Department of Art and Design, University of Alberta, 2012.

Bleakley, Alan. "Towards a 'Critical Medical Humanities.'" In *Medicine, Health, and the Arts: Approaches to the Medical Humanities*, edited by Victoria Bates, Alan Bleakley, and Sam Goodman, 17–26. New York: Routledge, 2014.

Brody, Howard. "Defining the Medical Humanities: Three Conceptions and Three Narratives." *Journal of Medical Humanities* 32, no. 1 (March 2011): 1–7.

Campo, Rafael. "'The Medical Humanities,' for Lack of a Better Term." *Journal of the American Medical Association* 294, no. 9 (September 2005): 1009–11.

Crawford, Paul, Brian Brown, Charley Baker, Victoria Tischler, and Brian Abrams. *Health Humanities.* New York: Palgrave Macmillan, 2015.

Gutierrez, Kevin J., and Sayantani DasGupta. "The Space That Difference Makes: On Marginality, Social Justice and the Future of the Health Humanities." *Journal of Medical Humanities* 37, no. 4 (December 2016): 435–48.

Jones, Therese, Michael Blackie, Rebecca Garden, and Delese Wear. "The Almost Right Word: The Move from Medical to Health Humanities." *Academic Medicine* 92, no. 7 (July 2017): 932–35.

Klugman, Craig M. "How Health Humanities Will Save the Life of the Humanities." *Journal of Medical Humanities* 38, no. 4 (December 2017): 419–30.

McManus, Ian C. "Humanity and the Medical Humanities." *Lancet* 349, no. 8983 (October 1995): 1143–45.

Pattison, Stephen. "Medical Humanities: A Vision and Some Cautionary Notes." *Medical Humanities* 29, no. 1 (June 2003): 33–36.

Shapiro, Johanna, Jack Coulehan, Delese Wear, and Martha Montello. "Medical Humanities and Their Discontents: Definitions, Critiques, and Implications." *Academic Medicine* 84, no. 2 (February 2009): 192–98.

Tsevat, Rebecca, Anoushka Sinha, Kevin Gutierrez, and Sayantani DasGupta. "Bringing Home the Health Humanities: Narrative Humility, Structural Competency, and Engaged Pedagogy." *Academic Medicine* 90, no. 11 (November 2015): 1462–65.

Viney, William, Felicity Callard, and Angela Woods. "Critical Medical Humanities: Embracing Entanglement, Taking Risks." *Medical Humanities* 41, no. 1 (June 2015): 2–7.

Wear, Delese. "The Medical Humanities: Toward a Renewed Praxis." *Journal of Medical Humanities* 30, no. 4 (December 2009): 209.

Medical Ethics Teaching

Barnard, David. "Residency Ethics Teaching: A Critique of Current Trends." *Journal of the American Medical Association* 148, no. 8 (August 1988): 1836–38.

Christakis, Dimitri A., and Chris Feudtner. "Ethics in a Short White Coat: The Ethical Dilemmas That Medical Students Confront." *Academic Medicine* 68, no. 4 (April 1993): 249–54.

Culver, Charles M., K. Danner Clouser, Bernard Gert, Howard Brody, John Fletcher, Albert Jonsen, Loretta Kopelman, Joanne Lynn, Mark Siegler, and Daniel Wikler. "Basic Curricular Goals in Medical Ethics." *New England Journal of Medicine* 312, no. 4 (January 1985): 253–56.

Delaney, Brendan, and Leslie Kean. "Attitudes of Medical Students to the Teaching of Medical Ethics." *Medical Education* 22, no. 1 (January 1988): 8–10.

Fox, Ellen, Robert M. Arnold, and Baruch Brody. "Medical Ethics Education: Past, Present, and Future." *Academic Medicine* 70, no. 9 (September 1995): 761–68.

Gillon, Raanan. "Editorial: Medical Ethics Education." *Journal of Medical Ethics* 13, no. 3 (September 1987): 115–16.

Goldie, John. "Review of Ethics Curricula in Undergraduate Medical Education." *Medical Education* 34, no. 2 (February 2000): 108–19.

Hafferty, Frederic W., and Ronald Franks. "The Hidden Curriculum, Ethics Teaching, and the Structure of Medical Education." *Academic Medicine* 69, no. 11 (November 1994): 861–71.

Johnston, Carolyn, and Peter Haughton. "Medical Students' Perception of Their Ethics Teaching." *Journal of Medical Ethics* 33, no. 7 (July 2007): 418–22.

Mattick, Karen, and John Bligh. "Teaching and Assessing Medical Ethics: Where Are We Now?" *Journal of Medical Ethics* 32, no. 3 (March 2006): 181–85.

Mattick, Karen, and John Bligh. "Undergraduate Ethics Teaching: Revisiting the Consensus Statement." *Medical Education* 40, no. 4 (April 2006): 329–32.

Miles, Steven H., Laura Weiss Lane, Janet Bickel, Robert M. Walker, and Christine K. Cassel. "Medical Ethics Education: Coming of Age." *Academic Medicine* 64, no. 12 (December 1989): 705–14.

Musick, David W. "Teaching Medical Ethics: A Review of the Literature from North American Medical Schools with Emphasis on Education." *Medicine, Health Care and Philosophy* 2, no. 3 (October 1999): 239–54.

Pellegrino, Edmund D. "Teaching Medical Ethics: Some Persistent Questions and Some Responses." *Academic Medicine* 64, no. 12 (December 1989): 701–3.

Perkins, Henry S. "Teaching Medical Ethics During Residency." *Academic Medicine* 64, no. 5 (May 1989): 262–66.

Perkins, Henry S., Helen P. Hazuda, and Cynthia M. A. Geppert. "Challenges in Teaching Ethics in Medical Schools." *American Journal of the Medical Sciences* 319, no. 5 (May 2000): 273–78.

Roff, Sue, and Paul Preece. "Helping Medical Students to Find Their Moral Compasses: Ethics Teaching for Second and Third Year Undergraduates." *Journal of Medical Ethics* 30, no. 5 (October 2004): 487–89.

Self, Donnie J., Fredric D. Wolinsky, and DeWitt C. Baldwin Jr. "The Effect of Teaching Medical Ethics on Medical Students' Moral Reasoning." *Academic Medicine* 64, no. 12 (December 1989): 755–59.

Siegler, Mark. "Training Doctors for Professionalism: Some Lessons from Teaching Clinical Medical Ethics." *Mount Sinai Journal of Medicine* 69, no. 6 (November 2002): 404–9.

Tysinger, James W., Leah K. Klonis, John Z. Sadler, and James M. Wagner. "Teaching Ethics Using Small-Group, Problem-Based Learning." *Journal of Medical Ethics* 23, no. 5 (October 1997): 315–18.

Veatch, Robert M., and Sharmon Sollitto. "Medical Ethics Teaching: Report of a National Medical School Survey." *Journal of the American Medical Association* 235, no. 10 (March 1976): 1030–33.

Medical Humanities Teaching

An, Jung Hee, Ivo Kwon, Soon Nam Lee, Jae Jin Han, and Jae Eun Jeong. "Study on the Medical Humanities and Social Sciences Curriculum in Korean Medical School: Current Teaching Status and Learning Subjects." *Korean Journal of Medical Education* 20, no. 2 (June 2008): 133–44.

Anderson, Ruric, and David Schiedermayer. "The Art of Medicine Through the Humanities: An Overview of a One-Month Humanities Elective for Fourth Year Students." *Medical Education* 37, no. 6 (June 2003): 560–62.

Barnard, David. "Making a Place for the Humanities in Residency Education." *Academic Medicine* 69, no. 8 (August 1994): 628–30.

Baum, Michael. "Teaching the Humanities to Medical Students." *Clinical Medicine* 2, no. 3 (May 2002): 246–49.

Belling, Catherine. "Commentary: Sharper Instruments: On Defending the Humanities in Undergraduate Medical Education." *Academic Medicine* 85, no. 6 (June 2010): 938–40.

Blasco, Pablo González, Graziela Moreto, and Marcelo R. Levites. "Teaching Humanities Through Opera: Leading Medical Students to Reflective Attitudes." *Family Medicine* 37, no. 1 (January 2005): 18–20.

Bleakley, Alan, and Robert Marshall. "Can the Science of Communication Inform the Art of the Medical Humanities?" *Medical Education* 47, no. 2 (January 2013): 126–33.

Calman, Kenneth C., Robin S. Downie, M. Duthie, and B. Sweeney. "Literature and Medicine: A Short Course for Medical Students." *Medical Education* 22, no. 4 (July 1988): 265–69.

Carson, Ronald A. "Teaching Ethics in the Context of the Medical Humanities." *Journal of Medical Ethics* 20, no. 4 (December 1994): 235–38.

Charon, Rita. "Commentary: Calculating the Contributions of Humanities to Medical Practice—Motives, Methods, and Metrics." *Academic Medicine* 85, no. 6 (June 2010): 935–37.

Clouser, K. Danner. "Humanities in Medical Education: Some Contributions." *Journal of Medicine and Philosophy* 15, no. 3 (June 1990): 289–301.

Darbyshire, Daniel, and Paul Baker. "A Systematic Review and Thematic Analysis of Cinema in Medical Education." *Medical Humanities* 38, no. 1 (January 2012): 28–33.

Dolan, Brian. "History, Medical Humanities and Medical Education." *Social History of Medicine* 23, no. 2 (April 2010): 393–405.

Donohoe, Martin, and Susan Danielson. "A Community-Based Approach to the Medical Humanities." *Medical Education* 38, no. 2 (February 2004): 204–17.

Doukas, David J., Laurence B. McCullough, and Stephen Wear. "Reforming Medical Education in Ethics and Humanities by Finding Common Ground with Abraham Flexner." *Academic Medicine* 85, no. 2 (February 2010): 318–23.

Evans, Martyn. "Reflections on the Humanities in Medical Education." *Medical Education* 36, no. 6 (June 2002): 508–13.

Evans, Martyn, and David Greaves. "Medical Humanities at the University of Wales Swansea." *Medical Humanities* 27, no. 1 (June 2001): 51–52.

Friedman, Lester D. "The Precarious Position of the Medical Humanities in the Medical School Curriculum." *Academic Medicine* 77, no. 4 (April 2002): 320–22.

Grant, Vincent J. "Making Room for Medical Humanities." *Medical Humanities* 28, no. 1 (June 2002): 45–48.

Green, Michael J. "Teaching with Comics: A Course for Fourth-Year Medical Students." *Journal of Medical Humanities* 34, no. 4 (September 2013): 471–76.

Halperin, Edward C. "Preserving the Humanities in Medical Education." *Medical Teacher* 32, no. 1 (January 2010): 76–79.

Hawkins, Anne Hunsaker, James O. Ballard, and David J. Hufford. "Humanities Education at Pennsylvania State University College of Medicine, Hershey, Pennsylvania." *Academic Medicine* 78, no. 10 (October 2003): 1001–5.

Hunter, Kathryn Montgomery, Rita Charon, and John L. Coulehan. "The Study of Literature in Medical Education." *Academic Medicine* 70, no. 9 (September 1995): 787–94.

Jones, Anne Hudson, and Ronald A. Carson. "Medical Humanities at the University of Texas Medical Branch at Galveston." *Academic Medicine* 78, no. 10 (October 2003): 1006–9.

Jones, Therese, and Abraham Verghese. "On Becoming a Humanities Curriculum: The Center for Medical Humanities and Ethics at the University of Texas Health Science Center at San Antonio." *Academic Medicine* 78, no. 10 (October 2003): 1010–14.

Kidd, Monica G., and Jason T. Connor. "Striving to Do Good Things: Teaching Humanities in Canadian Medical Schools." *Journal of Medical Humanities* 29, no. 1 (March 2008): 45–54.

Klugman, Craig M., Jennifer Peel, and Diana Beckmann-Mendez. "Art Rounds: Teaching Interprofessional Students Visual Thinking Strategies at One School." *Academic Medicine* 86, no. 10 (October 2011): 1266–71.

Kopelman, Loretta M. "Development of the Medical Humanities Program at East Carolina University." *Academic Medicine* 64, no. 12 (December 1989): 730–34.

Li, Peng, and Su-juan Ran. "Present Situation of Medical Humanities Quality Education in China." *Northwest Medical Education* 17, no. 5 (2009): 929–31.

Louis-Courvoisier, Micheline, and Aaron Wenger. "How to Make the Most of History and Literature in the Teaching of Medical Humanities: The Experience of the University of Geneva." *Medical Humanities* 31, no. 1 (June 2005): 51–54.

Macnaughton, Jane. "The Humanities in Medical Education: Context, Outcomes and Structures." *Medical Humanities* 26, no. 1 (June 2000): 23–30.

Meng, Kwang-ho. "Teaching Medical Humanities in Korean Medical Schools: Tasks and Prospect." *Korean Journal of Medical Education* 19, no. 1 (March 2007): 5–11.

Montgomery, Kathryn, Tod Chambers, and Douglas R. Reifler. "Humanities Education at Northwestern University's Feinberg School of Medicine." *Academic Medicine* 78, no. 10 (October 2003): 958–62.

Nazario, Rubén J. "Medical Humanities as Tools for the Teaching of Patient-Centered Care." *Journal of Hospital Medicine* 4, no. 8 (October 2009): 512–14.

Ousager, Jakob, and Helle Johannessen. "Humanities in Undergraduate Medical Education: A Literature Review." *Academic Medicine* 85, no. 6 (June 2010): 988–98.

Pellegrino, Edmund D., and Thomas K. McElhinney. *Teaching Ethics, the Humanities, and Human Values in Medical Schools: A Ten-Year Overview*. Washington, DC: Institute on Human Values in Medicine, Society for Health and Human Values, 1982.

Radwany, Steven M., and Bernard H. Adelson. "The Use of Literary Classics in Teaching Medical Ethics to Physicians." *Journal of the American Medical Association* 257, no. 12 (March 1987): 1629–31.

Self, Donnie J., and DeWitt C. Baldwin Jr. "Teaching Medical Humanities Through Film Discussions." *Journal of Medical Humanities* 11, no. 1 (March 1990): 23–37.

Shapiro, Johanna, and Lynn Hunt. "All the World's a Stage: The Use of Theatrical Performance in Medical Education." *Medical Education* 37, no. 10 (October 2003): 922–27.

Shapiro, Johanna, and Deborah Kasman. "Words and Wards: A Model of Reflective Writing and Its Uses in Medical Education." *Journal of Medical Humanities* 27, no. 4 (September 2006): 231–44.

Shapiro, Johanna, and Lloyd Rucker. "Can Poetry Make Better Doctors? Teaching the Humanities and Arts to Medical Students and Residents at the University of California, Irvine, College of Medicine." *Academic Medicine* 78, no. 10 (October 2003): 953–57.

Sirridge, Marjorie, and Kathleen Welch. "The Program in Medical Humanities at the University of Missouri-Kansas City School of Medicine." *Academic Medicine* 78, no. 10 (October 2003): 973–76.

Stempsey, William E. "The Quarantine of Philosophy in Medical Education: Why Teaching the Humanities May Not Produce Humane Physicians." *Medicine, Health Care and Philosophy* 2, no. 1 (July 1999): 3–9.

Thomasma, David C., and Patricia Marshall. "The Clinical Medical Humanities Program at Loyola University of Chicago." *Academic Medicine* 64, no. 12 (December 1989): 735–39.

Wear, Delese. "The Medical Humanities: Toward a Renewed Praxis." *Journal of Medical Humanities* 30, no. 4 (December 2009): 209.

Wetzel, Patti, John Hinchey, and Abraham Verghese. "The Teaching of Medical Humanities." *Clinical Teacher* 2, no. 2 (December 2005): 91–96.

Nursing Ethics Teaching

Allmark, Peter. "Uncertainties in the Teaching of Ethics to Students of Nursing." *Journal of Advanced Nursing* 22, no. 2 (August 1995): 374–78.

Aroskar, Mila, and Robert M. Veatch. "Ethics Teaching in Nursing Schools." *Hastings Center Report* 7, no. 4 (August 1977): 23–26.

Davis, Anne J., Verena Tschudin, and Louise de Raeve, eds. *Essentials of Teaching and Learning in Nursing Ethics: Perspectives and Methods*. Edinburgh: Elsevier, 2006.

Dinç, Leyla, and Refia Selma Görgülü. "Teaching Ethics in Nursing." *Nursing Ethics* 9, no. 3 (May 2002): 259–68.

Fry, Sara T. "Teaching Ethics in Nursing Curricula: Traditional and Contemporary Models." *Nursing Clinics of North America* 24, no. 2 (June 1989): 485–97.

Hanson, Stephen. "Teaching Health Care Ethics: Why We Should Teach Nursing and Medical Students Together." *Nursing Ethics* 12, no. 2 (March 2005): 167–76.

Holland, Stephen. "Teaching Nursing Ethics by Cases: A Personal Perspective." *Nursing Ethics* 6, no. 5 (September 1999): 434–36.

Krawczyk, Rosemary M. "Teaching Ethics: Effect on Moral Development." *Nursing Ethics* 4, no. 1 (January 1997): 57–65.

Lin, Chiou-Fen, Meei-Shiow Lu, Chun-Chih Chung, and Che-Ming Yang. "A Comparison of Problem-Based Learning and Conventional Teaching in Nursing Ethics Education." *Nursing Ethics* 17, no. 3 (May 2010): 373–82.

Numminen, Olivia, Arie van der Arend, and Helena Leino-Kilpi. "Nurse Educators' and Nursing Students' Perspectives on Teaching Codes of Ethics." *Nursing Ethics* 16, no. 1 (January 2009): 69–82.

Nursing Humanities Teaching

Bartol, Genevieve Marie. "Using the Humanities in Nursing Education." *Nurse Educator* 11, no. 1 (January 1986): 21–23.

Brown, Sylvia T., Mary K. Kirkpatrick, Dana Mangum, and Jeanette Avery. "A Review of Narrative Pedagogy Strategies to Transform Traditional Nursing Education." *Journal of Nursing Education* 47, no. 6 (June 2008): 283–86.

Callister, Lynn Clark. "The Use of Student Journals in Nursing Education: Making Meaning out of Clinical Experience." *Journal of Nursing Education* 32, no. 4 (April 1993): 185–86.

Casey, Briege. "Editorial: Arts-Based Inquiry in Nursing Education." *Contemporary Nurse* 32, no. 1–2 (April 2009): 69–82.

Darbyshire, Philip. "Lessons from Literature: Caring, Interpretation, and Dialogue." *Journal of Nursing Education* 34, no. 5 (May 1995): 211–16.

Darbyshire, Philip. "Nursing, Art, and Science: Revisiting the Two Culture." *International Journal of Nursing Practice* 5, no. 3 (September 1999): 123–31.

Darbyshire, Philip. "Understanding Care Through Arts and Humanities: A Medical/Nursing Humanities Approach to Promoting Alternative Experiences of Thinking and Learning." *Journal of Advanced Nursing* 19, no. 5 (May 1994): 856–63.

Davis, Cortney. "Nursing Humanities: The Time Has Come: Literature and Art Can Change Nurses' Work." *American Journal of Nursing* 103, no. 2 (February 2003): 13.

Davis, Sandra K. "Nursing and the Humanities: Health Assessment in the Art Gallery." *Journal of Nursing Education* 31, no. 2 (February 1992): 93–94.

Dellasega, Cheryl, Paula Milone-Nuzzo, Katherine M. Curci, J. O. Ballard, and Darrell G. Kirch. "The Humanities Interface of Nursing and Medicine." *Journal of Professional Nursing* 23, no. 3 (May–June 2007): 174–79.

Ehrhart, Patricia M., and Beth Furlong. "The Renaissance Nurse: Permeating Clinical Competence with the Humanities." *Nurse Educator* 18, no. 3 (May 1993): 22–24.

Ferrell, Betty, Rose Virani, Hollye Harrington Jacobs, Pam Malloy, and Kathe Kelly. "Arts and Humanities in Palliative Nursing Education." *Journal of Pain and Symptom Management* 39, no. 6 (May 2010): 941–45.

German, Carol P. "Using Literature to Teach Nursing." *Journal of Nursing Education* 25, no. 2 (February 1986): 84–86.

Halloran, Laurel. "Teaching Transcultural Nursing Through Literature." *Journal of Nursing Education* 48, no. 9 (September 2009): 523–28.

Hermann, Mary L., and Robert J. Wright. "The Current Nature of the Integration of the Humanities Within Baccalaureate Nursing Education." Paper presented at the Annual Meeting of the American Educational Research Association, New Orleans, LA, April 1–5, 2002. https://files.eric.ed.gov/fulltext/ED465702.pdf.

Hydo, Sharon K., Diane L. Marcyjanik, CeCelia R. Zorn, and Nicole M. Hooper. "Art as a Scaffolding Teaching Strategy in Baccalaureate Nursing Education." *International Journal of Nursing Education Scholarship* 4, no. 1 (January 2007): 1–11.

Inskeep, Sandra J., and Susan A. Lisko. "Alternative Clinical Nursing Experience in an Art Gallery." *Nurse Educator* 26, no. 3 (May 2001): 117–19.

Jackson, Debra, and Jennifer R. Sullivan. "Integrating the Creative Arts into a Midwifery Curriculum: A Teaching Innovation Report." *Nurse Education Today* 19, no. 7 (October 1999): 527–32.

Jensen, Alice, and Mary Curtis. "A Descriptive Qualitative Study of Student Learning in a Psychosocial Nursing Class Infused with Art, Literature, Music, and Film." *International Journal of Nursing Education Scholarship* 5, no. 1 (January 2008): 1–9.

Lazenby, Mark. "On the Humanities of Nursing." *Nursing Outlook* 61, no. 1 (January–February 2013): e9–e14.

MacDonnell, Judith A., and Geraldine (Jody) Macdonald. "Arts-Based Critical Inquiry in Nursing and Interdisciplinary Professional Education: Guided Imagery, Images, Narratives, and Poetry." *Journal of Transformative Education* 9, no. 4 (October 2011): 203–21.

Marnocha, Suzanne, and Mark Marnocha. "Windows Open: Humanities Teaching During Undergraduate Clinical Experiences." *Journal of Nursing Education* 46, no. 11 (November 2007): 518–21.

McCaffrey, Ruth, and Marguerite Purnell. "From Experience to Integration: The Arts in Nursing Education." *Nursing Education Perspectives* 28, no. 2 (March–April 2007): 72–76.

McIntyre, Marjorie, and Carol McDonald. "Contemplating the Fit and Unity of Nursing Theory and Nursing Scholarship Informed by the Social Sciences and Humanities." *Advances in Nursing Science* 36, no. 1 (January–March 2013): 10–17.

McKie, Andrew. "Using the Arts and Humanities to Promote a Liberal Nursing Education: Strengths and Weaknesses." *Nurse Education Today* 32, no. 7 (October 2012): 803–10.

McKie, Andrew, and John P. Gass. "Understanding Mental Health Through Reading Selected Literature Sources: An Evaluation." *Nurse Education Today* 21, no. 3 (April 2001): 201–8.

Moorman, Margaret. "The Meaning of Visual Thinking Strategies for Nursing Students." *Humanities* 4, no. 4 (October 2015): 748–59.

Moyle, Wendy, Alan Barnard, and Charne Turner. "The Humanities and Nursing: Using Popular Literature as a Means of Understanding Human Experience." *Journal of Advanced Nursing* 21, no. 5 (May 1995): 960–64.

Peden, Ann R., and Ruth R. Staten. "The Use of the Humanities in Psychiatric Nursing Education." *Journal of Nursing Education* 33, no. 1 (January 1994): 41–42.

Robb, Alna J. P., and Rowena Murray. "Medical Humanities in Nursing: Thought Provoking?" *Journal of Advanced Nursing* 17, no. 10 (October 1992): 1182–87.

Sakalys, Jurate A. "Literary Pedagogy in Nursing: A Theory-Based Perspective." *Journal of Nursing Education* 41, no. 9 (September 2002): 386–92.

Smith, Robyn L., Michelle Bailey, Sharon Kay Hydo, Margret Lepp, Sylvia Mews, Susan Timm, and CeCelia Zorn. "All the Voices in the Room: Integrating Humanities in Nursing Education." *Nursing Education Perspectives* 25, no. 6 (November–December 2004): 278–83.

Snyder, Melissa J. "Reconnecting with Your Passion: An Action Research Study Exploring Humanities and Professional Nursing." *Journal of Poetry Therapy* 25, no. 4 (December 2012): 239–43.

Stowe, Ann Coghlan, and Lorraine C. Igo. "Learning from Literature: Novels, Plays, Short Stories, and Poems in Nursing Education." *Nurse Educator* 21, no. 5 (September–October 1996): 16–19.

Wall, Barbra Mann, and Eileen K. Rossen. "Media as a Teaching Tool in Psychiatric Nursing Education." *Nurse Educator* 29, no. 1 (January 2004): 36–40.

Walsh, Sandra, Catharina Chang, Lee A. Schmidt, and Jan H. Yoepp. "Lowering Stress While Teaching Research: A Creative Arts Intervention in the Classroom." *Journal of Nursing Education* 44, no. 7 (June 2005): 330–33.

Whitman, Brenda L., and Wanda J. Rose. "Using Art to Express a Personal Philosophy of Nursing." *Nurse Educator* 28, no. 4 (July 2003): 166–69.

Wikström, Britt-Maj. "A Picture of a Work of Art as an Empathy Teaching Strategy in Nursing Education Complementary to Theoretical Knowledge." *Journal of Professional Nursing* 19, no. 1 (January–February 2003): 49–54.

Wikström, Britt-Maj. "Nursing Education at an Art Gallery." *Journal of Nursing Scholarship* 32, no. 2 (June 2000): 197–99.

Wikström, Britt-Maj. "Works of Art: A Complement to Theoretical Knowledge When Teaching Nursing Care." *Journal of Clinical Nursing* 10, no. 1 (January 2001): 25–32.

Young-Mason, Jeanine. "Health, Humanities, and the Arts." *Clinical Nurse Specialist* 15, no. 5 (September 2001): 210–11.

Yu, An-bang. "The Encounter of Nursing and the Clinical Humanities: Nursing Education and the Spirit of Healing." *Humanities* 3, no. 4 (November 2014): 660–74.

Public Health Ethics Teaching

Coughlin, Steven S., Wendy H. Katz, and Donald R. Mattison. "Ethics Instruction at Schools of Public Health in the United States." *American Journal of Public Health* 89, no. 5 (May 1999): 768–70.

Jennings, Bruce, Jeffrey Kahn, Anna Mastroianni, and Lisa S. Parker, eds. *Ethics and Public Health: Model Curriculum*. Rockville, MD: Health Resources and Services Administration; Washington, DC: Association of Schools of Public Health, 2003.

Kass, Nancy E. "An Ethics Framework for Public Health." *American Journal of Public Health* 91, no. 11 (November 2001): 1776–82.

Kessel, Anthony S. "Public Health Ethics: Teaching Survey and Critical Review." *Social Science and Medicine* 56, no. 7 (April 2003): 1439–45.

Moon, Sang-Eun, Yun-Jeong Kim, and Seon-Young Kim. "Current Condition of Humanities and Social Sciences Classes in the Public Health Curricula." *Journal of Korean Society of Dental Hygiene* 14, no. 6 (December 2014): 961–66.

Thomas, James C. "Teaching Ethics in Schools of Public Health." *Public Health Reports* 118, no. 3 (May 2003): 279–86.

Public Health Humanities Teaching

Saffran, Lise. "'Only Connect': The Case for Public Health Humanities." *Medical Humanities* 40, no. 2 (May 2014): 105–10.

Stewart, Kearsley A., and Kelley K. Swain. "Global Health Humanities: Defining an Emerging Field." *Lancet* 288, no. 10060 (November 2016): 2586–87.

Social Justice-Informed Health Humanities Teaching

Acosta, David, and Kupiri Ackerman-Barger. "Breaking the Silence: Time to Talk About Race and Racism." *Academic Medicine* 92, no. 3 (2017): 285–88.

Banner, Olivia. "Structural Racism and Practices of Reading in the Medical Humanities." *Literature and Medicine* 34, no. 1 (2016): 25–52.

Blackie, Michael, and Erin Gentry Lamb. "Courting Discomfort in an Undergraduate Health Humanities Classroom." In *The Health Humanities Reader*, edited by Therese Jones, Delese Wear, and Lester D. Friedman, 490–500. New Brunswick, NJ: Rutgers University Press, 2014.

Blanchet Garneau, Amélie, Annette J. Browne, and Colleen Varcoe. "Drawing on Antiracist Approaches Toward a Critical Antidiscriminatory Pedagogy for Nursing." *Nursing Inquiry* 25, no. 1 (2018).

Brondani, Mario A., and Randy Paterson. "Teaching Lesbian, Gay, Bisexual, and Transgender Issues in Dental Education: A Multipurpose Method." *Journal of Dental Education* 75, no. 11 (October 2011): 1354–61.

DasGupta, Sayantani, Alice Fornari, Kamini Geer, Louisa Hahn, Vanita Kumar, Hyun Joon Lee, Susan Rubin, and Marji Gold. "Medical Education for Social Justice: Paulo Freire Revisited." *Journal of Medical Humanities* 27, no. 4 (2006): 245–51.

Donald, Cameron A., Sayantani DasGupta, Jonathan M. Metzl, and Kristen L. Eckstrand. "Queer Frontiers in Medicine: A Structural Competency Approach." *Academic Medicine* 92, no. 3 (2017): 345–50.

Fitzgerald, Des, and Felicity Callard. "Entangling the Medical Humanities." In *The Edinburgh Companion to the Critical Medical Humanities*, edited by Anne Whitehead and Angela Woods, 35–49. Edinburgh: Edinburgh University Press, 2016.

Gutierrez, Kevin J., and Sayantani DasGupta. "The Space That Difference Makes: On Marginality, Social Justice and the Future of the Health Humanities." *Journal of Medical Humanities* 37, no. 4 (2016): 435–48.

Jones, Esther L. "Structural Competency and African Contexts: A Mixed Methodological Approach to Interrogating Strategies for Greater Health Equity." In *Diversity and Inclusion in Higher Education and Societal Contexts*, edited by Sunhee Kim Gertz, Betsy Huang, and Lauren Cyr, 189–210. Cham, Switzerland: Springer, 2018.

Pasco, John Carlo, Camille Anderson, and Sayantani DasGupta. "Visionary Medicine: Speculative Fiction, Racial Justice and Octavia Butler's 'Bloodchild.'" *Medical Humanities* 42, no. 4 (2016): 246–51.

Tsai, Jennifer, and Ann Crawford-Roberts. "A Call for Critical Race Theory in Medical Education." *Academic Medicine* 92, no. 8 (2017): 1072–73.

Viney, William, Felicity Callard, and Angela Woods. "Critical Medical Humanities: Embracing Entanglement, Taking Risks." *Medical Humanities* 41, no. 1 (2015): 2–7.

Wear, Delese. "The Medical Humanities: Toward a Renewed Praxis." *Journal of Medical Humanities* 30, no. 4 (2009): 209–20.

Wear, Delese, Joseph Zarconi, Julie M. Aultman, Michelle R. Chyatte, and Arno K. Kumagai. "Remembering Freddie Gray: Medical Education for Social Justice." *Academic Medicine* 92, no. 3 (2017): 312–17.

INDEX